MRI Atlas of the Brain

MRI Atlas of the Brain

William G Bradley, MD, PhD

Director
MR Imaging Laboratory
Huntington Memorial Hospital
Pasadena, CA

Graeme Bydder, MB, ChB

Professor of Diagnostic Radiology
Department of Diagnostic Radiology
Hammersmith Hospital
London

MARTIN DUNITZ

British Library Cataloguing-in-Publication Data

Bradley, William G
    MRI atlas of the brain.
    1. Man. Brain. Diagnosis. Magnetic
    resonance imaging
    I. Title   II. Bydder, Graeme.
    616.8'047575
    ISBN 0-948269-46-4

Laserset by Scribe Design, Gillingham, Kent
Origination by Adroit Photolitho, Birmingham
Printed and bound in Great Britain by Butler & Tanner Ltd, Frome, Somerset

Preface

In the past decade since its introduction into clinical practice, magnetic resonance imaging (MRI) has revolutionized the practice of medicine in general and radiology in particular. When compared to x-ray computed tomography (CT), MRI is both safer and provides more contrast for most imaging problems in the brain. This is due both to the multiplicity of variables on which the MR signal depends (eg proton density, T_1, and T_2 and to the wealth of pulsing sequences available (eg T_1 or T_2-weighted spin echo, inversion recovery, and gradient echo (partial saturation) sequences). In addition, MRI can easily produce images in any plane, while CT is generally constrained to the transaxial plane, plus or minus a few degrees of gantry angulation. In addition, because it does not rely on ionizing radiation, MR is safer than CT. Even the contrast agent used for MRI (Gadolinium-DTPA) is safer than the iodinated contrast agents used in CT. Therefore, it is not surprising that MRI has become the preferred radiological technique for imaging the brain.

When the authors began clinical imaging, there were only a handful of scanners in the world. As this book goes to press, the number of scanners around the world is approaching 2 000. In California alone (where there is no governmental intervention), over 250 scanners have been installed, reflecting primary physician demand. There is now even talk of malpractice if a referring physician orders a CT instead of an MRI to exclude early disease in the brain.

The authors of this book consider themselves fortunate to have been involved in the development of MRI at an early stage in the late 1970s: WGB at UCSF and then at the Huntington Medical Research Institutes, and GMB at Hammersmith Hospital, University of London. While we continue to be among the fortunate few who are able to spend most of their time involved with MRI, the propagation of this technology has resulted in a situation where many radiologists must now render MR interpretations with minimal previous experience while participating in MRI less than once a week. It is for such physicians that this book has been written.

The authors have a combined experience of over 20 years in MR education. Through longstanding Visiting Fellowships and Overreading Programs, we have attempted to make MR understandable to those just beginning in the field. We have organized Teaching Programs for the two MRI Societies (the SMRM and the SMRI) and were each serving as President as this book was being written.

Our intention has been to provide an easily understandable description of how MRI works without resorting to a detailed discussion of quantum mechanics. The discussion focuses on the end result, namely the change in signal intensity as a result of changing intrinsic MR parameters, which can be brought about by the various pulsing sequences in our armamentarium. This is provided both in the chapter on Fundamentals and in the multiple clinical examples which follow.

Since most radiologists will start from a basic of familiarity with pathophysiology of disease and a knowledge of cross-sectional imaging (at least in the transaxial plane), they are in a good position to recognize and diagnose many of the abnormalities we can currently see with CT. The appearance of these lesions on MRI is the basis for the majority of the images in this book. Specifically, chapters on Tumors, Infarcts and Ischemia, Demyelination and Infection,

Hydrocephalus, and Pediatrics feature multiple images displaying the MR appearance of many common lesions with minimal associated text. Instead of focusing on pathophysiology, attention is directed to the variable appearance of these disease states using various MR imaging techniques. Although the MR contrast agent, Gadolinium-DTPA, has similar behavior (physiologically) to meglumine diatrizoate in CT, the MR techniques which result in optimal visualization of enhancing lesions are nonintuitive and are discussed in a separate chapter. Similarly, the appearance of flowing blood and CSF and hemorrhage does not follow easily from a pre-existing CT base, therefore additional text has been devoted to these subjects.

For the future, new sequences continue to be developed which generate greater (or different) contrast with more signal-to-noise in less time. Many of these are discussed in the chapter on New Techniques and provide a basis for understanding the imaging techniques which will undoubtedly become routine during the next decade.

William G Bradley, MD, Phd
Graeme Bydder, MB, ChB

June 1989

Contents

1 **Fundamentals** 1
William G Bradley

2 **New techniques** 39
Graeme Bydder

3 **Flow phenomena** 68
William G Bradley

4 **Tumors** 112
Graeme Bydder

5 **Ischemia—infarction** 143
William G Bradley

6 **Demyelinating disease and infection** 182
Graeme Bydder

7 **Hemorrhage and vascular abnormalities** 201
William G Bradley

8 **Hydrocephalus** 265
William G Bradley

9 **Use of Gadolinium-DTPA** 302
Graeme Bydder

10 **Pediatric brain** 326
Graeme Bydder

Index 351

Acknowledgments

While it may appear to the casual observer that only two people were involved the writing of this book, such a project would not have been possible without the contributions of many people both in Pasadena and in London. On the Pasadena side, WGB thanks his stalwart MR technologists during the 1983–9 period: Jay Mericle, Terry Andrues, Leslee Watson, Ken Bishop, Jose Jimenez, Laurel Adler, and Sheri Gregory; our artist, Cathy Reichel-Clark; and our photographers, Sal Vallone and Gordon Galloway. Several MR Fellows have contributed significantly to the ideas which follow: Keith Kortman, MD, Jay Tsuruda, MD and Anthony Whittemore, MD, PhD. From the London side, GMB wishes to acknowledge the major contributions from Jacqueline Pennock and Ian Young.

The bulk of the work in the preparation of a manuscript such as this falls on the shoulders of those who do the typing and editing of the multiple drafts involved. On the Pasadena side, hearty thanks go out to Kaye Finley; from the London side to Patricia Hamilton and Dulcie Rodrigues.

A project such as this is greatly facilitated by a publisher who is accommodating and continues to gently push until completion. Such is the Martin Dunitz Organization. In addition to Martin himself we thank Mary Banks, Elizabeth Puttick and Lucy Hamilton.

We were all deeply saddened by the tragic death of Sally Jones at the age of 26 as the result of a skiing accident. She was the original editor of this book. Sally graduated in biology from Cambridge University and was responsible for the expansion of medical publishing at Martin Dunitz. She had an excellent eye for good design combined with a meticulous grasp of detail. She was determined, tactful, intelligent and a delightful person. We dedicate this book to her memory.

1

Fundamentals

William G Bradley

Introduction

Since its introduction to clinical imaging nearly a decade ago,[1-3] magnetic resonance imaging (MRI) has radically modified the practice of medicine in general and radiology in particular. Like its predecessor, X-ray computed tomography (CT), MRI is a computer-based imaging modality which displays the body in thin tomographic slices. Unlike CT, which requires ionizing radiation, MRI is based on an apparently safe interaction between radio waves and hydrogen nuclei in the body in the presence of a strong magnetic field. In addition to being generally safer than CT, MRI produces images which are often better than those of CT. This reflects not only better contrast between a lesion and its background but also the ability to display the lesion in multiple planes of projection. In CT, one must scan in the plane of the gantry, that is, axial or semi-coronal. In MRI, one is able to acquire images directly in any plane, that is, axial, sagittal, coronal, or oblique.

In both CT and MRI, physical characteristics of a volume element or 'voxel' of tissue are translated by the computer into a two-dimensional image composed of picture elements or 'pixels'. It is useful to compare the determinants of pixel intensity in CT and MRI to demonstrate differences in the imaging methods. The pixel intensity in CT reflects the electron density; in MRI it reflects the density of hydrogen, generally as water (H_2O) or fat. To be more exact, MR signal intensity reflects the density of mobile hydrogen nuclei modified by the chemical environment, that is, by the magnetic relaxation times, T_1 and T_2,[4] and by motion.[5-7]

The hydrogen nucleus is a single proton, as illustrated in Figure 1.1. Since it is charged (positively) and since it spins (like a top), it displays the phenomenon of nuclear magnetic resonance (NMR). Nuclear magnetic resonance has been used by chemists and physicists for over 40 years for chemical analysis. The equipment required to perform NMR consists simply of a strong magnet and a radio transmitter and receiver, as shown in Figure 1.2. When NMR is used for chemical analysis, the magnetic field across the test tube sample must be very, very uniform, often to one part in 100 million (0.01 ppm). When NMR is used for imaging, the magnetic field across the body-sized sample is intentionally made non-uniform by superimposing additional magnetic fields which can be turned on and off rapidly. Activation of these additional fields results in a net gradient in the strength of the magnetic field across the body which is necessary to perform imaging. Thus the essential components of an MR imaging system include (1) a large magnet which generates a uniform magnetic field, (2) smaller electromagnetic coils to generate magnetic field gradients for imaging, and (3) a radio transmitter and receiver and its associated transmitting and receiving antennae or coils. In addition to these fundamental components, a computer is necessary to coordinate signal generation and acquisition and image formation and display.

Having now briefly described the clinical utility of MRI and the equipment required, it will be useful to describe very simply how it works. When the body lies in the large magnet, it becomes temporarily magnetized. This state is achieved because the hydrogen nuclei in the body line up with the strong magnetic field. In this state, the body will respond in an interesting manner to exposure to radiowaves at a particular frequency. Imagine the following experiment. The body is exposed to a burst of radio waves at a particular frequency. The radio receiver then

1

immediately listens for a radio response from the body at that frequency. As multiple radio frequencies are scanned, nothing happens and then, at a particular frequency, a signal is returned by the body like an echo. For a given nucleus (for example, hydrogen), the frequency at which this 'spin-echo' phenomenon occurs is known as the Larmor frequency and it depends only on the strength of the magnetic field at that point. The phenomenon itself is known as 'resonance'.[8] A careful frequency analysis of the spin-echo signal indicates where each frequency component originated. The resonant frequency is intentionally made to be slightly different at each position by transiently superimposing an additional magnetic field, creating a magnetic field gradient. Thus spatial information in MRI is contained *in the frequency* of the signal, unlike X-ray-based imaging modalities such as CT.

Magnetization

The MR signal is proportional to a quantity called the magnetization.[8] The magnetization is a measurable property which results when the body is placed in a magnetic field and is temporarily magnetized. The most abundant element in the body is hydrogen. When the proton nucleus of the hydrogen atom spins, it generates a small magnetic spin field called a 'magnetic moment' (μ), as shown in Figure 1.1. The hydrogen nuclei behave like small bar magnets or compass needles and tend to align with a stronger magnetic field. Immediately after being placed in a magnetic field, there is an equal number of protons pointing north and south or 'parallel' and 'antiparallel' to the main magnetic field. Thus, initially the individual magnetic moments cancel and there is zero net magnetization. Within a few seconds (in biological substances), a redistribution occurs such that a slightly greater number of hydrogen nuclei align parallel to the field and the body is said to be 'magnetized'. Magnetization increases exponentially with a first-order exponential time constant known as the T_1 relaxation time, as shown in Figure 1.3. The magnetization plateaus at an equilibrium value which is dependent on the hydrogen density and the magnetic susceptibility, which is the ratio of the magnetic field temporarily induced in the substance to the applied magnetic field. Certain substances with unpaired electrons (paramagnetic, superparamagnetic, and ferromagnetic materials) have very high magnetic susceptibilities. The iron in hemosiderin is an example of such a superparamagnetic substance; a much stronger field is induced in tissues containing hemosiderin than in normal tissues.

Although at equilibrium the magnetization only points along the main z-axis of the static magnetic field, in general it can point in any direction. The magnetization is a vector quantity[8] which can be represented by a longitudinal component (along the z-axis of the main magnetic field) and by a second component perpendicular to the first, called the transverse magnetization, which is in the xy-plane, as in Figure 1.4. Transverse magnetization results from the application of short bursts of radiofrequency (RF) energy (radiowaves) called RF pulses.

A 90° RF pulse tips the longitudinal magnetization from the z-axis into the transverse xy-plane. This causes a total loss of longitudinal magnetization but produces transverse magnetization. The usual 'tip' or 'flip' angle initiating a spin-echo sequence is 90°; this means that the magnetization is tipped 90° from the z-axis so that it lies in the xy-plane. A 180° pulse causes 180° of rotation so that the longitudinal magnetization becomes directed along the −z-axis. Unlike a 90° pulse, a 180° pulse cannot generate transverse magnetization. As illustrated in Figure 1.5, the maximum transverse magnetization results from a 90° flip angle; flip angles less than 90° do not cause such a loss of longitudinal magnetization, but they also produce less transverse magnetization per flip.[9] However, since less time is needed for longitudinal recovery, they can be repeated rapidly, and may actually generate more transverse magnetization, that is, more signal per unit time. This is the basis for some of the fast scanning techniques which have been developed.[10]

Whenever transverse magnetization is present, it rotates about the z-axis at the resonance or Larmor frequency which is determined by the magnitude of the magnetic field and the gyromagnetic ratio of the nucleus. This is also the frequency of the spin-echo radio signal which is eventually processed into the MR image. Only the transverse component of magnetization rotates and thus can be detected; longitudinal magnetization does not rotate and cannot be detected.

Two types of MR signals can be produced by transverse magnetization. Immediately following an RF pulse, a signal is produced by the freely rotating transverse magnetization. This signal is called a 'free induction decay' or 'FID', illustrated in Figure 1.6. Transverse magnetization decays rapidly due to nonuniformities in the main magnetic field which cause protons to resonate at slightly different frequencies at slightly different positions within the voxel. As these protons get out of phase or 'lose coherence', transverse magnetization (and induced signal) is lost exponentially. The envelope of the decay curve is described by the expression $e^{-t/T_2^\star}$, hence the first-order time constant of decay is $T_2^\star$.

When a 90° pulse and a 180° pulse are applied sequentially, a spin-echo signal is generated,[8] also illustrated in Figure 1.6. The purpose of the 180° pulse is to 'refocus' the phase of the protons, causing them to regain coherence and thereby to recover transverse magnetization,[8] producing a spin echo. (Similar rephasing can be accomplished by symmetrically reversing the gradient fields, producing a 'gradient' or 'field' echo'.[9]) Following the spin echo, coherence is again lost as the protons continue to resonate at slightly different frequencies due to non-uniformities in the main magnetic field. If another 180° pulse is applied, coherence can again be established for a second spin echo. In fact, multiple spin-echo signals can be produced if the original 90° pulse is followed by multiple 180° pulses (or gradient reversals). This 'echo train' is illustrated in Figure 1.6.

Although the 180° pulses cause some rephasing to occur (that due to fixed non-uniformities in the main field), complete rephasing is not possible due to randomly fluctuating magnetic fields within the substance itself. Thus, the maximum intensity of the spin-echo signals in the echo train is limited by an exponentially decaying curve, as shown in Figure 1.6. The time constant of this decay curve is the second magnetic relaxation time T_2.[8]

To summarize, there are two types of decay of magnetization: reversible and irreversible.[8] Immediately following the initial 90° pulse, transverse magnetization decays rapidly (at rate $T_2^\star$) due to non-uniformities in the external magnetic field. As this transverse magnetization initially decays, an FID is produced, although this signal is rarely acquired on clinical MR imaging systems. Since the non-uniformities in the main magnetic field which caused this initial rapid decay are fixed, transverse magnetization can be partially restored by a 180° RF pulse, producing a spin echo. Transverse magnetization is also lost by magnetic non-uniformities within substance which result from randomly fluctuating internal fields. Unlike the reversible decay due to fixed non-uniformities in the main field, this decay is irreversible. Like radioactive decay, this is a first-order exponential decay process with time constant T_2.

In general, one must be careful to distinguish terms used to describe MR signals from those used to describe MR pulsing sequences. A traditional spin-echo signal and sequence results from a 90°/180° RF pulse pair. An FID signal results from a terminal 90° RF pulse. An inversion recovery (IR) sequence results from a 180°/90° pulse pair. Since the final pulse in the IR sequence is a 90° pulse, an FID signal is produced. By adding a terminal 180° pulse, ie, 180°/90°/180°, an IR sequence can produce a spin-echo signal. A traditional spin-echo signal results from rephasing both temporally (by the 180° pulse) and spatially (by gradient reversal). For particularly uniform static fields, echo formation can result from gradient reversal alone, producing a 'gradient' or 'field' echo.[11] Like the reduced flip angle, this is one of the basic features of the newer fast scanning techniques described more fully in Chapter 2.

In CT and MRI, certain parameters are fixed by the manufacturer, and other parameters are under operator control. CT parameters under operator control include voltage, time, current, and number of views. In MRI, the parameters of operation are less familiar and utilize a new vocabulary. Those which are generally determined by the manufacturer include field strength, acquisition technique (projection-reconstruction or Fourier transform), and acquisition signal (spin echo, gradient echo, or free induction decay). Factors under operator control include choice of pulsing sequence, sequence parameter times, matrix size, slice thickness and gap between slices, field of view, number of excitations, orientation of imaging plane, diameter and type of radiofrequency (RF) coil, and use of cardiac gating.

Improved spatial resolution in CT is generally associated with increased radiation dose. Spatial resolution in MRI can be calculated from matrix size and field of view and is determined by the strength of the gradient fields and the specific range of frequencies (bandwidth) which can be detected and discriminated. On a given MR imaging system, increased spatial resolution (at a given signal-to-noise ratio, S/N) requires longer acquisition times but does not increase patient risk.

The MR image differs from the CT image in several respects. The effect of the magnetic relaxation times on MR pixel intensity has no parallel in CT. Magnetic relaxation effects depend on the choice of pulsing sequences and the sequence parameter times.[3,4] Flowing blood appears different on MR than on CT.[5-7] On MR images, intraluminal blood can appear black, white or gray, depending on the pulsing sequence, orientation of the flowing blood to the imaging plane, and velocity. The intraluminal signal can yield information on velocity and characteristics of flow which is not available from CT. Flow phenomena are discussed more completely in Chapter 3.

Physical basis for T_1 and T_2

T_1 is variously called the 'longitudinal', 'thermal', and 'spin-lattice' relaxation time. It indicates the time required for a substance to become magnetized, as described in Figure 1.3, after first being placed in a magnetic field, or, alternatively, the time required to regain longitudinal magnetization following an RF pulse. T_1 is determined by thermal interactions between the resonating protons and other protons and other magnetic nuclei in the magnetic environment or 'lattice'. These interactions allow the energy absorbed by the protons during resonance to be dispersed to other nuclei in the lattice.

All molecules have natural motions due to vibration, rotation, and translation.[8] Smaller molecules like water generally move more rapidly, thus they have higher natural frequencies. Larger molecules like proteins move more slowly. When water is held in hydration layers around the protein by hydrophilic side groups, its rapid motion slows considerably as illustrated in Figure 1.7.[12]

The T_1 relaxation time reflects the relationship between the frequency of these molecular motions and the resonant Larmor frequency (which depends on the main magnetic field of the MR imager). When the two are similar, T_1 relaxation is efficient and rapid; when they are different, T_1 relaxation is prolonged.[12] The water molecule is small and moves too rapidly for efficient T_1 relaxation; large proteins move too slowly. Both have natural frequencies significantly different from the Larmor frequency and thus have long T_1 relaxation times. Cholesterol, a medium-sized molecule, has natural frequencies close to those used for MR imaging,[4] and has a short T_1 when it is in the liquid state, as illustrated in Figure 1.8. Thus the liquid cholesterol in craniopharyngiomas and intrapetrous epidermoids appears bright on T_1-weighted images. When cholesterol is in the solid form, however, no detectable signal is generated, thus most cisternal or intraventricular epidermoid tumors appear dark on T_1-weighted images (Figure 1.8).

Water in the bulk phase, like CSF, has a long T_1 relaxation time because the frequency of its natural motions is much higher than the range of Larmor frequencies used clinically.[12] However, when this same CSF is forced out into the periventricular white matter as interstitial edema due to ventricular obstruction, its T_1 relaxation time is much shorter, shown in Figure 1.9. The T_1-shortening reflects the fact that water is now in hydration layers rather than in the bulk phase (Figure 1.7). Proteinaceous solutions (such as abscesses and necrotic tumors) have a higher percentage of water in the hydration layer environment and thus have a shorter T_1 compared to 'pure' aqueous solutions like CSF, demonstrated in Figure 1.10.

As shown in Figure 1.11, subacute hemorrhage has a shorter T_1 than brain. This reflects the paramagnetic characteristics of the iron in methemoglobin.[13] T_1-shortening is produced by a dipole–dipole interaction between unpaired electrons on the paramagnetic iron and water protons in the solution. The short T_1 allows subacute hemorrhage to recover longitudinal magnetization very quickly relative to brain. Thus, subacute hemorrhage will generally appear brighter than brain, illustrated in Figure 1.12.

Some paramagnetic contrast agents function by a similar dipole–dipole interaction, shortening the T_1 of all mobile protons within several angstroms of the paramagnetic center,[14] increasing the signal. As the concentration of the paramagnetic substance is increased, however, T_2 is also shortened. Thus with increasing concentration, the intensity is initially increased due to accelerated T_1 recovery and then decreased due to accelerated T_2 decay as discussed below. This phenomenon is clearly demonstrated in Figure 1.13.

T_2 is called the 'transverse' or 'spin-spin' relaxation time. It is a measure of how long transverse magnetization would last in a perfectly uniform external magnetic field (Figure 1.14). Alternatively, it is a measure of how long the resonating protons remain coherent or precess 'in phase' following a 90° RF pulse. T_2 decay is due to magnetic interactions which occur between spinning protons. Unlike T_1 interactions, T_2 interactions do not involve transfer of energy, and only a change in phase which leads to loss of coherence.

T_2 relaxation depends on the presence of static internal fields in the substance.[8] These are generally due to protons on larger molecules. These stationary or slowly fluctuating magnetic fields create local regions of increased or decreased magnetic field, depending on whether the protons align with or against the main magnetic field, shown in Figure 1.15. Local field non-uniformity causes the protons to precess at slightly different frequencies. Thus following the 90° pulse, the protons lose coherence and transverse magnetization is lost. This results in both $T_2^\star$ and T_2 relaxation (Figure 1.6).

When paramagnetic substances with high magnetic susceptibility are stationary or compartmentalized, they cause rapid loss of coherence and have a short $T_2^\star$ and T_2. For example, Figure 1.16 illustrates that the magnetization induced inside a deoxygenated red blood cell is greater than in the plasma outside the red cell because the intracellular deoxyhemoglobin is paramagnetic.[15] This compartmentalization of substances with different degrees of induced magnetization leads to magnetic non-uniformity with shortened $T_2^\star$, causing the FID to decay more rapidly. Since gradient echo images are essentially rephased FID images, this also leads to signal loss on gradient echo images. Thus acute and early subacute hemorrhage (containing deoxy and intracellular methemoglobin, respectively) appear dark on $T_2^\star$-weighted gradient echo images (Chapter 7). The different magnetic field inside and outside red cells results in rapid dephasing of water protons diffusing across the red cell membrane in an acute hematoma with secondary T_2-shortening and loss of signal, as seen in Figure 1.17.

As the natural motional frequency of the protons increases, T_2 relaxation becomes less and less efficient. Rapidly fluctuating motions average out over a period of time on the order of the echo-delay time, leading to a more uniform internal magnetic environment. This results in a long T_2 relaxation time. It should be apparent that an environment which is efficient at one form of relaxation may not be efficient for another.

The hydration-layer water in brain edema has a shorter T_1 than bulk-phase water like CSF.[12] Yet the motion of the protons in brain edema is not so slow that T_2 relaxation is efficient, so T_2 remains long. This accounts for the intense appearance of the vasogenic edema associated with brain tumors on T_2-weighted MR images, as in Figure 1.18.

Spin echo

An MR pulsing sequence involves acquisition of multiple spin echo signals. For a 256×256 image with two excitations, 512 separate spin echoes are acquired. During the time between acquisitions, the longitudinal magnetization recovers or 'relaxes' along the z-axis. Longitudinal recovery is identical to the process of initial magnetization when the body was first placed in the magnet. When the body is in the magnet, the 'equilibrium state' is that of full magnetization. Therefore, longitudinal relaxation represents the recovery of magnetization along the z-axis which occurs between spin-echo acquisitions.[8]

In the first step of a spin-echo pulsing sequence, a 90° RF pulse flips the existing longitudinal magnetization from the z-axis 90° into the transverse xy-plane. Whenever transverse magnetization is present, it rotates at the Larmor frequency and induces an oscillating MR signal in a receiving coil. The magnitude of the transverse magnetization after the 90° pulse is approximately equal to the magnitude of the longitudinal magnetization which had recovered during the interval allowed between repetitions. This interval is called the repetition time TR and is one of the programmable sequence parameters.

In the process of flipping the magnetization 90° into the transverse orientation, the longitudinal component of magnetization is totally lost and must be allowed to recover before another signal can be generated. The amount of longitudinal magnetization which is recovered depends on the rate of recovery (T_1) and the time allowed for recovery to occur, that is TR, illustrated earlier in Figure 1.3.

The magnitude of the signal detected depends not only on longitudinal recovery between repetitions but also on how well the signal persists, or alternatively, on how slowly the transverse magnetization decays from its initial maximum value, as described in Figure 1.14. This decay depends on the T_2 of the substance. The amount of time allowed for decay to occur—the time between the initial 90° RF pulse and the detection of the spin echo—is called the echo-delay time (TE) and is another programmable sequence parameter.

Mathematically the intensity (I) of the spin-echo signal can be approximated:[2]

$$I = N(H)f(v)(1 - e^{-TR/T_1})e^{-TE/T_2}$$

where $N(H)$ is the NMR-visible, mobile proton density and $f(v)$ is an unspecified function of flow. This equation indicates that intensity of the MR signal increases as hydrogen density and T_2 increase and as T_1 decreases. It should also be noted that T_1 and T_2 influences are both relative to TR and TE, the programmable sequence parameters. Thus the effect of the T_1 and T_2 times of the substance on signal intensity is subject to the specific values of TR and TE selected before the image is acquired. Only mobile protons, that is, those associated with liquids, return an NMR signal. Solids have a very short T_2 and thus have no significant NMR signal.

When considered in the most simplistic terms, the spin echo is a two-step process. The first step (longitudinal recovery) determines the starting intensity for the second step (transverse decay). The starting intensity reflects the relationship between T_1 and TR, modified by the proton density. The subsequent decay from this starting intensity reflects differences in T_2 and TE. Consider the differentiation of brain and CSF shown in Figure 1.19. At TR = 0.5 seconds, the CSF signal starts to decay from a markedly decreased initial value. Despite the longer T_2 of CSF, the intensity remains less than that of brain over the range of echo-delay times shown. If the repetition time TR is lengthened to 2.0 seconds, the CSF signal starts to decay from a greater initial intensity and still decays more slowly than the signal from brain. Thus the two signals will become isointense at approximately 50 msec. At longer TE, the CSF is more intense than brain, illustrated in Figure 1.20. The MR appearance of the CSF-filled ventricular and subarachnoid spaces on long TR/long TE sequences can simulate a CT study with the intrathecal contrast.

The difference in T_1 values between brain parenchyma (shorter T_1) and CSF (longer T_1) can be used to enhance contrast between the two. This is important when seeking abnormalities at the brain–CSF interface. As shown in Figure 1.3, a short TR time allows a shorter T_1 substance (such as brain) to recover signal between repetitions to a much greater extent than a longer T_1 substance (such as CSF). The contrast in short TR/short TE sequences is based primarily on differences in T_1; they are called 'T_1-weighted' images. Note that substances with low values of T_1 have the highest signal intensity on T_1-weighted images.

As the TR is prolonged, all substances fully recover longitudual magnetization between repetitions and the pixel intensity becomes independent of T_1. At short TE, the effect of T_2 decay is minimized and one is left with an image which depends primarily on differences in proton density, that is, a 'proton density-weighted' image.

The effect of variable T_1- and proton density-weighting is demonstrated in Figure 1.21. At long TR, the white matter in the corpus callosum is less intense than the gray matter due to the lower mobile proton density in white matter,[4] shown in Figure 1.22. When the TR is shortened, however, the relative signal from the corpus callosum increases because white matter has a shorter T_1 than gray matter.

Substances with longer T_2 times will generate stronger signals than substances with shorter T_2 times, if both are acquired at the same TE and if proton density and T_1 are comparable as illustrated in Figure 1.14. When multiple spin echoes are acquired, the signal strength generally decreases as TE is lengthened due to T_2 decay, as shown earlier in Figure 1.6. As discussed in Chapter 3, an exception to this statement may occur in slow laminar blood flow where the intraluminal signal may be greater on the second-echo image than on the first due to even-echo rephasing.[6]

Increasing the TE increases the differences in the T_2 relaxation times between substances, increasing the T_2-weighting. Images obtained with a sufficiently long TR and TE such that the CSF is more intense than brain are regarded as 'heavily T_2-weighted'. Figure 1.20 also displays 'moderately T_2-weighted' images, where brain and CSF are isointense.

A typical edematous or cystic lesion has a longer T_1 and T_2 than brain, illustrated in Figures 1.23 and 1.24. On T_1-weighted images such a lesion will appear dark, ie it will have negative contrast. On T_2-weighted images it will appear bright and will thus have positive contrast. If a short TR/long TE sequence is inadvertently chosen, the tendencies towards positive and negative lesion contrast will cancel and the lesion may not be detected, as seen in Figure 1.23b.

In general, the strongest signal is detected from those substances with the highest proton densities (high water content), shortest T_1 times (rapid recovery) and longest T_2 times (slowest decay). The high signal from short T_1 substances, for example, liquid cholesterol (Figure 1.8), fat (Figure 1.25), subacute hemorrhage (Figure 1.26), and gadolinium-enhanced brain tumor[16] (Figure 1.27) is enhanced on short TR/short TE images. The high signal from long T_2 substances, such as mucus (Figure 1.28), subacute hemorrhage (Figure 1.29), and CSF (Figure 1.24) is enhanced on long TR/long TE spin-echo images or on short TR/low flip angle gradient-echo images (Figure 1.30). The weakest MR signals come from tissues with low proton density, long T_1 values (slow recovery), short T_2 values (rapid decay), and rapidly flowing blood (Figure 1.29). Air (Figure 1.28), dense calcification (Figure 1.31), and cortical bone (Figures 1.29 and 1.32) have low mobile hydrogen density. Acute hemorrhage (Figure 1.17) and early subacute hemorrhage (Figure 1.26) have low signal on long TR/long TE images.

To summarize: the spin-echo MR signal is greatest when the T_1 is short and the T_2 and proton density are high; it is decreased if the T_1 is long and the T_2 and proton density are small. The differentiation of lesions from normal tissues can be enhanced if one is aware of the differences in the proton density and magnetic relaxation times and selects the sequence times accordingly.

A comment on the measurement of T_1 and T_2 relaxation times in current MR imagers: although they are useful in a qualitative sense, the absolute values have little meaning. With most MR imaging systems, there is significant RF non-uniformity throughout the imaging volume.[17] This is because the double-saddle RF coil cannot produce an exact 90° pulse at each point in a large imaging volume. At some points it overshoots and at others the flip angle is less than 90°. The result is a non-uniform MR signal from otherwise comparable tissue throughout the volume. Because apparent T_1 and T_2 times can be calculated from these intensities, the calculated values are also position-dependent. In addition, the particular TR and TE times chosen to calculate the T_1 and T_2 relaxation times affect the measured values. Since the tissue is generally heterogeneous and, therefore, a single exponential model may be inaccurate.[18] Thus, even in the same imager, a substance may appear to have different relaxation times, depending on the position in the coil and the particular values of TR and TE being used. Similarly there will be differences in measured T_1 and T_2 relaxation times between different MR imaging systems because of differences in RF coil design and RF power input and gain settings even if they operate at the same field. For imagers operating at different field strengths, T_1 increases as the field strength increases (T_2 remains essentially constant).[8]

Measured values of T_2 vary, not only because of RF non-uniformity, but also because of differing strengths of the gradient fields. For bulk-phase liquids in particular, self diffusion during the time gradients are applied ·leads to additional dephasing and T_2-shortening.[19] The measured T_2 also depends on the chosen value of TE since longer interpulse intervals (the time TE/2 between the 90° and 180° pulses) allow more time for dephasing due to self-diffusion. T_2 measurements will therefore be different for different imagers and will vary when different TE times and gradients are used in the same imager.

Forming an MR image

The generation of an MR image requires the combination of spatial and intensity information. As discussed above, spatial information is encoded in the frequencies which comprise the spin-echo signal.[8] The frequency of resonance depends on the local value of the magnetic field. Although the main magnetic field is designed to be quite uniform, additional magnetic fields can be temporarily superimposed on the main static field. This creates spatial variation in the net magnetic field, resulting in a magnetic field gradient. At each position along this gradient, there is a slightly different resonant frequency. By knowing the exact value of the magnetic field at each point, one can predict the local resonant frequency. Thus the various frequencies in the spin echo indicate the position of the resonating protons which generated that signal. Since three coordinates (x, y, and z) must be specified to localize a point in space, MR images require three separate gradient fields. In practice these fields are generated by electromagnetic coils which can be turned on and off rapidly.

An MR image is the result of a complicated interplay between RF pulses and intermittently activated gradient fields, all of which are under computer control.[20] Depending on the programming, signal can be acquired from the whole volume simultaneously (three-dimensional (3D) acquisition) or from slices or planes within the volume (two-dimensional (2D) acquisition). A particularly efficient method to generate images from multiple slices within the volume of interest involves sequential acquisition of adjacent slices.[2] Thus while protons in one slice are recovering during the repetition time between pulses, other slices can be imaged by selective exposure to RF pulses containing very specific frequencies. Such selective pulses must be applied in the presence of a slice-selecting gradient so that only protons within the intended slice resonate.[8]

Two algorithms are generally used for image reconstruction. Projection-reconstruction techniques (2DPR or 3DPR) are similar to the method used in CT and are thus prone to the same streak and motion artifacts present in CT. Spatial resolution is related to the number of different projections or angles used. Fourier transform techniques (2DFT or 3DFT) are less sensitive to motion artifacts and are now the most commonly used for reconstruction. Spatial resolution in such techniques is determined by the number of phase-encoded projections for a given field of view (FOV) and by the relationship between the strength of the gradient and the range of frequencies (bandwidth) which are detected, shown in Figure 1.33a.

There are two axes in a 2DFT image: the 'readout' axis and the 'phase-encoded' axis. For a transaxial image in the traditional orientation (z-axis along the main magnetic field), the z-gradient is used to select the slice. The y-gradient may be used for 'phase-encoding' and the x-gradient for 'frequency encoding' or 'readout' (or vice versa).

During readout, the spin echo signal is 'sampled' a certain number of times. This reduces the analog signal to a string of digital numbers which can be handled by the computer. The number of times the spin echo is sampled is equal to the number of 'projections' along the readout or frequency encoded axis, for example, typically 256. The total period of time the echo is sampled is called the 'echo sampling time' and is of the order of 20 milliseconds. The interval between samplings of the spin echo is called the sampling interval or 'dwell time'. Dwell times are typically of the order of 100 microseconds. The bandwidth is defined as the inverse of the dwell time. Thus, for 256 readout projections and echo sampling time of 25.6 milliseconds, the dwell time would be 100 microseconds and the bandwidth 10 kHz. Since the bandwidth is the inverse of the dwell time, it is also equal to the number of readout projections divided by the echo sampling time.

To determine the spatial resolution one must now set the gradient strength:

spatial resolution = 1/(readout projections × dwell time × gradient strength)

Thus for 256 readout projections, a dwell time of 100 microseconds and a gradient strength of 0.1 gauss/cm (420 Hz/cm), the spatial resolution would be 1 mm.

Since the field-of-view (FOV) is the product of the number of readout projections and the spatial resolution, the above relationship can be modified to show that the bandwidth is equal to the product of the FOV and the gradient strength. (In fact, some confusion exists as to whether the polarity of the gradient should be considered in bandwidth measurements or not. The convention used in Figure 1.33 is that used by most manufacturers when they quote a value of bandwidth. For purposes of calculating FOV, the 'full bandwidth' should be used, which does not take polarity into account and is twice that shown in Figure 1.33.

If a constant range of frequencies is received (bandwidth constant), increasing the gradient reduces the field of view along a particular axis, increasing the spatial resolution. Alternatively if the gradient is held constant and the bandwidth is reduced, spatial resolution is improved. Reduced bandwidth techniques have the benefit that they reduce noise (since noise is proportional to the square root of the bandwidth), and thus increase the signal-to-noise ratio.[20]

The only 'penalty' for increasing spatial resolution along the readout axis is that there are fewer protons resonating in the smaller voxels which decreases the signal-to-noise ratio.[21] An increase in spatial resolution along the phase-encoded axis requires an increase in the number of phase-encoded projections, N, each with a different strength of the phase-encoding gradient. When the strength of the readout gradient and the strength of the strongest phase-encoded gradient are the same (and the bandwidths are the same), spatial resolution is comparable along the two axes.

Like the sequence parameter times (TR and TE), spatial resolution must be set prospectively during clinical operation of an MR imager. This is accomplished by specification of the size of the acquisition matrix and the field of view. Larger matrices (covering the same area or volume) result in better spatial resolution, but not necessarily in greater lesion detectability. In addition, larger matrices (larger N) may require longer acquisition times since the acquisition time is equal to the product TR $\times$ n $\times$ N, where n is the number of excitations. Spatial resolution can be increased along the readout axis without increasing the acquisition time. This may be useful when the aspect ratio of the image is other than 1:1 such that the readout direction corresponds to the longer side in the rectangular image. For example, a sagittal spine image might well be longer along the axis of the spine than from front to back in the patient. If the aspect ratio of the image were 1:2, then a 128 $\times$ 256 acquisition matrix could produce square pixels. Assignment of the longer axis to the readout direction would result in greater spatial resolution (compared to dividing the same signal into 128 bins) without increasing the acquisition time. If such an asymmetric acquisition matrix is used for a square field of view, non-square pixels result.

Other considerations may influence the assignment of phase-encoding and readout gradients to particular axes in addition to the image aspect ratio. Motion artifacts in a 2DFT image occur along the phase-encoded axis,[22] regardless of the direction of motion. Using a sagittal image of the spine as an example, one might assign the phase-encoded direction to the shorter anterior-posterior axis. However, on heavily T_2-weighted images, this might result in projection of motion artifacts from the high-intensity flowing CSF onto the spinal cord itself. When such artifacts are unacceptable, they can be eliminated by phase encoding along the axis of the spine (although the longitudinal field of view would be reduced).

Other artifacts may arise when the object is larger than the field of view.[23] These are known as 'wraparound' or 'aliasing' artifacts, illustrated in Figure 1.34. Increasing the field of view or changing the direction of the phase-encoded and readout axes may also modify these artifacts.

Signal-to-noise ratio (S/N)

The 'resolving power' as defined by Rose is a useful measure of the machine-determined ability to discriminate a lesion from its background.[24] Resolving power increases with increasing spatial resolution, S/N, and object contrast. The S/N from a pixel is proportional to the product of the voxel volume V and the square root of the product of the number of excitations n and the number of phase-encoded projections N:[1]

$$S/N \propto V\sqrt{nN}$$

Voxel volume is the product of the square of the in-plane pixel dimension and the slice thickness, assuming symmetric matrices. Spatial resolution is determined by the FOV divided by the number of pixels along a particular axis in the image. For purposes of further discussion, the matrix will be considered to be square with equal numbers of square pixels along both axes.

Thinner slices and higher spatial resolution carry an S/N penalty. When higher spatial resolution is achieved by increasing N (rather than decreasing the FOV), there is also a time penalty since the acquisition time t is the product of TR, N, and n:

$$t = \text{TR} \times N \times n$$

The signal-to-noise ratio improves as the square root of the number of excitations. This is because as the two (or more) spin echoes of identical acquisitions are 'averaged' together, the noise adds randomly and increases only as $\sqrt{n}$ while the signal adds linearly with n; the net result is thus $n/\sqrt{n} = \sqrt{n}$ increase in S/N. Similarly, as N increases, the noise in the multiple spin echoes added together sums randomly (as $\sqrt{N}$) while the signal adds linearly for a similar net result of $N/\sqrt{N} = \sqrt{N}$ increase in S/N (ignoring the separate effect of a smaller voxel volume on S/N).

As an example, consider the net effect on S/N per pixel when the spatial resolution is improved by increasing from a 128^2 to a 256^2 matrix at constant bandwidth, FOV, TR, TE, slice thickness, and number of excitations:

$$\frac{(S/N)_1}{(S/N)_2} = \frac{V_1}{V_2}\sqrt{\frac{n_1}{n_2}}\sqrt{\frac{N_1}{N_2}}$$

If subscript 1 refers to the high resolution 256^2 image and subscript 2 to the 128^2, then:

$$\frac{(S/N)_1}{(S/N)_2} = \frac{1}{4}\sqrt{\frac{1}{1}}\sqrt{\frac{2}{1}} = 0.35$$

thus the S/N per pixel of the high-resolution image is 35 per cent of the low-resolution image.[21] (Also, the acquisition time is twice as long since $N_1 = 2N_2$ and TR and n are the same.) If the acquisition time is to be held constant, then the number of excitations must be halved in the high resolution images. In this case, the S/N ratio per pixel is:

$$\frac{(S/N)_1}{(S/N)_2} = \frac{1}{4}\sqrt{\frac{1}{2}}\sqrt{\frac{2}{1}} = 0.25$$

thus for equal acquisition times, the S/N of the high resolution image is one-quarter that of the low resolution image.[21]

While S/N per pixel determines edge discrimination which is necessary to detect small lesions, S/N per unit area is a more appropriate quantity to use for the vomparison of large lesions.[21] The eye tends to integrate the pixels in a given area, 'averaging' the signals in a manner similar to the effect of multiple excitations of the spin-echo sequence. The ratio of pixels per unit area is N_1^2/N_2^2 and S/N per unit area increases as the square root of this quantity:

$$\sqrt{N_1^2/N_2^2} = N_1/N_2$$

For the example above, this will double the relative S/N of the high-resolution images. In practice, the comparison of S/N in two images is between that predicted for S/N per pixel and that predicted for S/N per unit area, depending if one is trying to detect small or large lesions, respectively.

It should be noted that spatial resolution along the frequency-encoded (readout) axis can be improved in two ways: by doubling the strength of the readout gradient and sampling twice as fast (bandwidth increased) or by leaving the gradient unchanged and by sampling twice as long (bandwidth constant). The above analysis utilizes the latter technique which leaves bandwidth (and thus S/N) unchanged.[23]

Perception, like many other biologic processes, is logarithmic, as the eye does not respond linearly to stimuli but rather is more sensitive at low levels and less sensitive at higher levels of S/N.[21] The perceived image quality is a logarithmic function of S/N. If there is a high intrinsic S/N (due to high fields or reduced-bandwidth techniques), then reducing the S/N to 25–35 per cent of its previous value may be tolerated without a significant perceptual loss in image quality. However, at lower S/N, such losses not only result in a 'grainy' appearance to a normal image but in loss of contrast-to-noise such that small lesions may be missed.[21]

To illustrate the effect of varying spatial resolution on image quality as a function of changing baseline S/N, consider Figures 1.35–1.37. These figures demonstrate progressive comparison of image quality in patients with multiple sclerosis (MS) using 128^2 and 256^2 images on our Diasonics unit from 1983 to 1986 as system upgrades improved S/N. They are considered typical of such improvements on medium-field units over this period of time. Multiple sclerosis was chosen as the typical low-contrast lesion and detectability was compared after each major upgrade. As is obvious, it was not until both reduced-bandwidth technology and quadrature detection were implemented that a 256^2/5 mm thick/two-excitation image was felt to be diagnostically superior to the 128^2/5 mm/four-excitation image.

Partial-volume effects

The detectability of a small, low-contrast lesion is also markedly affected by the slice thickness. While thicker slices have greater S/N (due to larger voxel volumes), small, low-contrast lesions can easily go undetected due to overwhelming partial-volume effects. To quantitate this effect, a computer study was performed,[25] moving a lesion of given inherent contrast through a slice and the gap between slices. Figure 1.38 demonstrates the effect of slice thickness on lesion detectability. Clearly, a higher percentage of large, high-contrast lesions are detected when the gap is minimized. However, for low-contrast lesions with a high filling factor detection threshold, the lesion must be large or almost entirely within the slice to be detected. Small lesions entirely within the slice may never be detected due to partial-volume effects if the slice is too thick. As the slice thickness decreases, the filling factor increases for a lesion of given size, increasing its chances of being detected. Figure 1.38 compares 5 and 10 mm slices with the same 1 mm spatial resolution in a patient with MS. The MS plaques cannot be seen on the 1 cm slices due to overwhelming partial-volume effects. The lesions are only seen on the 5 mm slice where they occupy a greater percentage of a voxel and have a higher filling factor.

Chemical-shift artifact

Although the majority of the NMR signal comes from the hydrogen nuclei of water molecules, lipid protons in fatty tissues can also contribute.[26] Fat and water protons do not resonate at exactly the same frequency. Fat protons resonate at a slightly higher frequency, the *difference* of which is usually described as a fraction of the resonant frequency. Since the difference in frequencies (or the 'chemical shift') is very small, it is expressed as 'parts per million' or 'ppm'. Fat protons resonate at 3 ppm higher frequency than water protons. The absolute frequency difference depends on the strength of the main magnetic field (which determines the Larmor frequency). Thus at 0.35 Tesla (15 MHz resonant frequency) a 3 ppm chemical shift will result in fat resonating at 45 Hz (15 MHz × 3 ppm) higher frequency than water. At 1.5 Tesla (64 MHz) fat resonates at 192 Hz higher frequency than water.

Spatial information in the MR image is encoded in the specific frequencies comprising the spin echo. Such frequency discrimination is provided through the use of gradient fields. The minimum strength of the gradient field is determined by the degree of non-uniformity of the main magnetic field, that is, the net variation in field strength from point to point due to the gradient must be greater than that due to the random non-uniformity in the static field. Stronger static fields with comparable uniformity (such as 20 ppm) require stronger gradient fields.

If a 0.2 gauss/cm (2 mT/m) gradient is applied across a 25 cm object, there will be a field difference of 5 gauss across the object and a frequency difference of:

$$(5 \text{ gauss} \times 42 \text{ MHz/Tesla} \times \text{Tesla}/10^4 \text{ gauss}) = 21 \text{ kHz}$$

from one end of the object to the other, 10.5 kHz on the positive side of midline and 10.5 kHz on the negative side. (The bandwidth in this instance is 10.5 kHz.) If the object is divided into 256 pixels, there will be a frequency difference of 82 Hz (21 000/256) per pixel. If fat and water are both present in the pixel, they will resonate at frequencies which are separated by 45 Hz at 0.35 Tesla and by 192 Hz at 1.5 Tesla. Thus the frequency difference due to the chemical shift between fat and water is comparable to the frequency difference across 2.4 (195/82) pixels at 1.5 Tesla and one-half pixel at 0.35 Tesla. Therefore, at high field the fat image will be shifted 2.4 pixels along the readout (frequency-encoded) axis relative to the water image. This chemical-shift artifact (illustrated in Figure 1.25) is most noticeable at interfaces between tissues containing different amounts of fat and water.

Although the chemical-shift artifact may be more noticeable at high field, it is also increased when the strength of the gradient is reduced. As the intrinsic uniformity of lower field magnets has improved, weaker gradients can be used without sacrificing frequency discrimination. Weaker gradients narrow the bandwidth which reduces the noise, increasing the S/N, but have the disadvantage of increasing the chemical-shift artifact.

While chemical-shift artifact is a potential problem in most parts of the body, it is generally not in the brain, although fatty marrow can shift over the brain, creating a pseudo-subdural hematoma. Fat in the normal brain is not NMR-visible, thus there is no chemical-shift artifact, either at high field or on intermediate field systems using reduced bandwidth techniques. When chemical-shift artifact is present and bothersome, it can be eliminated by increasing the strength of the gradient fields (at a cost in S/N).

References

1 HOLLAND GN, HAWKES RC, MOORE WS, Nuclear magnetic resonance (NMR) tomography of the brain: coronal and sagittal sections, *J Comput Assist Tomogr* (1980) **4**: 429–33.

2 CROOKS LE, ARAKAWA M, HOENNINGER JC et al, NMR whole body imager operating at 3.5 kgauss, *Radiology* (1982) **143**: 169.

3 BYDDER GM, STEINER RE, YOUNG IR et al, Clinical NMR imaging of the brain: 140 cases, *AJR* (1982) **139**: 215–36; *AJNR* (1982) **3**: 459–80.

4 WEHRLI FW, MACFALL J, NEWTON TH, Parameters determining the appearance of NMR images. In: Newton TH, Potts DG, eds. *Advanced imaging techniques*, Vol II. (Clavadel Press: San Francisco 1983) 81–118.

5 BRADLEY WG, WALUCH V, Blood flow: magnetic resonance imaging, *Radiology* (1985) **154**: 443–50.

6 WALUCH V, BRADLEY WG, NMR even echo rephasing in slow laminar flow, *J Comput Assist Tomogr* (1984) **8**(4): 594–8.

7 BRADLEY WG, WALUCH V, FERNANDEZ E et al, The appearance of rapidly flowing blood, *AJR* (1984) **143**: 1167–74.

8 BRADLEY WG, CROOKS LE, NEWTON TH, Physical principles of NMR. In Newton TH, Potts DG, eds. *Advanced imaging techniques*, Vol II. (Clavadel Press: San Francisco 1983), 15–62.

9 NALCIOGLU O, CHO ZH, LEE SY et al, Fast hybrid 3D imaging by small tip angle excitation, *Magn Reson Imaging* (1986) **4**: 103.

10 FRAHM J, HAASE A, MATTHAEI D et al, FLASH MR imaging, *Magn Reson Imaging* (1986) **4**: 104.

11 BYDDER GM, YOUNG IR, Clinical use of the partial saturation and saturation recovery sequences in MR imaging, *J Comput Assist Tomogr* (1985) **9**(6): 1020–32.

12 FULLERTON GD, CAMERON IL, ORD VA, Frequency dependence of magnetic resonance spin-lattice relaxation of protons in biological materials, *Radiology* (1984) **151**: 135–8.

13 BRADLEY WG, SCHMIDT PS, The effect of methemoglobin formation on subarachnoid hemorrhage, *Radiology* (1984) **153**: 166.

14 BRASCH RC, Methods of contrast enhancement of NMR imaging and potential applications, *Radiology* (1983) **147**: 781–8.

15 GOMORI JM, GROSSMAN RI, GOLDBERG HI et al, Intracranial hematomas: imaging by high-field MR, *Radiology* (1985) **157**: 87–93.

16 GRAIF M, GYDDER GM, STEINER RE et al, Contrast-enhanced MR imaging of malignant brain tumors, *AJNR* (1985) **6**: 855–62.

17 ROSEN BR, PYKETT IL, BRADY TJ, Spin-lattice relaxation time measurements in two dimensional NMR imaging: corrections for plane selection and pulse sequence, *J Comput Assist Tomogr* (1984) **8**: 195–9.

18 LE JEUNE JJ, GALLIER J, RIVET P et al, Is an interpretation model for proton relaxation times in biological tissue possible? (abstract), *Magn Reson Med* (1984) **1**: 192.

19 WESBEY GE, MOSELEY ME, EHMAN RL, Translational molecular self-diffusion in magnetic resonance imaging: effects and applications. In James TL, Margulis AR, eds. *Biomedical magnetic resonance*. (University of California Press: San Francisco 1984) 63–78.

20 FEINBERG DA, CROOKS LE, HOENNINGER JC et al, Continuous thin multisection MR imaging by two-dimensional Fourier transform techniques, *Radiology* (1986) **158**: 811–17.

21 BRADLEY WG, KORTMAN KE, CRUES JV et al, Central nervous system high-resolution magnetic resonance imaging: effect of increasing spatial resolution on resolving power, *Radiology* (1985) **156**: 93–8.

22 WOOD M, HENKELMAN R, MR image artifacts from periodic motion, *Med Phys* (1985) **12**(2): 143–51.
23 BRADLEY WG, TSURUDA J, MR sequence parameter optimization: an algorithmic approach, *AJR* (1987) **149**: 815–23.
24 ROSE AA, *Vision: human and electronic* (Plenum Press: New York 1973) Chapter 1.
25 BRADLEY WG, GLENN BJ, The effect of variation in slice thickness and interslice gap on MR lesion detection, *AJNR* (1987) **8**: 1057–62.
26 BABCOCK EE, BRATEMAN L, WEINREB JC et al, Edge artifacts in MR images: chemical shift effect, *J Comput Assist Tomogr* (1985) **9**(2): 252–7.

Bibliography

ABRAHAM A, *The principles of nuclear magnetism*, International series of monographs on physics, (Clarendon Press: Oxford 1961).

ANDREW ER, *Nuclear magnetic resonance*, (Cambridge University Press: Cambridge 1969).

BLOEMBERGEN M, *Nuclear magnetic relaxation*, (WA Benjamin: New York 1970).

BRADLEY WG, ADEY WR, HASSO AN, *Magnetic resonance imaging of the brain, head and neck: a text atlas*, (Aspen Publications: Rockville 1985).

BRANT-ZAWADZKI M, NORMAN D, *Magnetic resonance imaging of the central nervous system*, (Raven Press: New York 1987).

CARRINGTON A, MCLACHLIN AD, *Introduction to magnetic resonance*, (Harper and Row: New York 1967).

FARRAR TC, BECKER ED, *Pulse and Fourier transform NMR: introduction to theory and methods*, (Academic Press: New York 1971).

FUKUSHIMA E, ROEDER SBW, *Experimental pulse NMR. A nuts and bolts approach*, (Addison-Wesley Publishing Company: Reading, Mass. 1981).

GADIAN DG, *NMR and its applications to living systems*, (Clarendon Press: Oxford 1982).

HIGGINS CB, HRICAK H, *Magnetic resonance imaging of the body*, (Raven Press: New York 1978).

JAMES TL, MARGULIS AR, eds, *Biomedical magnetic resonance*, (University of California Press: San Francisco 1984).

KAUFMAN L, CROOKS LE, MARGULIS AR, eds, *Nuclear magnetic resonance in medicine*, (Igaku-Shoin: Tokyo 1981).

NEWTON TH, POTTS DG, eds, *Modern Neuroradiology: advanced imaging techniques*, Vol II, (Clavadel Press: San Francisco 1983).

PARTAIN CL, PRICE RR, PATTON JA et al, eds, *Magnetic resonance (MR) imaging*, (WB Saunders Co: Philadelphia 1983).

SCHUMACHER RT, *Introduction to magnetic resonance*, (WA Benjamin: New York 1970).

SLICHTER CP, *Principles of magnetic resonance*, (Harper and Row: New York 1963).

STARK DD, BRADLEY WG, *Magnetic resonance imaging*, (CV Mosby Publications: St Louis 1988).

WONG WS, TSURUDA JS, KORTMAN KE, BRADLEY WG, *Practical magnetic resonance imaging: a case study approach*, (Aspen Publications: Rockville 1987).

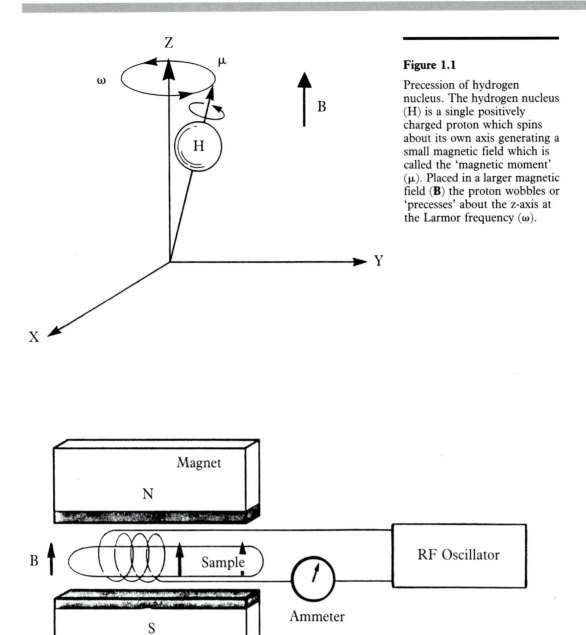

Figure 1.1

Precession of hydrogen nucleus. The hydrogen nucleus (H) is a single positively charged proton which spins about its own axis generating a small magnetic field which is called the 'magnetic moment' (μ). Placed in a larger magnetic field (**B**) the proton wobbles or 'precesses' about the z-axis at the Larmor frequency (ω).

Figure 1.2

Simple NMR spectrometer. When a sample or patient lies in a strong magnetic field (**B**) surrounded by a coil of wire (transmitting and receiving antenna), NMR can be performed by exposure to radio waves at a specific frequency (generated by the RF transmitter or oscillator). The spin-echo signal emitted by the sample induces a current in the receiving antenna which is detected by the radio receiver (ammeter).

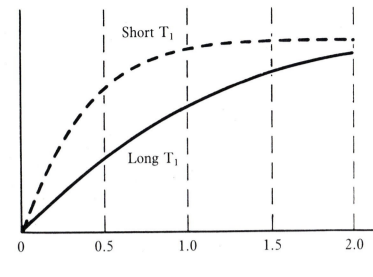

Starting Intensity

Short T$_1$

Long T$_1$

TR (sec)

Figure 1.3

T$_1$-relaxation. Following placement in a magnetic field or recovery from an RF pulse, magnetization recovers exponentially with a first-order time constant T$_1$, the 'spin-lattice' relaxation time. As the repetition time TR is prolonged, the magnetization increases, increasing the starting intensity of the second (decay) step in the spin echo.

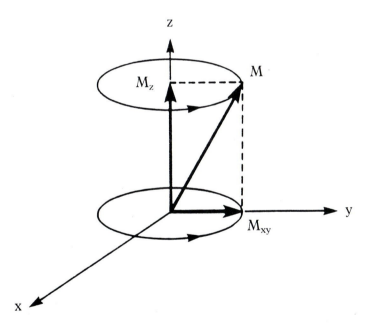

Figure 1.4

Magnetization. At equilibrium, only longitudinal magnetization (M_z) is present and points along the z-axis. When the magnetization (**M**) is tipped away from the z-axis, it can be described by a longitudinal component (**M**$_z$) along the z-axis and a transverse component (**M**$_{xy}$) in the transverse (xy) plane. Whenever transverse magnetization **M**$_{xy}$ is present, it rotates about the z-axis at the Larmor frequency and generates a radio signal.

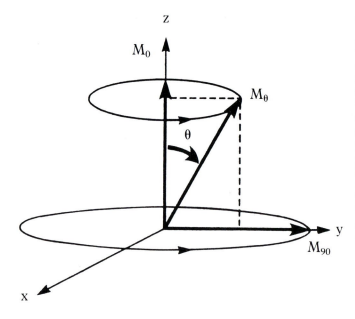

Figure 1.5

Magnetization. Equilibrium magnetization M_0 points along the z-axis and does not rotate. When the magnetization M_θ is displaced an angle θ away from the z-axis it begins to precess about that axis, generating a radio signal at the Larmor frequency. Flip angles θ less than 30° are often used for fast scanning techniques. Notice that such low flip angles result in one-half to one-third the normal transverse magnetization with minimal loss of longitudinal magnetization. When the magnetization is tipped 90°, completely into the xy-plane (M_{90}), the maximum transverse magnetization is generated, however, at a cost of total loss of longitudinal magnetization. The 90° flip angle is typically used to initiate a traditional spin-echo sequence.

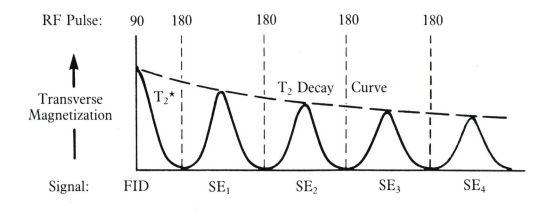

Echo Delay Time (TE)

Figure 1.6

Multiple spin echo train. Transverse magnetization decays rapidly following the initial 90° pulse due to both fixed and fluctuating nonuniformities in the magnetic field as well as to diffusion between these areas of differing magnetic field strength. The first order exponential time constant of the FID (free induction decay) is $T_2^\star$. The height of the peaks of the multiple spin echoes produced following each 180° pulse is limited by a more slowly decaying curve with time constant T_2, reflecting random field fluctuations and diffusion. T_2 is longer than $T_2^\star$ because dephasing due to the fixed nonuniformities in the main field and those due to local iron deposition are negated by the 180° pulse.

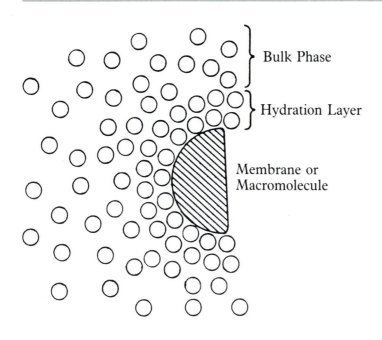

Bulk Phase

Hydration Layer

Membrane or Macromolecule

Figure 1.7

Molecular environment of water. Water in the bulk phase has natural motional frequencies much higher than the operating (Larmor) frequencies used for MR imaging. Water in hydration layers around macromolecules (such as proteins) moves at frequencies much closer to the Larmor frequency. Water protons in this environment have shorter T_1 times.

Figure 1.8

Cholesterol. When cholesterol is in the liquid state, it gives high signal intensity due to its short T_1. Craniopharyngiomas and intrapetrous epidermoids (cholesteatomas) generally demonstrate such high-signal intensity, particularly on T_1-weighted images. When cholesterol is in the solid form in subarachnoid or intraventricular epidermoid tumors, the signal intensity on T_1-weighted images is markedly reduced. On T_2-weighted images, signal intensity increases not as a result of more signal from the cholesterol but due to improved visualization of the water in the interstices of the tumor. (**a**) Craniopharyngioma (SE 1000/28). (**b**) Intrapetrous epidermoid tumor, ie, cholesteatoma, in the coronal plane (SE 500/30). (**c**) Intrapetrous cholesteatoma in the axial plane (SE 500/40). (**d**) Cerebellopontine angle epidermoid showing decreased signal (arrow) on T_1-weighted image (SE 500/30). (**e–f**) Signal intensity of epidermoid (arrow) increases with increasing T_2-weighting due to water content (SE 3000/40 and 80).

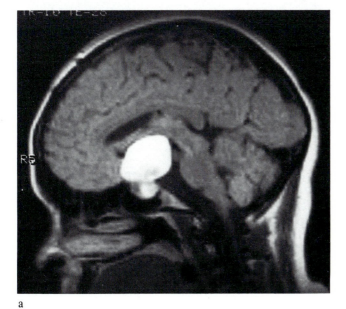

a

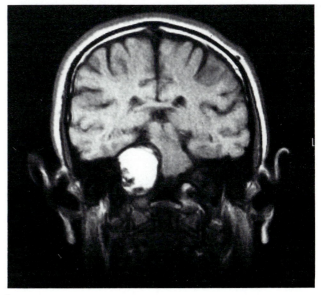

b

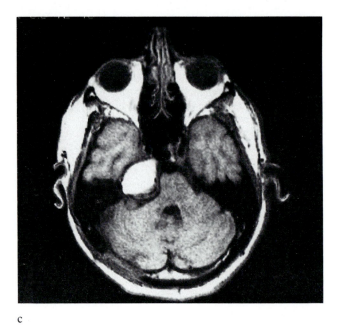

c

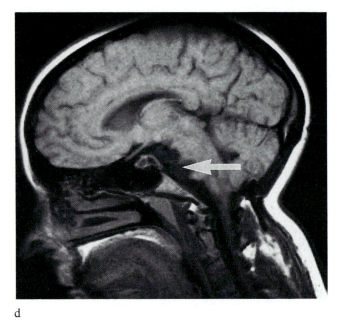

d

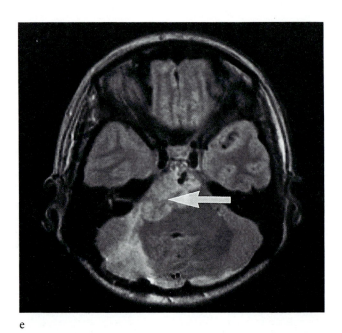

e

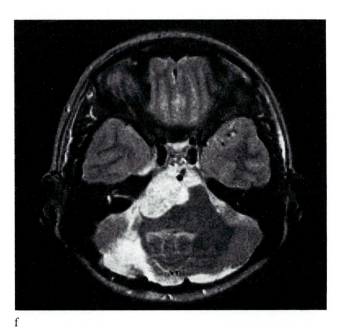

f

Figure 1.8 *continued*

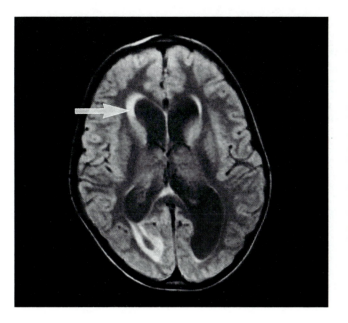

Figure 1.9

Interstitial edema. Water in the bulk phase as intraventricular CSF has a long T_1 relaxation time and thus appears dark on T_1-weighted images. When that same CSF is forced through the ependyma, it becomes partially bound by the myelin protein which shortens its T_1 relaxation time, increasing its intensity. Thus on MR images, water in the form of interstitial edema (arrow) appears different from water in the form of CSF.

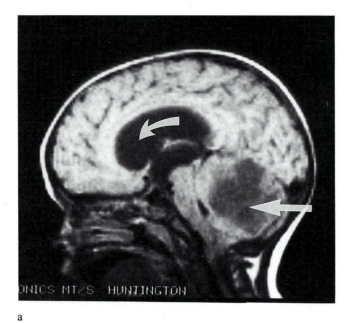

a

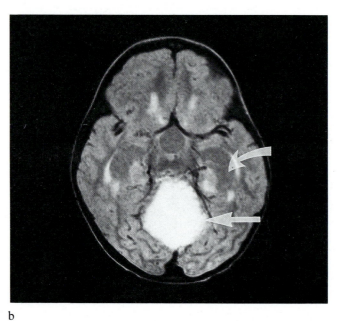

b

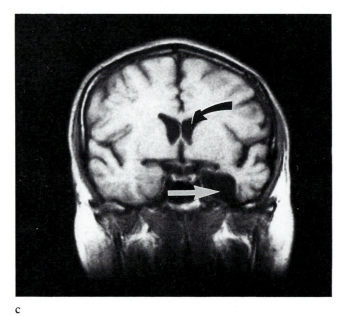

c

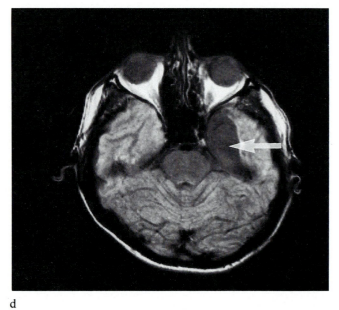

d

Figure 1.10

Effect of protein content on T_1. The proteinaceous fluid in cystic astrocytomas (**a–b**) has a higher percentage of hydration layer water and therefore a shorter T_1 relaxation time than the pure CSF in an arachnoid cyst (**c–d**). (**a**) T_1-weighted sagittal image of cystic astrocytoma demonstrating higher signal intensity in proteinaceous fluid (straight arrow) than in ventricle (SE

500/40) (curved arrow). (**b**) Moderately T_2-weighted axial section through cystic astrocytoma demonstrates higher signal intensity in cyst fluid (straight arrow) than in obstructed ventricles (curved arrow) due to T_1-shortening in former (SE 3000/40). (**c**) T_1-weighted coronal section (SE 500/30) through arachnoid cyst demonstrates signal intensity (straight arrow) approaching

that of intraventricular CSF (curved arrow). (Although the signal intensities should be identical since they have the same low protein content, there is further decrease in signal intensity within the ventricles due to CSF motion.) (**d**) T_2-weighted axial section (SE 2000/300) through arachnoid cyst (arrow) demonstrating signal intensity expected for intraventricular CSF.

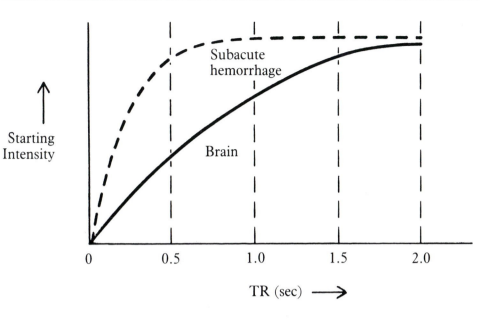

Figure 1.11

MR differentiation of brain and hemorrhage. Subacute hemorrhage has a very short T_1 which enhances its return to equilibrium magnetization relative to the longer T_1 of brain. This contrast is enhanced at short values and lost at long values of TR.

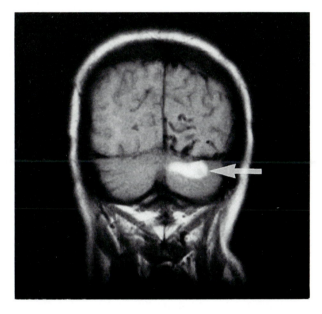

Figure 1.12

Subacute hemorrhage. One week following right occipital hemorrhage, hematoma (arrow) has higher intensity than surrounding brain parenchyma. This is accentuated on a T_1-weighted image which brings out the short T_1 character of the paramagnetic methemoglobin.

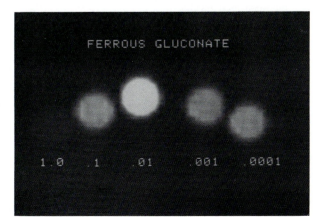

Figure 1.13

Effect of concentration of paramagnetic agent on T_1 and T_2 shortening. Serial dilutions of a paramagnetic substance (ferrous gluconate) are scanned using mildly T_2-weighted technique (SE 2000/28). At low concentrations, there is initially T_1-shortening and, as the ferrous gluconate is increased to full strength, T_2-shortening. The T_1-shortening increases the signal intensity due to the enhanced return to equilibrium magnetization during longitudinal recovery. Although there is full recovery of longitudinal magnetization at high concentrations of the paramagnetic solute, the increased T_2 decay results in loss of signal during the 28 msec required (in this case) for spin-echo formation.

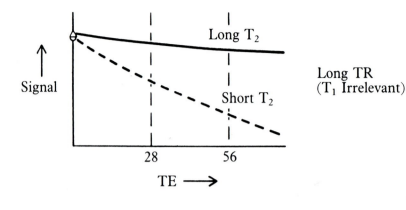

Figure 1.14

T$_2$ decay. At long repetition time TR, individual T$_1$-relaxation times become irrelevant and full magnetization is achieved between repetitions. If it is assumed that two substances have comparable proton density, then they will begin to decay from the same equilibrium magnetization. A substance with a long T$_2$ will decay more slowly than one with a short T$_2$. The decay curves are 'sampled' by acquiring spin-echo signals at variable echo delay times TE. Two such echo delay times, 28 and 56 msec, are indicated for a standard dual-echo sequence.

3D Molecular View of Tissue Lattice

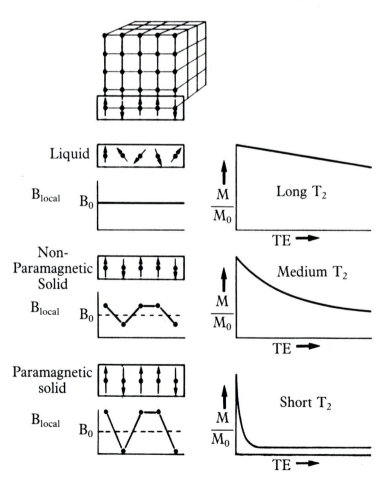

Figure 1.15

Effect of local magnetic non-uniformity on T$_2$ relaxation. When the small magnetic fields or 'moments' associated with individual protons are aligned with or against the main magnetic field (B$_0$) magnetic non-uniformity is created. This leads to slightly different proton precessional rates within a voxel which results in loss of coherence and faster T$_2$ decay. This is most marked in solids (particularly paramagnetic solids) where the magnetic moments are relatively fixed in their alignment with or against the main field. While individual magnetic moments are present in liquids, they fluctuate at high frequencies and, over the time course of an echo, contribute little to the net value of the local magnetic field. Coherence is therefore maintained for a longer period of time in liquids than in solids and T$_2$ decay is consequently slower.

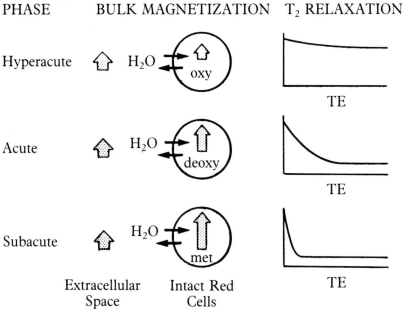

TEMPORAL
PHASE   BULK MAGNETIZATION   T₂ RELAXATION

Hyperacute

Acute

Subacute

Figure 1.16

T₂ shortening in fresh hematomas. (Vertical arrows are proportional to the bulk magnetization, ie, to the strength of the local magnetic field. As long as the red cells remain intact, there are potentially two different magnetic environments, ie, that within the red cell and that outside it. Deoxyhemoglobin and methemoglobin are both paramagnetic and thus have a higher magnetic susceptibility than the nonparamagnetic plasma outside the red cells. Water molecules diffusing in and out of the red cell thus experience a magnetic field *gradient* which results in dephasing and T₂ shortening. These heterogeneities in magnetic susceptibility also lead to T₂* shortening which causes additional signal loss on gradient echo images. Since methemoglobin has five unpaired electrons and deoxyhemoglobin only has four, the greatest dephasing and T₂ shortening occurs in the early subacute phase, prior to red cell lysis. Since oxyhemoglobin is not paramagnetic, the magnetic susceptibility inside the red cell is the same as outside, therefore there is no significant T₂ shortening. For this reason, CT remains the imaging modality of choice to detect hemorrhage during the hyperacute phase when the oxyhemoglobin form predominates.

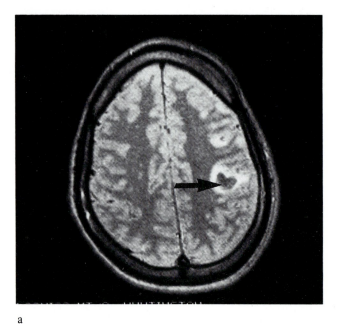

a

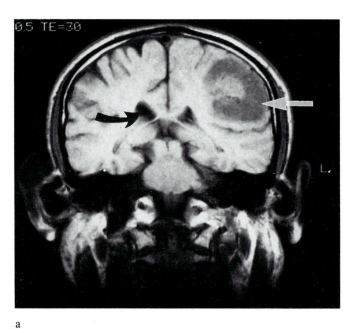

a

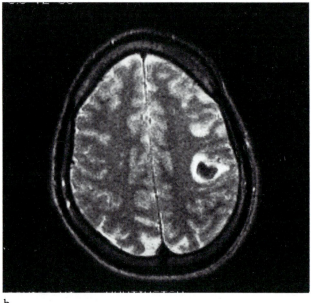

b

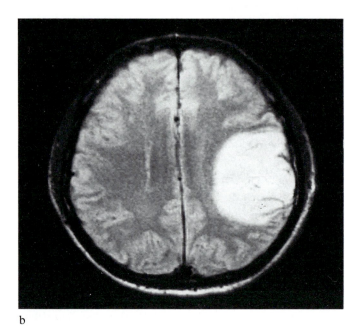

b

Figure 1.17

Acute hematoma two days following trauma. Paramagnetic, magnetically susceptible deoxyhemoglobin within intact red cells causes local magnetic non-uniformity leading to T_2-shortening and loss of signal (arrow). Note additional decrease in signal intensity on second echo which is evident even at 0.35 Tesla. (**a**) First echo (SE 3000/40). (**b**) Second echo (SE 3000/80).

Figure 1.18

Brain tumor. (**a**) On a T_1-weighted image this astrocytoma has intermediate signal (straight arrow) between the higher signal brain and the lower signal CSF in the ventricles (curved arrow) (SE 500/30). (**b**) With increased T_2-weighting (SE 2000/30), the tumor and surrounding edema become hyperintense relative to both brain and CSF due to the combination of an intermediate T_1 and long T_2, reflecting the elevated water content.

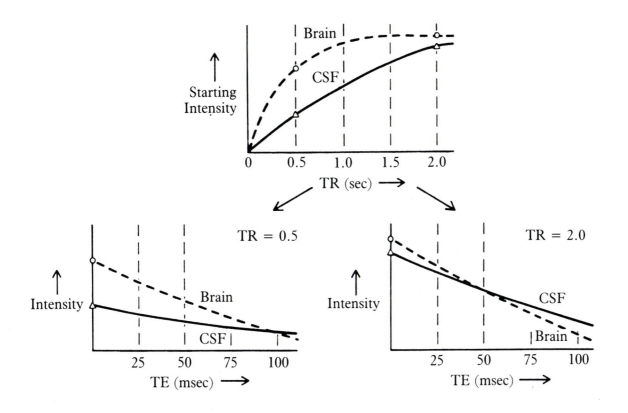

Figure 1.19

Differentiation of brain and CSF by MR. The differential rates of recovery of brain and CSF reflect their relative T_1 relaxation times as illustrated in the top half of the figure. The amount of time allowed for relaxation is the repetition time TR. Two cases (TR = 0.5 sec and TR = 2.0 sec) are illustrated in the lower two figures. In both cases, the small triangle and circle indicate the amount of recovery that occurs by time TR. This then determines the starting point for the second (decay) step for CSF and brain, respectively. Brain recovers magnetization more rapidly initially but decays more rapidly (due to its shorter T_1 and T_2 relaxation times respectively compared to CSF). Notice that brain is more intense than CSF at TR = 0.5 sec and TE < 100 msec. When the TR is increased to 2.0 sec, brain and CSF become isointense at 50 msec and then CSF becomes more intense than brain at longer TE.

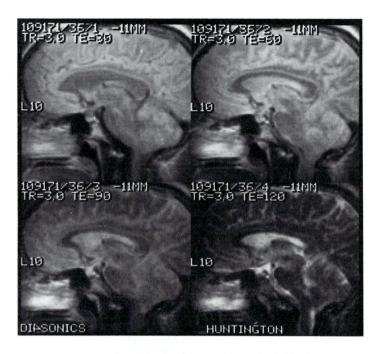

Figure 1.20

Effect of variable echo-delay time on T_2 contrast. Progressive prolongation of echo-delay time (TE) from 30 msec to 60, 90, and 120 msec demonstrates progressive increase in intensity of long T_2 CSF compared to brain. On an SE 3000/60 image, the signal intensity of brain and CSF is similar so that it is difficult to define the fourth ventricle. This is known as a 'moderately' T_2-weighted image. Images in which the CSF is brighter than brain at longer TE are 'heavily' T_2-weighted.

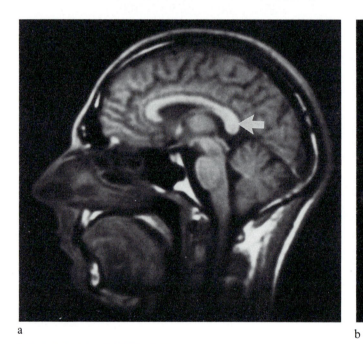

a

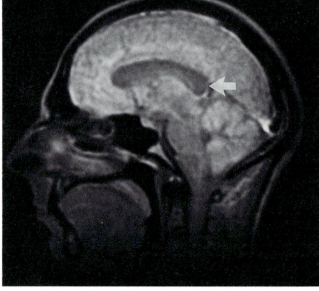

b

Figure 1.21

Effect of variable TR on T_1 contrast. (**a**) At TR = 0.25 sec, CSF is dark relative to brain parenchyma due to T_1 differences. The short T_1 white matter in the corpus callosum (arrow) is also more intense than the adjacent gray matter. (**b**) On TR = 4.0 sec image, the white matter in the corpus callosum now appears dark (arrow) relative to adjacent gray matter due to lower proton density.

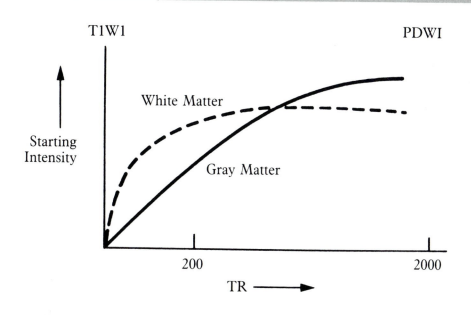

Figure 1.22

Effect of TR on gray/white differentiation. At short values of TR most of the contrast between gray and white matter reflects differences in the T_1 relaxation times. Since white matter has the shorter T_1 it is more intense than gray matter at short TR. (Repetition times less than 200 msec may become less T_1-weighted due to steady-state free precession, as is noted in fast scan techniques.) At long TR, the contrast between gray and white matter reflects differences in proton density. Since white matter has a lower mobile proton density than gray matter it appears darker.

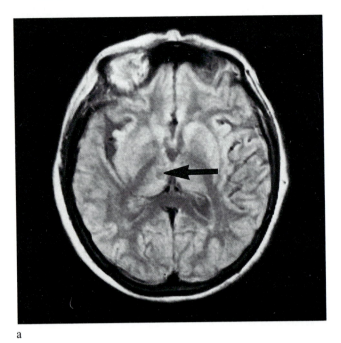

a

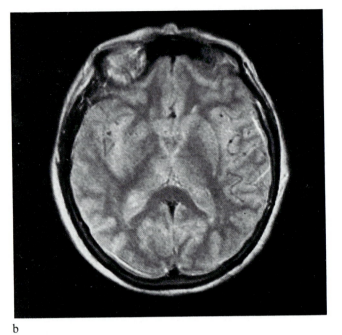

b

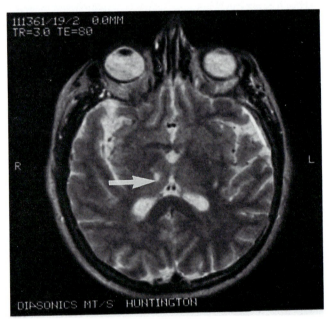

c   d

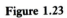

Figure 1.23

Tradeoffs in T_1 and T_2 contrast. (**a–b**) Right thalamic infarct (arrow) is poorly visualized at SE 2000/30 and invisible on SE 2000/60 images. This is due to the competing effects of T_2 contrast (which make the lesion brighter) and T_1 contrast (which make the lesion darker). (**c**) When T_1 contrast is increased (SE 500/40), the lesion has lower intensity than brain due to its longer T_1 (arrow). (**d**) When T_2-weighting is increased (SE 3000/80), the lesion (arrow) appears brighter than brain due to its longer T_2 relaxation time.

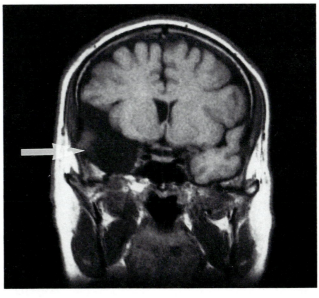

a

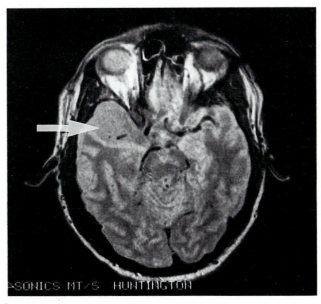

b

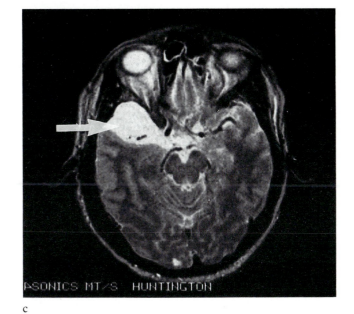

c

Figure 1.24

Opposing T_1 and T_2 contrast in
an arachnoid cyst. (**a**) On T_1-
weighted image, long T_1
arachnoid cyst (arrow) appears
dark relative to normal brain
(SE 500/30). (**b**) On heavily T_2-
weighted image long T_2
arachnoid cyst (arrow) is bright
relative to brain (SE 3000/80).
(**c**) On moderately T_2-
weighted image (SE 3000/40),
cyst (arrow) is isointense with
brain due to offsetting T_1 and
T_2 influences.

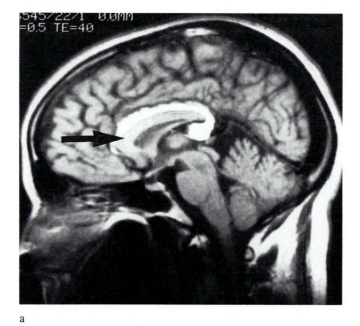

a

Figure 1.25

Lipoma. The fat in this lipoma has high-signal intensity due to its short T_1 relaxation time. This is enhanced on short TR/ short TE images. (**a**) Sagittal section demonstrating lipoma (arrow) and partial agenesis of the corpus callosum (SE 500/ 40). (**b**) Coronal section demonstrating chemical-shift artifact in the frequency-encoded direction (arrowhead).

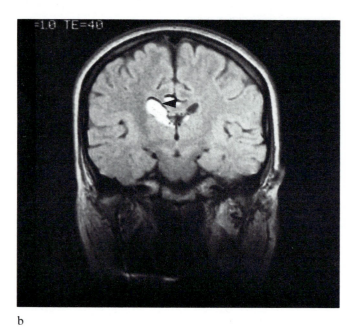

b

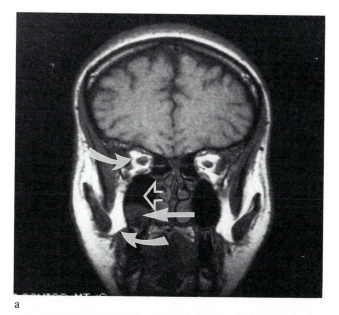

a

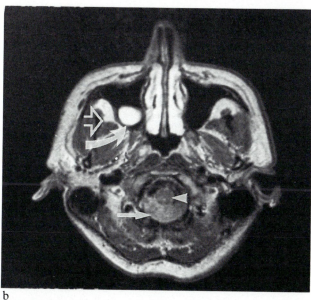

b

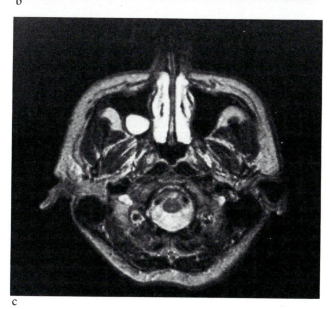

c

Figure 1.28

Mucus. (**a**) T_1-weighted coronal section through the maxillary sinuses demonstrates intermediate signal in the mucous retention cyst (straight arrow), low-signal intensity of the air in the maxillary sinus (open arrow) and high signal in the orbital and infratemporal fat (curved arrows) (SE 500/40). (**b**) On moderately T_2-weighted image (SE 3000/40), cord (arrowhead) and CSF (arrow) are isointense. The mucus retention cyst (curved arrow) has now increased in signal intensity so it is equal to that of the infratemporal fat (open arrow). (**c**) On heavily T_2-weighted image (SE 3000/80), mucus retention cyst is now higher in intensity than infratemporal and subcutaneous fat due to longer T_2 of the former. CSF is now hyperintense relative to cord.

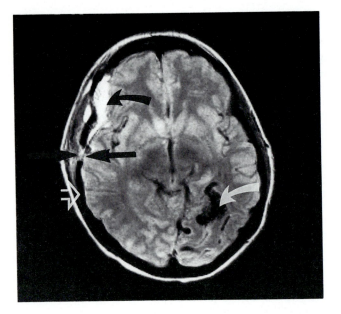

Figure 1.29

Arteriovenous malformation. Note loss of signal intensity (curved white arrow) due to rapidly flowing blood in AVM. Low intensity is also noted in cortical bone of calvarium (open arrow) except where craniotomy has been performed (straight arrow). Note also postoperative subacute epidural hematoma (curved black arrow) which has high-signal intensity due to methemoglobin.

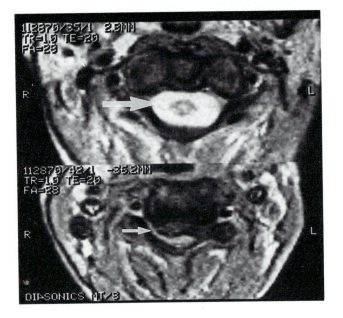

Figure 1.30

Partial flip angle, gradient-echo image. CSF in upper cervical subarachnoid space (arrow) has high-signal intensity due to T_2^*-weighting at a flip angle of 28°. Top image is entry slice in this multislice acquisition demonstrating additional high signal due to flow-related enhancement. Bottom section is interior slice demonstrating herniated disc and decreased signal intensity from CSF in remaining subarachnoid space (arrowhead) in lateral recess.

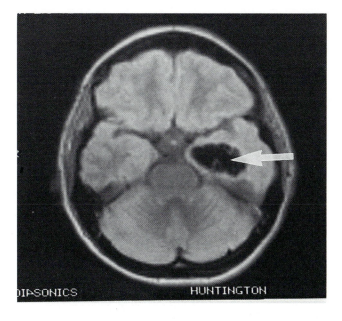

Figure 1.31

Dense calcification. Densely
calcified extra-axial mass
(arrow) has low-signal intensity
on mildly T_2-weighted image
(SE 2000/28).

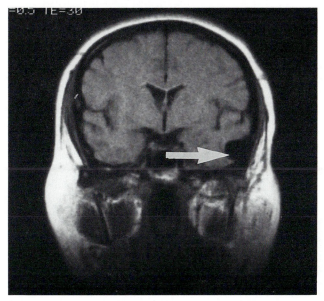

a

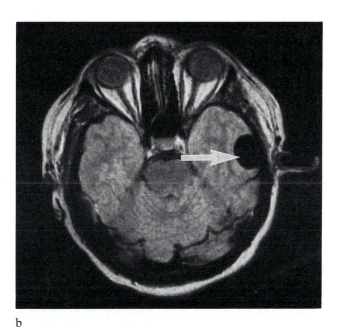

b

Figure 1.32

Osteoma. Cortical bone in
osteoma (arrow) appears dark
in both T_1- and T_2-weighted
images. (**a**) Coronal T_1-
weighted section (SE 500/30).
(**b**) Axial T_2-weighted image
(SE 2000/40).

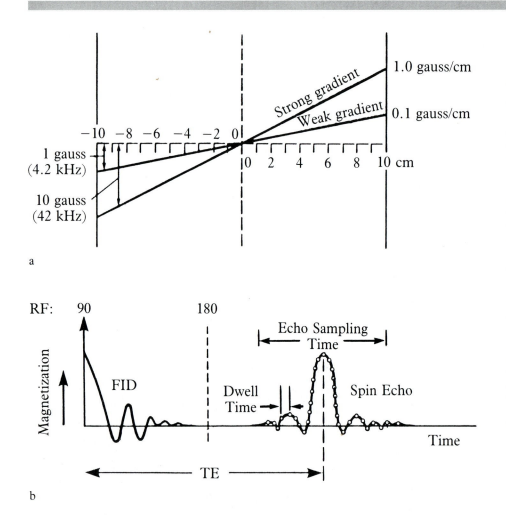

a

b

Figure 1.33

Bandwidth. (**a**) Effect of gradient strength on bandwidth. The bandwidth is the range of frequencies comprising the spin-echo signal. The bandwidth can be thought of as a 'frequency window' which lets in noise. Since noise is proportional to the square root of bandwidth, reduced bandwidth techniques decrease the noise, increasing the signal-to-noise ratio. Bandwidth can be decreased by decreasing the strength of the gradient as shown here. A relatively weak gradient (0.1 gauss/cm) leads to a bandwidth of 4.2 kHz for the 20 cm field of view. The gradient strength of 1 gauss/cm may be required for high spatial resolution or thin slices; however, the bandwidth is increased to an inefficient value of 42 kHz. (**b**) Echo Sampling Time. The spin echo is sampled typically 256 times. The interval between samplings is the dwell time. The bandwidth is the inverse of the dwell time.

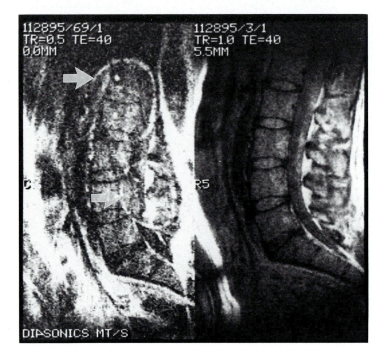

Figure 1.34

Aliasing artifact in the left-hand image which was produced with a body coil. The size of the body is larger than the selected field of view and the forearms (arrows) have wrapped around on the lumbar spine. When a surface coil is used with the same field of view, there is less sensitivity to the more anterior forearms and thus the artifact is eliminated.

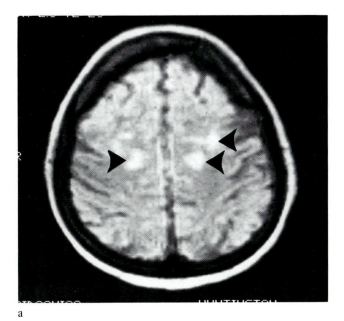

a

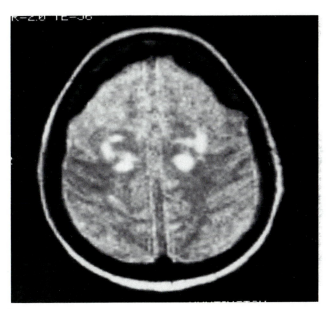

b

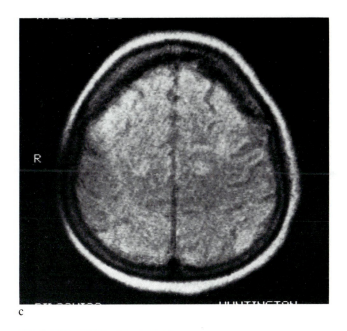

c

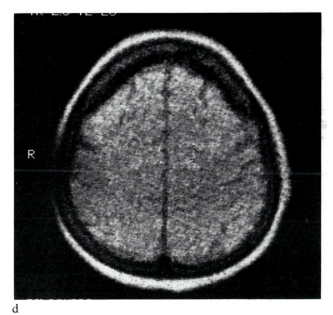

d

Figure 1.35

Image quality in 1983 before use of reduced-bandwidth technology or quadrature-detection head coil in patient with multiple sclerosis (MS). (**a**) 128 × 128 acquisition matrix (1.7 mm spatial resolution), SE 2000/28, four excitations, 7 mm slice thickness (17 min acquisition time). Several demyelinated plaques are evident (arrowheads). (**b**) Second-echo image (TE = 56 msec) of **a** in which MS plaques are more obvious because of additional T_2-weighting. (**c**) 256 × 256 matrix (0.85 mm spatial resolution), four excitations, 7 mm slice thickness (34 min acquisition). Conspicuity of MS plaques is diminished relative to (**a**) because of decreased signal-to-noise (despite better spatial resolution requiring longer imaging time). (**d**) 256 × 256 matrix (0.85 mm spatial resolution), two excitations, 7 mm slice thickness (17 min acquisition). Adjusted for comparable acquisition time, quality of 'high-resolution' image is significantly worse than that of (**a**) because of 75% decrease in signal-to-noise ratio per pixel.

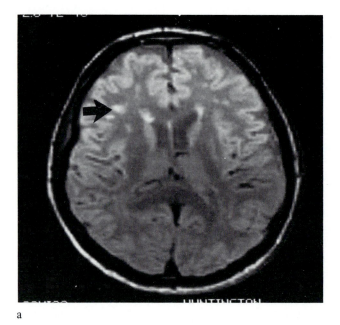

a

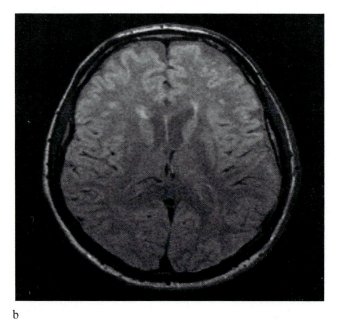

b

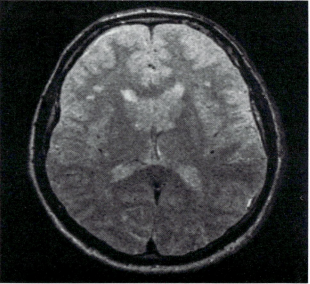

c

d

Figure 1.36

Image quality in early 1986 following implementation of reduced bandwidth technology in a patient with multiple sclerosis. (**a**) 128 × 128 acquisition matrix (1.7 mm spatial resolution), SE 2000/40, four excitations, 5 mm slice thickness (17 min acquisition time). Several plaques are evident (arrowheads). (**b**) 256 × 256 acquisition matrix (0.95 mm spatial resolution), two excitations (17 min acquisition). The plaques (arrows) are less obvious than **a**. (**c**) 128 × 128 matrix, second echo image (SE 2000/80) demonstrating plaques with greater contrast than in high resolution equivalent shown in **d**. (**d**) 256 × 256, two excitations (17 min acquisition) SE 2000/80 image.

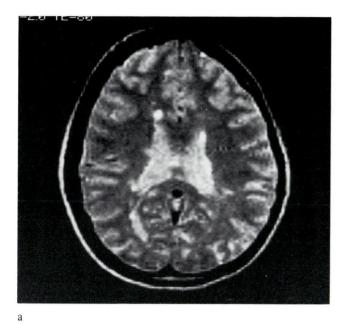

a

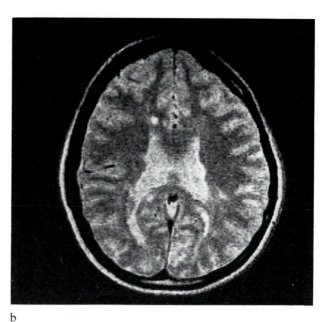

b

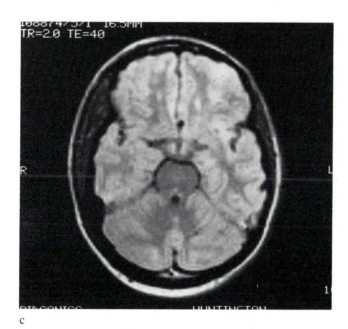

c

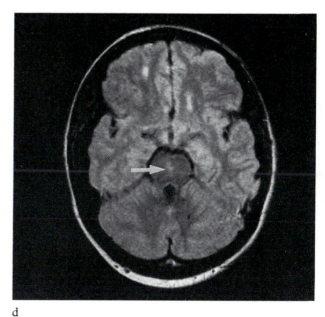

d

Figure 1.37

Image quality in late 1986 implementation of both reduced-bandwidth technology and quadrature detection in head coil. This resulted in addition 40 per cent improvement in signal-to-noise ratio over images in Figure 1.36. (**a**) 128 × 128 (1.7 mm spatial resolution, 5 mm thick), four excitations, SE 2000/80 (17 min acquisition) through lateral ventricles shows multiple sclerosis plaques (arrow). (**b**) 256 × 256 acquisition (0.95 mm spatial resolution, 5 mm thick), two excitations (17 min acquisition) through lateral ventricles. Multiple sclerosis plaques better seen now because of improved edge detection and adequate signal-to-noise ratio. (**c**) 128 × 128 (1.7 mm spatial resolution), SE 2000/40 (17 min acquisition) through midbrain, where no lesion is definitely seen. (**d**) 256 × 256 acquisition (0.95 mm spatial resolution), two excitations, 5 mm slice thickness (17 min acquisition) through midbrain. Multiple sclerosis plaque identified (arrow) because of decreased partial-volume effects with adequate signal-to-noise ratio.

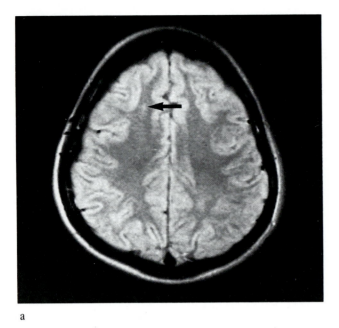

a

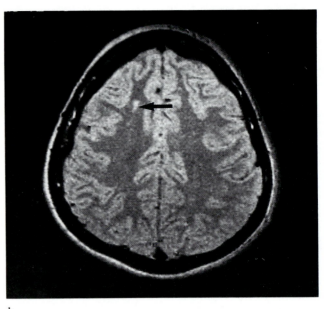

b

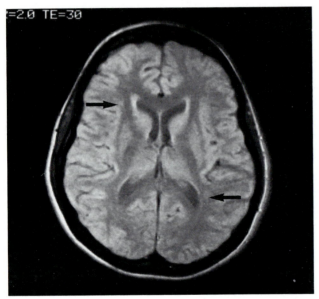

c

d

Figure 1.38

Partial-volume effects. Multiple sclerosis (MS) plaques which are well seen on 5 mm sections cannot be detected on 10 mm sections due to partial voluming of low-intensity white matter. (**a**) Section through the centrum semiovale demonstrating questionable abnormality (arrow) in the anterior right centrum semiovale, originally interpreted as gyrus from slice above. (**b**) 5 mm section through the same level as **a** unequivocally demonstrates MS plaque (arrow) which is higher signal than gray matter. (**c**) Section through the lateral ventricles demonstrates questionable abnormality lateral to the right frontal horn (arrow). (**d**) 5 mm section through the same level as **c** demonstrates definite abnormalities (arrows) lateral to the right frontal horn and atrium of the left lateral ventricle which were not detected on **c**.

2

New techniques

Graeme Bydder

Introduction

In this chapter, a scheme for understanding MR images is outlined and the role of pulse sequences in linking changes in the MR image parameters to changes in voxel signal intensity seen on an image is emphasized. This background is used to discuss recent developments in each of these three common pulse sequences: partial saturation (PS), spin echo (SE), and inversion recovery (IR).

The role of the pulse sequence in MRI

Figure 2.1 is designed to illustrate differences between the physics of image interpretation in X-ray computed tomography (CT) and that in magnetic resonance imaging (MRI). In X-ray CT, the signal intensity of different voxels is studied in order to make inferences about the properties of the tissues within these voxels. If the signal intensity is high (light on the image), the linear X-ray attenuation μ is high. The parameter μ is usually scaled relative to water and air, and expressed as an integer, the Hounsfield number H. For practical purposes, there is a linear relationship between signal intensity (or image brightness) and the value of H. Values of H for various tissues are known and it is possible to make inferences about the nature of the tissue and, in particular, whether it is abnormal or not, based at least in part on values for H. For example, a very high value of H implies calcification, whereas a very low value implies the presence of air. These

processes became so automatic in CT image interpretation that the inferences are often made without reference to the values of H themselves.

The situation with MRI is much more complex. Instead of the single image parameter used with unenhanced X-ray CT, at least ten image parameters are involved with MRI, as shown in Figure 2.1. Many of these parameters are quite new to physicians and the effects of some of them on signal intensity are still not fully understood. In fact, the development of clinical MRI can be traced through the application and understanding of these parameters. Pathological appearances in the first clinical cases described in 1980 were largely interpreted in terms of proton density.[1] In 1981 clinical IR sequences were used and T_1 was introduced as a major image parameter.[2,3] The clinical use of SE sequences followed in 1982,[4-6] introducing T_2 as another major parameter. Phase-contrast chemical-shift results were first described in 1983,[7] and clinical-flow techniques were first used and understood in 1984.[8-10] Clinical susceptibility effects were identified in 1985[11] and 1986,[12,13] and work is currently being performed in studying $T_{1\rho}$,[14] diffusion, and perfusion effects.[15] So far, radiofrequency absorption (RFA) has mainly been of interest from the point of view of safety.

In addition to the large number of image parameters, another concept is necessary in MRI—the pulse sequence. From an imaging point of view, the pulse sequence determines the dependence of the image voxel signal intensity on the ten image parameters. Thus it is possible to increase or decrease the dependence of a particular image on any one of the ten image parameters and thus change the contrast observed on the image. There are three common clinical sequences, which in order of increasing complexity are PS (90°/data collection), SE (90°/180°/data collection), and IR (180°/90°/data collection). There are also many other sequences such as the steady-state free precession (SSFP) and echoplanar imaging (EPI). The list of sequences increases each year. To date, most clinical imaging has been performed with the first three sequences mentioned above and, of these, the SE sequence has been far and away the most commonly used.

In order to establish a sound basis for image interpretation, it is necessary to work through both the left-hand side (the patient side) and the right-hand side (the machine side) of Figure 2.1. Thus on the left-hand side it is necessary to think through the properties of all tissues in terms of the ten imaging parameters and derive rules to recognize how, for example, tissue T_1 and T_2 change in common pathological processes. On the right-hand side, it is necessary to be able to relate the observed signal intensity to each of the ten image parameters via the pulse sequence and to know in detail how alteration of one of the pulse sequence parameters alters the dependence of the resulting image on each of the basic image parameters. This particular process will be discussed for the PS sequence in the next section.

Manipulation of image contrast with the PS sequence

For efficient clinical use of any pulse sequence, it is essential to manipulate the pulse sequence parameters to obtain the desired dependence on the image parameters. In this section, the first six image parameters in Figure 2.1 are emphasized. Perfusion is considered in the following section. Listed beside the first six image parameters in Table 2.1 are the important pulse sequence parameters for the PS sequence. The object of this section is to summarize the working rules necessary to control image contrast for the PS sequence by manipulation of the pulse sequence parameters.

In many ways, proton density (ρ) is the simplest image parameter of all since for each of the three common pulse sequences signal intensity is proportional to ρ (this is strictly true only if the inversion recovery sequence processing is phase corrected). Thus, with the PS sequence, a zero value of ρ corresponds to no signal intensity.

For the dependence of signal intensity on T_1, a useful rule is that the contrast between two tissues of different T_1 is maximized when TR is about equal to the average of the two values of T_1. This follows from

Table 2.1 Image and pulse sequence parameters

Image parameters	Pulse sequence parameters
ρ	TR
T_1	TE
T_2	α
δ	Spoiler pulses
flow	
χ	Rephasing pulses
	2DFT/PR
	Number of averages
	Spatial resolution 128×128, 256^2, etc
	Length of data collection and bandwidth
	Motion artifact suppression techniques
	Phase cycling, for example ROPE
	Cardiac gating
	Single slice/multislice/volume
	Phase mapping technique

considering the exponential recovery of T_1. If TR is either smaller or greater than this value, then T_1-dependent contrast is reduced.

TE has a major effect on the dependence of the PS sequence on three imaging parameters: T_2, chemical shift (δ), and susceptibility (χ). A working rule for maximizing the T_2-dependent contrast between two tissues with different values of T_2 is to make TE about equal to the average T_2 value of the two tissues of interest. This is derived from considering the properties of an exponential decay.

The situation for chemical-shift effects is different. The important consideration in proton images is the chemical shift between protons in water and protons in $-CH_2$ lipid bonds. The chemical shift between these two species is about 3.5 ppm. It is easy to show that the echo time TE_0 required for the MRI signals from protons in water and protons in lipid to become 180° out of phase is given by

$$TE_o = \frac{1}{2f\delta}$$

where f is the resonant frequency in MHz and δ is the chemical shift in ppm. Using Larmor's equation and substituting in the above

$$TE_o \text{ (msec)} = \frac{3.3}{B_o \text{ (Tesla)}}$$

so that the TE_0 at 0.15 Tesla (the field used for all the images in this chapter) is 22 msec while TE_0 is 2.2 msec at 1.5 Tesla.

Thus, if TE is chosen to have the value of TE_0, 'cancellation' effects arise within voxels which contain approximately equal proportions of protons in water and protons in triglycerides (mainly $-CH_2$). If a value of twice TE_0 is used, the signals from protons in water and lipid come back into phase and cancellation effects will not occur. Thus, choice of TE_0 or odd multiples of this value will result in cancellation effects, whereas use of even multiples will not produce these effects.

Susceptibility effects are also caused by dephasing. If protons within a voxel are in slightly different magnetic fields, their resonant frequencies are different and they progressively dephase. This effect increases with increasing TE. It also increases with increasing magnetic field strength (B_0). Differences in tissue susceptibility are commonly seen at air–tissue interfaces and in pathological circumstances they are associated with paramagnetic breakdown products of hemoglobin produced following hemorrhage. By increasing field (B_0) or TE (or both) these effects become more obvious. They are less well shown with conventional SE sequences since, to a first approximation, dephasing due to differences in tissue susceptibility is reversed by the 180° RF pulse.

The influence of flip angle (θ) is of considerable interest. The initial reason for reducing flip angle was to increase the signal-to-noise ratio obtainable per unit time as has been the practice in spectroscopy for many years. However, as θ is reduced from 90° with typical sequences, the T_1 dependence of the sequence is decreased. This is illustrated in Figure 2.2 where the magnetization, M, is excited through 30°. In this situation, half the transverse magnetization ($\sin 30°$) is available when compared with a 90° pulse. However $\cos 30°$, that is 85 per cent of the magnetization, remains in the longitudinal direction. Any T_1 dependence affects only this 15 per cent of the magnetization and T_1-dependent contrast is much reduced. The rules for T_2-dependent contrast remain the same, although with only half the available signal. When θ is increased beyond 90° then the T_1-dependent contrast is increased (up to a point). The analogy here is with the IR sequence, although PS sequences with θ greater than 90° are generally little used. Detailed treatment of the T_1 and T_2 dependence of the PS sequence has been published by Buxton et al.[16]

Spoiler pulses are used to try and destroy all coherent magnetization. To achieve this in imaging, a non-slice-selected 90° pulse is usually applied and this is followed by a large z-gradient (in the transverse plane). Immediately after the 90° pulse, no magnetization remains in the longitudinal direction and when the z-gradient is applied it dephases the transverse magnetization so that, to a first approximation, all coherent magnetization is destroyed. The tissue is said to be saturated and recovery following this can be described as saturation recovery (SR) in the sense used in the American College of Radiology convention. Assuming that a large whole-body transmitter coil has been used, all tissues in the field of the coil will be saturated and recovery then depends on T_1. There is very little flow-related enhancement since the 90° pulse is not slice-selective and all flowing blood within the field of the transmitter coil is saturated. There is thus no difference in tissue properties depending on whether they were included in the previous slice or not. The dephasing pulse also has a secondary effect in improving the quality of the slice. From a clinical point of view, SR sequences differ from PS sequences principally in their flow effects.

Rephasing pulses may be used to restore phase coherence after the phase-encoding gradient. Their general effect is an improvement in image quality when very small values of TR are used.

The PS sequence is normally described in its two-dimensional Fourier transform (2DFT) version, although it is possible to obtain the same effects with projection-reconstruction (PR) techniques. The slice-selecting gradient Gz results in an echo formation, that is rephasing due to z-gradients. Following this a constant gradient is applied in the Gx and Gy directions for each projection. These gradients can be reversed to rephase the signal again, or the rephasing from the Gz slice-selecting gradient can be used in combination with non-linear sampling techniques to collect data. The PR technique generally permits an earlier data collection than 2DFT, since the phase-encoding gradient is not needed after the 90° pulse. This technique may therefore be of particular value in detecting tissues with short T_2 components.

The use of averaging to improve signal-to-noise (S/N) ratio applies to the PS sequence in the same way as for other sequences. There is a square-root improvement in signal-to-noise ratio for a doubling in imaging time.

The PS sequence lends itself to use of increased data collection times with decreased receiver bandwidth. The PS data collection is not delayed until after a 180° pulse as it is with the SE sequence, and so may begin much earlier. With longer data collection it is possible to reduce bandwidth and thus reduce image noise. The advantage is offset to some extent by the fact that the sensitivity of the sequence to motion artifact is increased when longer data collection times are used.

A series of motion artifact suppression techniques can be applied with the PS sequence. These include respiratory-ordered phase encoding (ROPE),[17] as well as gradient-moment-nulling techniques[18] and phase-cycling techniques where the direction of the RF pulse is reversed on alternate excitations and the signal is averaged. Cardiac gating also helps control artifact.

The effects of fluid flow are complex, but the simplicity of the PS sequence has meant that it is frequently used to illustrate the principles involved and the published literature contains a number of examples obtained with this sequence. When unsaturated blood flows into a slice, it may provide a higher signal than tissues or fluids remaining in the slice when the next 90° pulse is applied. This produces a high-signal intensity. However, the signal is dephased when the fluid flows in the presence of a gradient, leading to a reduction in signal. The net result depends on the rate and direction of flow as well as the specific details of the pulse sequence.

Images also differ according to whether they are obtained from a single slice or volume set. With a multislice or volume set, blood may have been excited before it enters the slice of interest. It may be saturated to a greater or lesser extent and thus produce less signal than in the case of a single-slice acquisition. In this respect, multislice and volume PS sequences may resemble SR images.

A recent development is the field-echo even-echo rephasing (FEER) sequence,[19] which is the equivalent of a second-echo SE sequence. The second gradient echo frequently produces a higher signal from uniformly flowing blood.

Instead of simply using the magnitude of the signal to reconstruct the image, it is possible to obtain phase information as well. This is often used in the form of phase differences. Here one image is obtained as a reference and a second image is obtained with the same basic technique as the first, but with different delay times or additional gradients. When the phases of the two images are compared, it is possible to obtain phase difference maps which specifically reflect field inhomogeneities[13] or fluid flow.[20,21]

In addition to the effect of the sequences themselves, other factors influence the signal intensity on the image. These include the geometry of the receiver coils, whether uniform or non-uniform (as in surface coils), and inhomogeneities in B_0 due to shimming or metallic objects. The effect of the latter in producing image degradation is greater with PS sequences than it is with SE sequences of the same TR and TE values.

The various rules for manipulating and analysing the contrast available with PS sequences are summarized in Table 2.2. It can be seen that not all options are possible with any one sequence. However, even the relatively simple PS sequence offers a wide variety of approaches to clinical problems. In the following sections, the use of the PS and SR sequences in some clinical situations is illustrated.

Clinical applications of the PS sequence

Hemorrhage

The PS sequence provides interesting insights into the pathological features involved in hemorrhage, illustrated in Figure 2.3. Low-signal regions in and around hematomas are seen with higher sensitivity with PS sequences than those with the corresponding SE

Table 2.2   Pulse sequence parameters and contrast manipulation

Pulse sequence parameters	Rules for contrast manipulation
	SI is proportional to ρ
TR	To maximize T_1 contrast make TR $\simeq T_1$ average
TE	To maximize T_2 contrast make TE $\simeq T_2$ average
	Chemical shift cancellation occurs at $TE_0 = 3.3/B_0$
	Dephasing due to susceptibility and increases with TE and B_0
α	Decreasing α decreases T_1 dependence
Spoiler pulse	Reduce the effect of flow
2DFT/PR	PR may permit early data collection for short T_2 components
Number of averages	S/N increases as the square root of number of averages
Length of data collection and bandwidth	Long data collection and reduced bandwidth increases S/N
Motion artifact	ROPE, gradient moment nulling, phase cycling help control artifact
Single slice/multislice/volume	Mainly change flow effects and S/N
FEER	Rephases flow signal
Difference phase maps	Used for susceptibility maps and flow

sequences, indicating that there is a significant contribution from the susceptibility effects.[12] This is seen in acute, subacute, and chronic intracerebral hematomas. The stages of evolution seen with PS sequences follow in a general way the pattern defined with SE sequences at 1.5 Tesla,[11] but there are often differences.

The pattern of hematoma in trauma follows that seen with large extracerebral and intracerebral hematomas from other causes. In addition, low-signal areas are often seen within the brain with the PS sequences when they are not apparent with SE sequences, as shown in Figure 2.4. This is probably due to petechial or subarachnoid hemorrhage. It may be seen at times remote from the original injury and this feature may be relevant to the post-traumatic syndrome.

Susceptibility mapping performed by comparison of the phase difference between the two PS sequences with different values of TE has shown changes in all cases of intracerebral hemorrhage examined to date, although the images are initially difficult to evaluate because of broad black and white bands representing changes in field due to inhomogeneities in B_0 superimposed on the susceptibility changes. The changes present in the local field are produced by breakdown products of hemoglobin such as deoxyhemoglobin, methemoglobin, and hemosiderin.

Following hemorrhage, susceptibility change appears to persist in some cases for very long periods. In one case of probable neonatal intraventricular hemorrhage, evidence of paramagnetic blood breakdown products was seen around the ventricles 23 years later.

In the neonatal period, hemorrhage is particularly obvious. The brain has a longer T_2 than in adults so that there is less loss of signal in the infant brain for the same value of TE. The paranasal sinuses in children are less well developed than in adults so that artifacts at their tissue interfaces are less of a problem. The normal neonatal brain does not contain detectable iron until about six months of age. Hemorrhage is common in the neonatal period and the sensitivity of the PS sequence is high.

Tumors

Studies of cerebral tumors have provided a useful clinical test for the development of faster sequences. With a reduced flip angle, the T_1-dependent contrast is reduced. If low values of TR and TE are used, a fast but low-contrast sequence results. This sequence is sensitive to mass effects but does not compare in sensitivity to highly T_2-dependent SE sequences. In order to achieve contrast comparable with this type of sequence, the TE of the PS sequence must be increased. Using this T_2-dependent SE sequence,

lesion contrast similar to highly T_2-dependent SE sequences can be developed with an order of magnitude saving in time, illustrated in Figure 2.5. The disadvantages of this approach are that the PS sequences are more vulnerable to motion artifact and to artifact from the presence of metallic objects. A further problem may arise with T_2-dependent PS sequences in developing adequate T_2-dependent contrast whilst keeping the signal from CSF less than that of the surrounding brain. This can be done consistently at low fields (0.15 Tesla) using an SE sequence such as SE 1500/80, but it is more difficult to achieve with PS sequences. In some circumstances, SR sequences may have an advantage because they reduce signal from CSF.

Using PS sequences, hemorrhage is not infrequently detected in or around tumors. This presents as a low-signal area which may be shown with the T_2-dependent SE but is generally less well demonstrated. These regions usually display changes in susceptibility maps.

Vascular disease

Apart from hemorrhage, the next most interesting group of vascular disease to be imaged with PS sequences is arteriovenous malformation. Flow-related enhancement may allow a specific diagnosis to be made, as in Figure 2.6, although care is necessary to ensure that the increased signal intensity is not due to blood clot.

The technique can be extended further by the use of phase-mapping techniques to quantify blood flow. Two images are taken with the rephasing of the gradient slice-selective pulse slightly delayed in the second case. The resulting phase map shows velocity as directly proportional to phase, allowing direct measurements to be made. Similar techniques have been applied to the CSF flow for quantification purposes.

Differences between PS and SR sequences can also be shown with reference to CSF flow. The CSF signal as seen with the PS sequences is frequently enhanced as a result of fluid flow into the slice. The effect is reduced with the SR sequences and the boundaries of the spinal cord are then seen more clearly.

Other disease of the brain

A wide variety of disease has now been imaged with PS sequences. In general, the T_2-dependent PS sequence provides the highest sensitivity. The sequence is rapid and sensitive to susceptibility effects, but it is less tolerant to movement than the corresponding SE sequence. The PS sequence has been of value in multiple sclerosis and can be used to demonstrate periventricular lesions. T_1-dependent forms of the PS sequence (with $\theta > 90°$ and short TE) are more satisfactory for anatomical detail. T_1-dependent sequences display a moderate sensitivity to contrast enhancement with Gd-DTPA. The SR sequence shows similar properties to the PS sequence and may have advantages when it is important to suppress the signal from flowing blood or CSF. Chemical-shift effects have been observed with lipid-containing tumors in the brain with the PS sequence. The PS sequence may be used with an SE sequence with the same values of TR and TE to obtain 'water' and 'lipid' fractions within lesions in a manner analogous to that used by Dixon[7] with the asymmetrical SE sequence.

Use of SE sequences to produce phase maps for assessment of brain perfusion

Although a number of MRI techniques are now available for the measurement of blood flow,[9,22–26] less attention has been directed towards the assessment of tissue perfusion. Le Bihan et al have described a technique in which the signal amplitudes obtained from two SE sequences are compared in order to provide an assessment of intravoxel incoherent motion (IVIM).[27] This section describes the same basic technique, with the exception that the phases rather than amplitudes of the two SE sequences are compared. The information provided by this latter technique can be termed intravoxel coherent motion (IVCM).

Initially a reference SE image is used to calculate a phase map. A second SE sequence containing a pair of unipolar gradients on either side of the 180° pulse is then performed and a further phase map is calculated. A map of the phase differences between the first two phase images is then constructed. The phase difference Φ for each voxel on this map is given by

$$\Phi = \gamma \, G \, \delta \, \Delta \, V$$

where γ is the gyromagnetic ratio, G is the gradient strength, δ is the time during which the gradient is applied, Δ is the time between the leading edges of the two unipolar gradients, and V is the velocity of the moving nuclei in the direction of the gradient.[9]

In blood-flow work the additional sensitization gradient is relatively small, giving a full-scale range for velocity measurement of the order of ±1000 mm/sec. In perfusion studies, the gradient pulse duration is typically 10, 15, or 20 msec at full amplitude of 16 milliTesla/m in the transverse plane. Depending on the gradient pulse duration, the sequence can be sensitized to flow rates of ±0.5, ±1.0, or ±2.0 mm/sec (full scale). These gradients are sensitized to in-plane perfusion in the x and y directions and through-plane perfusion in the z direction, respectively.

In order to reduce the effects of pulsatile motion of the brain and CSF, the sequences were gated to the R wave signal from the electrocardiograph with a delay of 300 to 500 msec from the 90° pulse of the SE sequence.

The results are shown as phase-difference maps, representing the point-by-point differences of voxel phase between the SE images acquired with and without flow sensitization. The gray scale on these images is saw-tooth, so that any flow greater than those listed above results in a repetition of the saw-tooth scale, with an abrupt change of signal intensity.

Clinical results from SE phase mapping

With the use of phase maps sensitized to flow rates of ± 1 mm/sec, differences between normal gray and white matter are seen in adults. In infants (less than 2 years of age), central and peripheral phase changes are observed rather than the gray/white matter pattern seen in adults.

Marked changes in CSF flow are regularly seen. Complex patterns of flow are observed with the CSF in the ventricular system moving in different directions. These often appear off the saw-tooth scale for the perfusion sensitivity in use. The extent of flow changes can be expanded by an increase in the gradient strength. When the gradients are reversed, the brain and CSF changes are also reversed. The flow-sensitized sequences are vulnerable to motion artifact. This problem increases with gradient strength, and may result in severely degraded images.

In cases of chronic infarction with well defined areas of infarction seen with CT, SE 1500/80 and SE 1500/200 images, abnormal perfusion patterns have been demonstrated with flow-sensitized phase maps, as shown in Figure 2.7. Deep white matter infarction was seen with SE 1500/80 images, but more extensive changes may be apparent with flow-sensitized images than with SE 1500/80 images.

A patient with epilepsia partialis continua is illustrated in Figure 2.8.

A patient with an arteriovenous malformation in the left cerebellopontine angle showed perfusion changes which reversed with reversed gradient sensitivity, as illustrated in Figure 2.9.

All malignant tumors examined to date have shown some change. Because of the increase in T_2 of the tumor, the phase contribution for the static fraction of the tumor is relatively greater and this produces an alteration in the appearance of the lesion, shown in Figure 2.10.

Cerebral blood flow is complex and can be divided into a static component (which will show no phase change in the phase-difference image) and a mobile component. The latter is likely to be smaller but the single-phase measurement for each voxel contains contributions from both static and mobile components. Full analysis is complex and involves consideration of diffusion effects, macroscopic incoherent flow and macroscopic coherent flow.

Comparison of images with gradients reversed provides an internal validation of the technique, demonstrated in Figure 2.11, as does the use of a graduated series of gradient strengths.

Differences have been seen between gray and white matter as well as between central and peripheral zones in infants. This distribution of perfusion differences has been described in positron emission tomography (PET) studies.[28] While this MRI technique does not provide a measure of blood perfusion in terms of ml/100g tissue per minute, it does provide directional information and it should be possible to construct a vector map representing tissue perfusion.

One of the main advantages of this technique is that it can be performed as an 'add on' to existing MRI procedures without the need for any additional equipment. Hence MRI can be used directly for both the basic examination and for perfusion studies in a totally non-invasive manner. This is not the case with single photon emission tomography (SPECT) and positron emission tomography (PET) studies.

The IR sequence

The dependence of signal intensity seen with the IR sequence on proton density, T_1, and T_2 has been described in mathematical terms,[29,30] but a qualitative description of the IR sequence will be used in this section. The proton magnetization induced in the patient by the static magnetic field can be represented by a vector **M**. The component of the magnetization in the transverse plane at any given time is then represented by M_{xy}, and that in the longitudinal direction at the same time by M_z. The effect of a 90° pulse is to rotate M_z into the transverse plane to become M_{xy}, illustrated in Figure 2.12.

Following a 90° pulse, M_z increases exponentially from zero with time constant T_1 (Figure 2.13a) and M_{xy} decays exponentially with time constant T_2 (Figure 2.13b). At the following 180° pulse, M_z is inverted to become $-M_z$ and recovers with a time constant T_1, but at twice the rate for the earlier longitudinal recovery after the 90° pulse. At the next 90° pulse, M_z is rotated to become M_{xy}, which then decays exponentially with time constant T_2. Using a gradient-echo or free induction decay (FID) data collection, signal is collected at a mean time, TE, after the 90° pulse and the cycle is repeated.

A composite diagram is shown in Figure 2.14, which first follows M_z then M_{xy} after the second 90° pulse, and can be used to represent the 'potential signal intensity' at various stages in the sequence in order to understand how this may be varied.

The size of the received signal and ultimately the signal intensity or pixel value in the image is proportional to M_{xy} at the time of the data collection. M_{xy} is also proportional to tissue proton density.

The times TI and TE as used in the American College of Radiology convention are shown in Figures 2.12 and 2.13. TR is the duration of each cycle of the sequence, TI is the inversion time between the inverting 180° pulse and the following 90° pulse and TE is the time from the last 90° pulse to the following echo.

Using Figure 2.14 as a model of the IR sequence, we can compare the signal intensities of white matter (a tissue with a relatively short T_1), gray matter (a tissue with a longer T_1) and CSF (which has a very long T_1). The signal intensity observed is proportional to the height of M_{xy} and it can be seen that the shorter T_1 of white matter results in a higher signal intensity than for gray matter. The very long T_1 of CSF is a low signal intensity which may be negative, as in Figure 2.14. The last segment of the decay converges towards zero for both gray and white matter with their positive signal intensities, as well as for CSF with its negative signal intensity. Display of the resultant image after phase-corrected processing gives white for white matter, gray for gray matter, and black for CSF. The signal for gray matter is slightly greater than that for white matter at the time of the 180° pulse because of its greater proton density. Differences between gray matter and tumor are shown in Figure 2.15.

In the following sections, the effects of changing TR, TI, TE, imaging processing technique, and other parameters on the signal intensity at the time of data collection are considered.

Effect of changes in TR

The general rule is that a time of at least $3T_1$ should be allowed for recovery of the longitudinal magnetization between the 90° pulse of the last pulse cycle and the following 180° pulse of the next pulse cycle to allow a high level of recovery of M_z, although, in practice, it is possible to use times less than this.

Reducing TR produces a reduction in signal intensity for tissues with a long T_1, although there is less effect on tissues with a short T_1 where TR is still greater than $3T_1$. Reducing TR is therefore used to reduce the relative signal intensity of tissues or fluids such as CSF which have a very long T_1.

There is little advantage in increasing TR beyond 3 to $5T_1$.

Effect of changes in TI

It is useful to consider three variants of the IR sequence according to their values of TI:

(a) Short TI (TI of the order 0–250 msec)
(b) Medium TI (TI of the order 250–700 msec)
(c) Long TI (TI of the order 700 msec and longer)

These TI categories are applicable at 0.15 Tesla. Tissue T_1 increases with field strength. Thus to achieve the same effects at higher fields, TI and TR must be multiplied by the appropriate factors. Table 2.3 lists the factors for a number of tissues and field strengths.[31]

Short TI

The values of TI included here are in the range 0–250 msec. In the limit where TI equals zero (or, from a practical point of view about 1 msec) the 90° and 180° pulses add to give a 270° pulse which is equivalent to a −90° pulse. This is equivalent to a 90° pulse and the sequence in Figure 2.14 becomes 90°/data collection, or the PS sequence. Thus the PS sequence can be regarded as a limiting case of the IR sequence with TI = 0. The same reasoning applies when an SE data collection is used and the IR sequence (with TI = 0) becomes equivalent to an SE sequence. Using magnitude reconstruction with TI in the range of 0 to about 250 msec, an IR image of the brain appears like an SE image, although with greater gray/white matter contrast. The magnetization curves can be represented as shown in Figure 2.16. Note that following the final 90° pulse, the T_1 and T_2 contrast are additive. Thus, an increase in the T_1 of a tissue increases the tissue's relative signal intensity, as does an increase in its T_2. (This is not the case in Figure 2.14, which illustrates medium values of TI.) The short TI IR (STIR) sequence is sensitive to changes in T_1 and T_2 and can be used as a screening sequence in the brain in a similar way to the SE sequences with long TE and long TR, such as SE 1500/80. To reduce the signal intensity of CSF to less than that of white matter, TR can be shortened, as suggested in the previous section, to 1000 msec with a sequence such as IR 1000/44/100.

Since many pathological lesions produce an increase in both T_1 and T_2, the addition of these two types of contrast with the STIR sequence produces a high net tissue contrast. This type of sequence also enables some T_1-dependent decay to be substituted for the T_2-dependent decay in the equivalent SE sequence. This is of particular value where the T_1 and T_2 decays of the tissues differ and explains why the gray/white

Table 2.3   Ratio of T_1 at different fields to that at 0.15 Tesla for various tissues.[31]

Tissue	*Field strength (Tesla)*				
	0.15	*0.3*	*0.5*	*1.0*	*1.5*
Gray matter	1	1.24	1.45	1.79	2.03
White matter	1	1.27	1.52	1.93	2.23
Cardiac muscle	1	1.28	1.55	1.99	2.30
Liver	1	1.30	1.58	2.05	2.39
Spleen	1	1.24	1.49	1.88	2.15
Kidney	1	1.19	1.35	1.60	1.77
Skeletal muscle	1	1.34	1.66	2.22	2.63
Fat	1	1.13	1.24	1.39	1.50

matter contrast of this sequence is greater than the equivalent SE sequence.

It is also possible to choose particular values of TI so that the signal intensity of a particular tissue is zero at the time of the 90° pulse, as shown in Figure 2.16. (This occurs at a value of TI typically between 0.56 and 0.69 T_1 for TR > 3T_1.) Values of about 100 msec are suitable to eliminate the fat signal, while 255 msec is adequate for white matter. In this situation, the tissue signal is said to be 'suppressed'. Suppression or partial suppression of the fat signal is of particular value in the orbit.

Medium TI

The working rule to obtain an image with good contrast between two tissues of different T_1 values is to choose a value of TI intermediate between the two tissues of interest (neglecting the effects of proton density and T_2), so that satisfactory contrast between white matter (T_1 = 350 msec) and gray matter (T_1 = 450 msec) is achieved with a TI of about 400 msec. Note that the signal intensity is not maximal at this point so the image appears noisier than that obtained with, for example, TI = 500 msec, where the signal is higher (although the gray/white matter contrast is less). In theory, maximum contrast is obtained when TI is about 0.63 times the average of the T_1 between the two tissues, but the signal levels in this case are close to zero, so maximizing the appearance of the noise of the image. Note that the TI for optimum contrast between gray matter and a tumor (which has an increased T_1) is greater than that for gray and white matter.

There are two additional modifying factors. The increased mobile proton density of gray matter relative to white matter results in slightly less tissue contrast. More important is the fact that the T_2-dependent period following the 90° pulse and prior to data collection may produce a reduction in tissue contrast. This is particularly so for lesions which follow the common pattern and have both T_1 and T_2 increased. The T_2-dependent decay, in the last component of the sequence, reduces the T_1 contrast developed earlier in the sequence.

The method of image reconstruction and the type of data collection affect TE. TE can generally be shorter with projection-reconstruction than with two-dimensional Fourier transformation (2DFT), since a single vector-encoding gradient is used, without the need for a previous phase-encoding gradient as with 2DFT. A gradient-echo data collection can be completed earlier than an SE collection with the same bandwidth, although the former is more vulnerable to B_0 field inhomogeneities.

With the brain (T_2 about 100 msec), the T_2 dependence of the IR sequence is not such a big problem as it is in the body, where values of T_2 are typically about half those in the brain, making the same IR sequence much more T_2-dependent than when it is used in the brain. The use of short values of TE to control this problem then becomes important. The alternative is to use short values of TI so that the T_1 and T_2 contrast after the 90° pulse is additive as outlined in the previous section.

Long TI

For reasons outlined above, these sequences may be useful in separating tumor from edema (where both have increased values of T_1). Sequences designed for this purpose require an increase in the value of TR. They are also useful in pediatrics where the T_1 of normal brain may be increased 300–400 per cent compared with adults. Another use is suppression of long T_1 fluids such as CSF, urine, and bowel contents, where values of TI of 800–1200 msec can be used.

Effect of changes in TE

Increasing TE increases the T_2 dependence of the IR sequence. This is useful for short TI sequences, generally not useful for medium TI sequences, and of limited value for long TI sequences.

Short TI

The rule of maximum contrast for SE sequences is to use TE half-way between the T_2 values of the two tissues of interest (neglecting proton density and T_1 effects). It is most useful to increase TE when imaging tissues with a long T_2, such as brain. For STIR sequences, TE values rather less than this are often used because of the additional T_1-dependent contrast.

Additional echoes can be usefully added to this type of sequence.

Medium TI

In general, TE should be reduced to a minimum. Projection-reconstruction with a field-echo data collection was used for this purpose in earlier studies.

Long TE

TE can be increased with this type of sequence to increase the relative T_2 dependence, although the contrast may be ambiguous unless TI is quite long.

Effects of methods of processing

There are two types of image reconstruction available: phase-corrected, where positive values of signal intensity are shown positive and negative values appear negative, and magnitude reconstruction where the magnitude of the signal is used irrespective of its sign. For STIR sequences, using phase-corrected processing white matter is white and gray matter is gray, but the reverse is so with magnitude processing. For medium TI sequences, the CSF appears dark with phase-corrected processing but may show a 'rebound' with a lighter central area with magnitude processing. The signal intensities follow directly from considering (Figures 14–16).

Effects of multislice or single-slice imaging

The 90° pulse in the IR sequence is always slice-selective, although for single slice scans the 180° pulse(s) need not be. However, when the IR sequence is used to obtain an interleaved set of slices, 180° pulse(s) must be slice-selected. When the 180° pulse is slice-selected, it is possible for flowing blood to experience only part of the IR sequence depending on where it is at the times of the inversion pulses. For example, blood flowing into a slice may only experience a 90° pulse and behave as though it is being imaged with a PS sequence producing a high-signal intensity due to flow-related enhancement, rather than the usual low-signal intensity.

Clinical illustrations using the IR sequence

Many of the applications of the IR sequence follow directly from considerations in the previous section and have been well demonstrated by a variety of groups.[32–35]

STIR sequences can be used for disease detection. TR and TI can be adjusted so that one version of the sequence generates images with the signal intensity of CSF slightly less than that of white matter so that periventricular lesions can be recognized without confusion from partial-volume effects, and the other version generates images with the CSF signal greater than that of brain, as in Figure 2.17c. Use of the two types of image processing is also illustrated in Figure 2.17.

Separation of tumor from edema may also be accomplished as shown in Figure 2.18, and additional lesions may also be seen in vascular disease, illustrated in Figure 2.19. Medium TI images provide localization of disease, assessment of mass effects, and developmental information in older infants. Contrast enhancement is usually maximal with these sequences, as in Figure 2.20. The sequence also provides a better technique for computing T_1 maps than by using two SE sequences.

'Short T_1 and T_2 tumors, including some acoustic neuromas and some meningiomas are well demonstrated with medium TI IR sequences (Figures 2.21 and 2.22 respectively), as are subacute hemorrhage and MS lesions in the brainstem.

Long TI IR sequences may be useful in distinguishing tumor from edema as well as in pediatric applications.

A disadvantage of IR is the fact that, with medium and long TI IR sequences, it is more difficult to construct an interleaved multislice set because of the relatively isolated 180° inverting pulse, than it is for a comparable SE multislice set. This limitation does not apply to short TI IR sequences to the same extent.

There are some more specific problems with particular variants of the IR sequence which are worth listing:

(a) Partial-volume effects with medium TI IR sequences between gray and white matter of the brain may simulate brain lesions. This can be reduced or avoided by using short TI variants.

(b) The phase-corrected version of the medium TI image displays zero signal intensity in the mid-gray region. This signal may simulate tissue in the sinuses, etc. This is not a problem with STIR sequence.

(c) Increased time may be needed for a low-resolution phase-calibrating image for the phase-corrected version of the IR sequence. We use a 64×64 matrix SE 544/44 scan which adds about 30 seconds to the imaging time.

(d) Radiofrequency pulse calibration needs to be precise for the IR sequence, since errors in the angle of rotation of the magnetization produce a greater loss of tissue contrast than is the case with SE images. This is a greater problem at high field where the loading of the transmitter coil is greater than that at low field.

(e) The field-echo data acquisition method is more susceptible to magnetic field inhomogeneity than the SE one. Again this problem is greater at high field and limits the value of the short TE field-echo data collection.

Several particular applications of the IR sequence are worthy of emphasis; and will be discussed in the following sections.

Disease detection in the brain

The STIR sequences have a similar sensitivity to the corresponding SE sequence with IR 1500/44/100 approximately equivalent to SE 1500/80. Although the IR sequences show greater gray/white matter contrast than the SE ones, the signal from CSF can be kept lower than that from brain by reducing TR or TI. Where the lesion is not periventricular and there is no problem with having the CSF signal greater than the brain (or a benefit in having it greater), longer values of TE, TR, and TI can be used.[34]

Localization of lesions and mass effects

Although the T_2 dependence of most medium TI IR sequences reduces their sensitivity in disease detection, the high level of gray/white matter contrast provides a series of interfaces of value in the localization of lesions and assessment of mass effects.

Pediatrics

The medium or long TI IR sequences provide excellent demonstrations of normal myelination as well as delays or deficits in this process. In addition, the fact that the T_2 of the neonatal and infant brain is longer than that of adults means that IR sequences are less T_2-dependent and therefore of more value in disease detection. The high water content of the infantile brain (85 to 95 per cent) means that edema is often not so obvious and that edema detection alone with an SE sequence is a less rewarding strategy in infants than adults. Age-adjusted IR sequences are useful, although in follow-up studies a dilemma arises when a decision has to be made either to keep the sequence constant or adjust it for age.

Contrast enhancement

Paramagnetic contrast agents produce the opposite effect to most disease processes: they decrease both T_1 and T_2. The most sensitive sequence for detecting contrast enhancement is the medium TI IR sequence (with TI intermediate between the lesion T_1 before and after contrast enhancement), with the short TE and short TR SE next best and the long TE and long TR SE least sensitive. This may create a problem when long TE and long TR SE sequences are used for screening purposes since contrast agents (such as Gd-DTPA) may not produce enhancement with this type of sequence. It is therefore necessary to perform an additional pre-enhancement scan of a different type if a contrast agent is used, so increasing the total time of examination.

Note that with sequences like the medium TI IR, and the SE with a short TE and short TR, there is usually an increase in signal intensity as the concentration for paramagnetic contrast is increased and this is followed by a decrease as the concentration is increased further.

Meningiomas and other 'short T_1 short T_2' tumors

There are a number of tumors, including meningiomas, which may have a normal or only slightly increased T_2 and a normal or low proton density. They usually have a higher T_1 than white matter. With SE sequences, there is very little T_2 contrast to be exploited; with medium TI IR sequences, however, the low to normal proton density and slightly increased T_1 both tend to reduce signal intensity, producing lesion contrast with normal brain and providing better visualization than with SE sequences. In addition, this group of tumors may show a high level of contrast enhancement and this is best shown with medium TI IR sequences. Since meningiomas have a ubiquitous presentation and are important to exclude, this result has considerable significance in the design of a routine screening strategy for MRI. The T_2 dependence of the medium TI IR sequences, which is usually a significant disadvantage with malignant tumors, is not such a disadvantage with the type of tumor described above, since its T_2 is normal or only slightly increased. The same general considerations apply to other tumors of this type.

Conclusion

Different aspects of each of the given pulse sequences have been described, and simplified approaches to understanding the contrast developed by each of them have been outlined. Considerable effort has been expended in evaluating pulse sequences and adopting them for a particular purpose. In many respects, the most surprising thing has been the degree to which the results can be predicted from very simple models.

References

1 HAWKES RC, HOLLAND GN, MOORE WS et al, Nuclear magnetic resonance (NMR) tomography of the brain: a preliminary

clinical assessment with demonstration of the pathology, *J Comput Assist Tomogr* (1980) 4:577–86.

2 SMITH FW, MALLARD JR, NMR imaging in liver disease, *Br Med Bull* (1984) 40(2):194–6.

3 YOUNG IR, HALL AS, PALLIS CA et al, Nuclear magnetic resonance imaging of the brain in multiple sclerosis, *Lancet* (1981) ii:1063–6.

4 BAILES DR, YOUNG IR, THOMAS DJ et al, NMR imaging of the brain using spin-echo sequences, *Clin Radiol* (1982) 33:395–414.

5 CROOKS LE, ARAKAWA M, HOENNINGER J et al, Nuclear magnetic resonance whole body imager operating 3.5 kgauss, *Radiology* (1982) 143:169–74.

6 BYDDER GM, STEINER RE, YOUNG IR et al, Clinical NMR imaging of the brain: 140 cases, *AJR* (1982) 139:215–36.

7 DIXON WT, Simple proton spectroscopic imaging, *Radiology* (1984) 153: 189–94.

8 AXEL L, Blood flow effects in MRI, *AJR* (1984) 143:1157–66.

9 BRYANT DJ, PAYNE JA, FIRMIN D et al, Measurement of flow with NMR imaging using a gradient pulse and phase difference technique, *J Comput Assist Tomogr* (1984) 8:588–93.

10 WALUCH V, BRADLEY WG, NMR even echo rephasing in slow laminar flow, *J Comput Assist Tomogr* (1984) 8:594–8.

11 GOMORI J, GROSSMAN RI, GOLDBERG HI et al, Intracranial hematomas: imaging by high field MR, *Radiology* (1985) 157:87–93.

12 EDELMAN RR, JOHNSON KE, BUXTON R et al, MR of hemorrhage: a new approach, *AJNR* (1986) 7:751–6.

13 YOUNG IR, KHENIA S, THOMAS DGT et al, Clinical magnetic susceptibility mapping of the brain, *J Comput Assist Tomogr* (1987) 11(1):2–6.

14 SEPPONEN RE, POHJENEN JA, TANTTU JI, Method of T_1 MR imaging, *J Comput Assist Tomogr* (1985) 9:1007–11.

15 LE BIHAN B, BRETON E, LALLEMAND D et al, MR imaging of intravoxel incoherent motion: application to diffusion and perfusion in neurological disorders, *Radiology* (1986) 161:401–7.

16 BUXTON RE, EDELMAN RR, ROSEN BR et al, Contrast in rapid MR imaging: T_1 and T_2 weighted imaging, *J Comput Assist Tomogr* (1987) 11(1):7–16.

17 BAILES DR, GILDERDALE DJ, BYDDER GM et al, Technical note. Respiratory ordered phase encoding ROPE: a method for reducing respiratory motion artefacts in MR imaging, *J Comput Assist Tomogr* (1985) 9:835–8.

18 PATTANY PM, PHILLIPS JJ, CHIU LC et al, Motion artefact suppression technique (MAST) for MRI imaging, *J Comput Assist Tomogr* (1987) 11:369–77.

19 NAYLOR GL, FIRMIN DH, LONGMORE DB, Blood flow imaging by cine magnetic resonance, *J Comput Assist Tomogr* (1986) 10:715–22.

20 RIDGWAY JP, SMITH M, A technique for velocity imaging using MRI, *Br J Radiol* (1986) 59:603–7.

21 YOUNG IR, BYDDER GM, PAYNE JA, Flow measurement by the development of phase differences during slice formation in MR imaging, *Magn Reson Med* (1986) 3(1):175–9.

22 STEJSKAL EO, TANNER JE, Spin diffusion measurements: spin-echos in the presence of a time-dependent field gradient, *J Chem Phys* (1965) 42:288–92.

23 PACKER KJ, The study of slow coherent molecular motion by pulsed nuclear magnetic resonance, *Mol Phys* (1969) 17:355–69.

24 MORAN PR, A flow velocity zeugmatographic interleave for NMR imaging in humans, *Magn Reson Imaging* (1982) 1:197–203.

25 WEEDEN VJ, ROSEN BR, BRADY TJ, Magnetic resonance angiography. In: Kressel HY, ed. *Magnetic resonance annual.* (Raven Press: New York 1987) 113–178.

26 DUMOULIN CL, HART HR, Magnetic resonance angiography, *Radiology* (1986) 161:717–20.

27 LE BIHAN D, BRETON E, LALLEMAND D et al, MR imaging of intravoxel incoherent motions: appliction to diffusion and perfusion in neurologic disorders, *Radiology* (1986) 161:401–7.

28 CHUGANI HT, PHELPS ME, Maturational changes in cerebral function in infants determined by ^{18}FDG positron emission, *Tomogr Sci* (1986) 231:840–3.

29 YOUNG IR, BAILES DR, BURL M et al, Initial clinical evaluation of a whole body NMR tomograph, *J Comput Assist Tomogr* (1982) 6:1–18.

30 WEHRLI FW, MACFALL JR, SHUTTS D et al, Mechanisms of contrast in NMR imaging, *J Comput Assist Tomogr* (1984) 8:369–80.

31 BOTTOMLEY PA, FOSTER TH, ARGSINGER RE et al, A review of normal tissue hydrogen NMR relaxation time and relaxation mechanisms from 1–100 mHz; dependence on tissue type, NMR frequency, temperature species, exercise and age, *Med Phys* (1984) 11:425–48.

32 DWYER AJ, FRANK JA, SANK VJ et al, Short-TI inversion recovery pulse sequence: analysis and initial experience in cancer imaging, *Radiology* (1988) 168:827–36.

33 SCHNAPF DJ, SEN S, FRANK JA et al, MRI of joints: evaluation of the short TI pulse sequence, *Magn Reson Imaging* (1988) 6(1):103.

34 PORTER BA, SHIELDS AF, OLSON DO, Magnetic resonance imaging of bone marrow disorders, *Radiol Clin North Am* (1986) 24:269.

35 MILLER DH, JOHNSON G, MCDONALD WI et al, Detection of optic nerve lesions in optic neuritis with magnetic resonance imaging, *Lancet* (1988) i:1490–1.

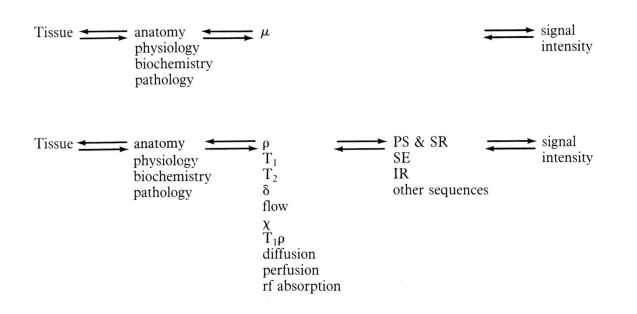

Figure 2.1

Scheme for the image interpretation with CT (above) and MRI (below). In both situations, the radiologist observes the signal intensity on an image and attempts to make inferences about the tissue observed. In unenhanced CT, only a single image parameter (the X-ray attenuation coefficient μ) is involved. With MRI, ten image parameters: proton density (ρ), T_1 and T_2, chemical shift (δ), flow, susceptibility (χ), T_1 in the rotating frame ($T_1\rho$), diffusion, perfusion, and radiofrequency absorption (RFA) are involved. The pulse sequences—partial saturation (PS) and saturation recovery (SR), spin echo (SE), and inversion recovery (IR)—are also needed to relate the image parameters to signal intensity for each voxel.

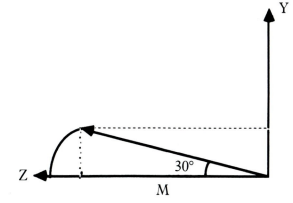

Figure 2.2

Variation of flip angle. The diagram illustrates the magnetization (M) in the patient. When this is rotated through 30 degrees, half the transverse magnetization is available and 85 per cent of the longitudinal magnetization remains.

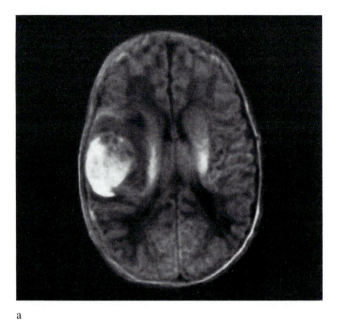

a

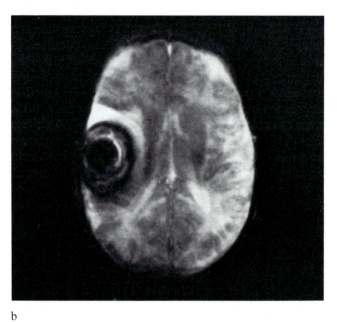

b

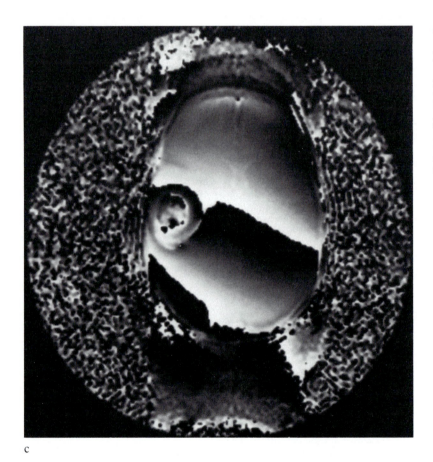

c

Figure 2.3

Acute intracerebral
hemorrhage IR 1800/44/600
(**a**), PS 500/193/30 degrees (**b**)
and phase difference map (**c**).
The intracerebral hemorrhage
has a low-signal intensity (**b**)
and shows marked
susceptibility changes (**c**).

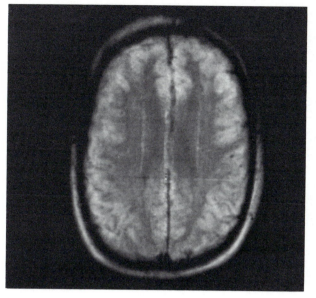
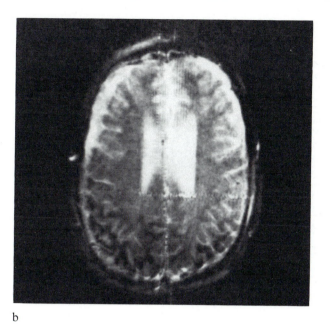

a

b

Figure 2.4

Acute head trauma: SE 1500/80
(**a**) and PS 250/120/30 degrees
(**b**) scans. Changes are seen in
both occipital lobes in (**b**) but
not in (**a**).

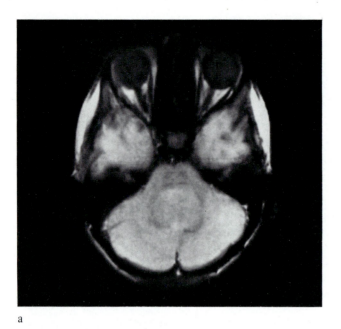

a

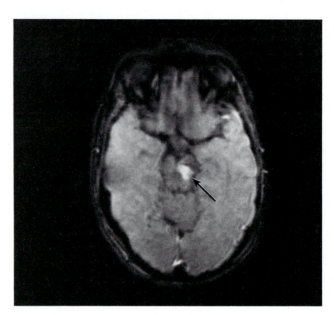

Figure 2.6

Arteriovenous malformation
(PS 500/22). Blood flow into the
lesion in the brainstem is
highlighted (arrow).

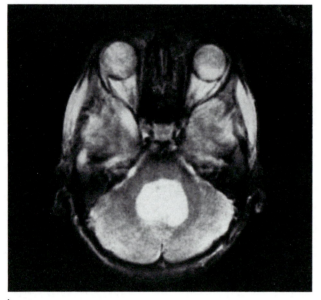

b

Figure 2.5

Low grade astrocytoma: PS
250/59/90 degrees (**a**) and PS
250/50/30 degrees (**b**)
sequences. Low contrast is seen
in (**a**). This is increased by
reducing the flip angle in (**b**).

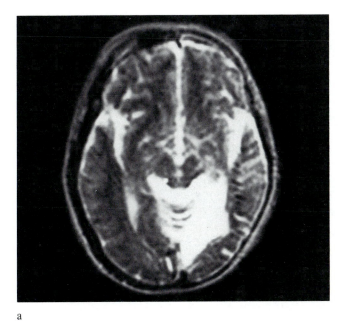

a

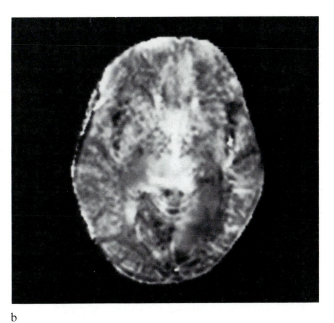

b

Figure 2.7

Cerebral infarction SE 1500/
200 (**a**) and phase map with
sensitization +1 mm/sec (**b**) and
−1 mm/sec (**c**). The medial
portion of the occipital lobe is
abnormal in both phase maps.
Note the gray/white matter
differences within the
remaining brain and the
reversal of the CSF pattern
between (**b**) and (**c**).

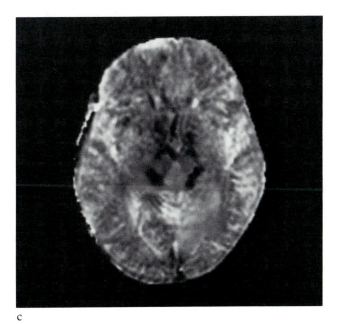

c

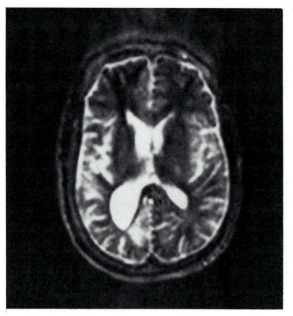

a

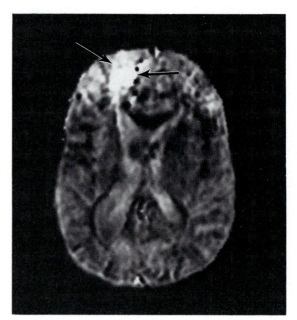

b

Figure 2.8

Epilepsia partialis continua: SE
1500/200 (**a**) and phase map
with sensitization to +1 mm/sec
(**b**). No abnormality is seen in
the frontal lobe in (**a**) but
perfusion changes are seen in
(**b**) (arrows).

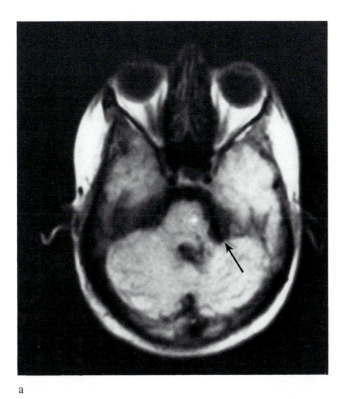

a

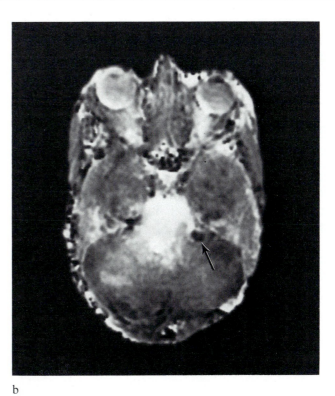

b

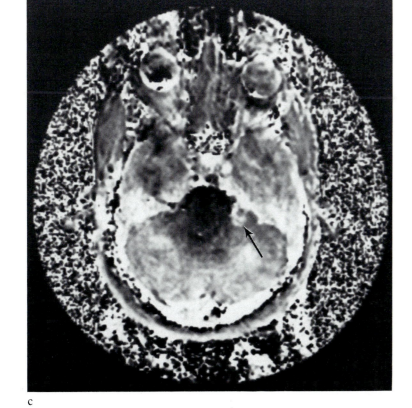

c

Figure 2.9

Arteriovenous malformation in the left cerebellopontine angle: SE 544/22 (**a**) and phase-sensitive maps +1 mm/sec (**b**) and −1 mm/sec (**c**). The central part of the lesion is shown (arrows). The perfusion pattern in the pons and cerebellum is also seen and reverses when the gradient is changed (**b**) and (**c**).

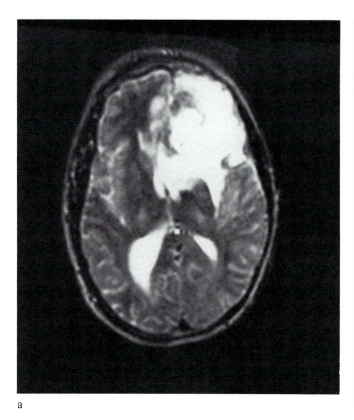

a

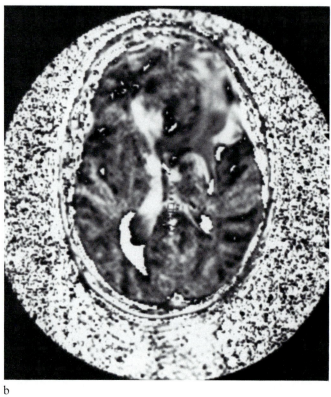

b

Figure 2.10

Astrocytoma grade III: SE
1500/200 (**a**) and sensitized
phase map +1 mm/sec (**b**) and
IVIM image (**c**). Differences in
perfusion are seen within the
tumor and surrounding brain.

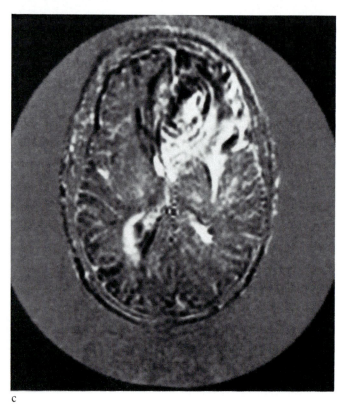

c

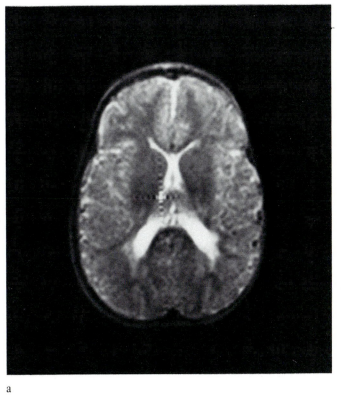

a

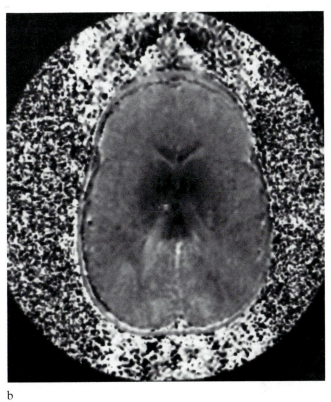

b

Figure 2.11

Periventricular leukomalacia:
SE 1500/200 (**a**) and phase
maps with sensitization +1 mm/
sec (**b**) and −1 mm/sec (**c**).
Changes are seen between the
central and peripheral regions
in (**b**). These are reversed in
(**c**).

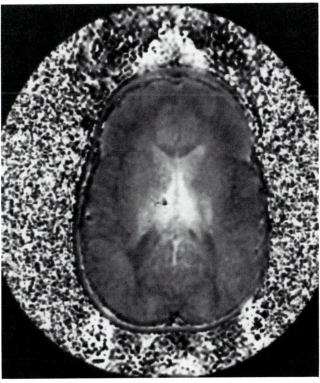

c

A

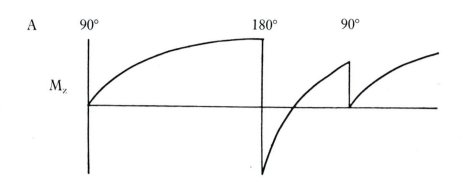

M_z

B

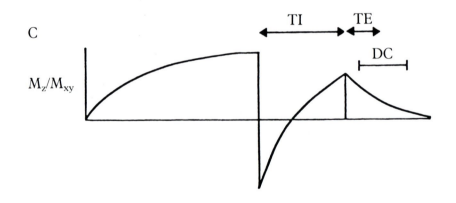

M_{xy}

C

M_z/M_{xy}

Figure 2.12

Changes in M_z (**a**) and M_{xy} (**b**) with time in the IR sequence (medium TI) using a field-echo data collection (DC). (**c**) shows M_z in the first two segments then M_{xy} in the last segment.

A

90° 180°   180°   90° 180°

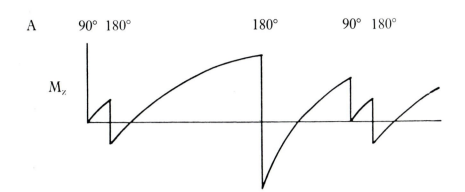

M_z

B

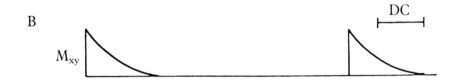

M_{xy}

DC

C

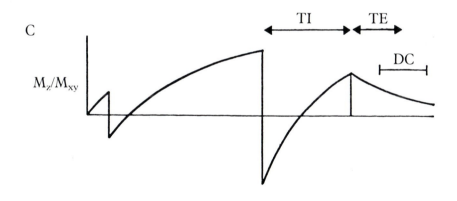

M_z/M_{xy}

TI   TE

DC

Figure 2.13

Changes in M_z (**a**) and M_{xy} (**b**) with time in the IR sequence (medium TI) using a spin-echo data collection (DC). (**c**) shows M_z initially then M_{xy} in the last segment.

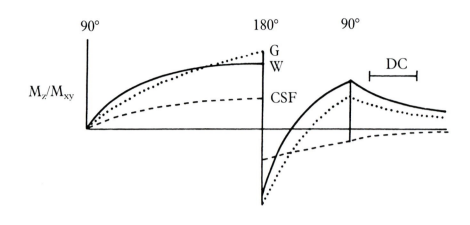

Figure 2.14

Changes in M_z/M_{xy} with time in the IR sequence (medium TI) for white matter (W), gray matter (G), and CSF using a field-echo data collection (DC).

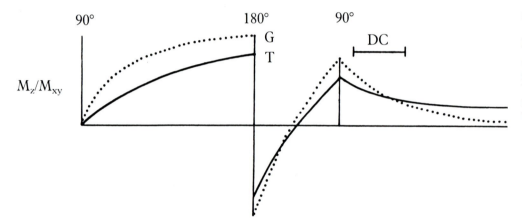

Figure 2.15

Changes in M_z/M_{xy} with time for a medium TI IR sequence. The magnitude of the signal from gray matter (G) is greater than that for tumor (T).

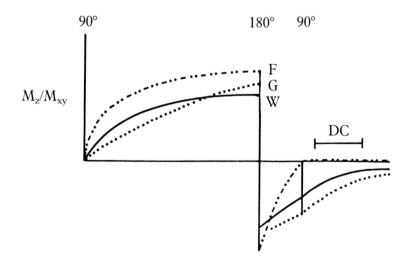

Figure 2.16

Changes in M_z/M_{xy} with time for fat (F), white matter (W), and gray matter (G) using a fat-suppressed STIR sequence. The signal from gray matter is greater than that from white matter. Fat gives no signal.

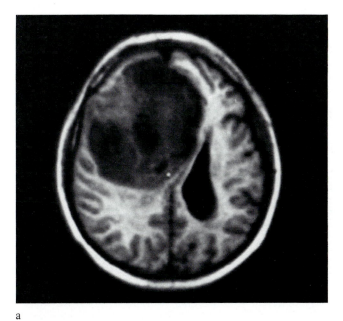

a

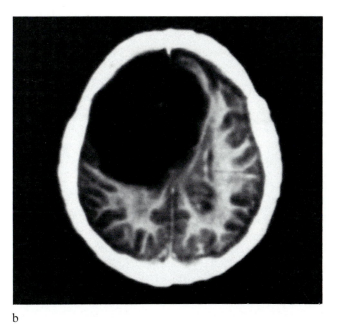

b

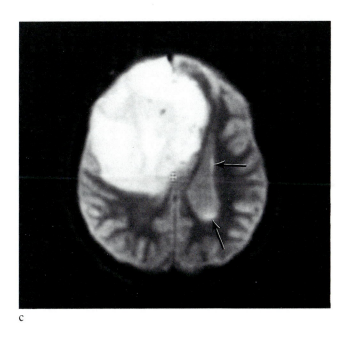

c

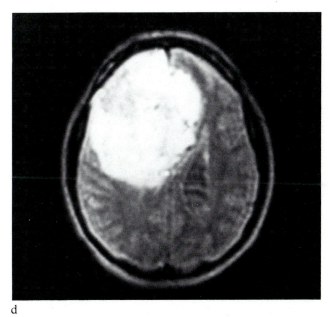

d

Figure 2.17

Astrocytoma grade I in the frontal lobe: phase corrected IR 1500/44/500 (**a**), magnitude-processed IR 1500/44/100 (**b**), magnitude-processed IR 1500/44/100 (**c**), and SE 1500/80 (**d**) images. The tumor is clearly seen on all four images. Note the gray/white matter reversal in (**c**) and the lesions at the periventricular margin (arrows).

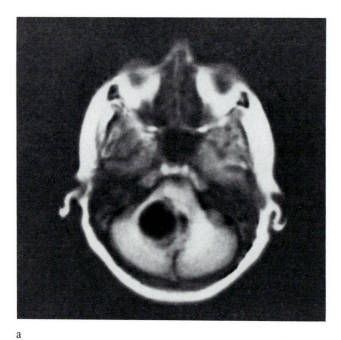

a

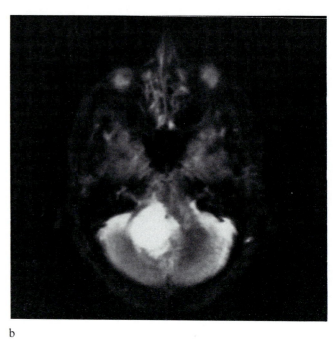

b

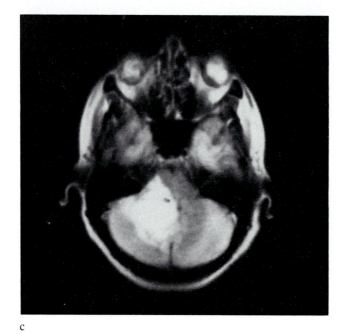

c

Figure 2.18

Astrocytoma grade II: IR 1500/
44/500 (**a**), IR 2000/44/100 (**b**),
and SE 1500/80 (**c**) images.
Separation of tumor from
edema is better with the IR
images. The CSF signal is
greater than brain in (**b**).

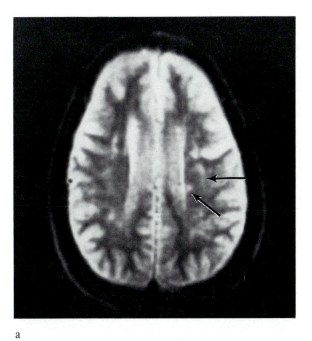

a

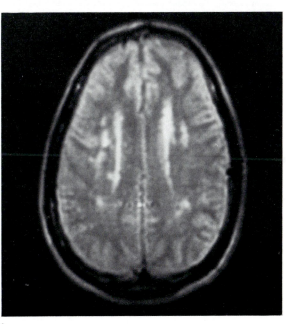

b

Figure 2.19

Vascular disease: IR 1500/44/
100 (**a**), and SE 1500/80 (**b**)
images. The lesions identified
on (**a**) with arrows in the left
centrum semiovale are better
seen in (**b**).

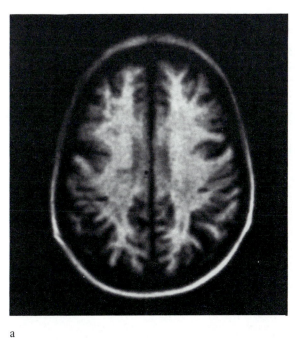

a

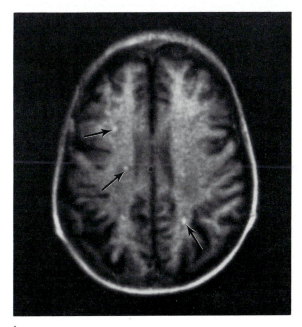

b

Figure 2.20

Metastases: IR 1500/44/500
scans before iv Gd-DTPA (**a**)
and after enhancement (**b**). The
lesions are more obvious in (**b**)
(arrows).

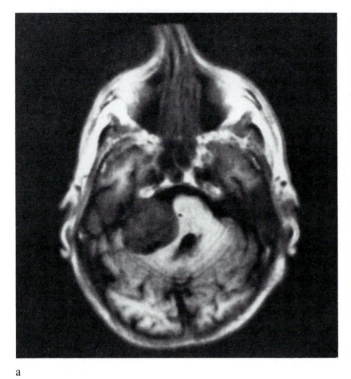
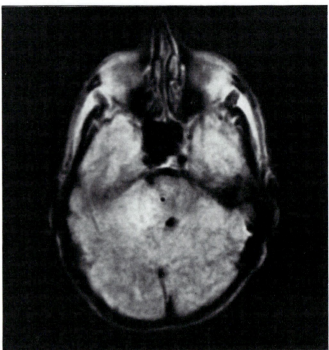

a   b

Figure 2.21

Acoustic neuroma: IR 1500/44/
500 (**a**) and SE 1500/80 (**b**)
images. The tumor is better
defined in (**a**).

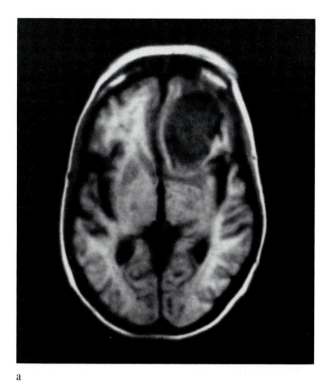

a

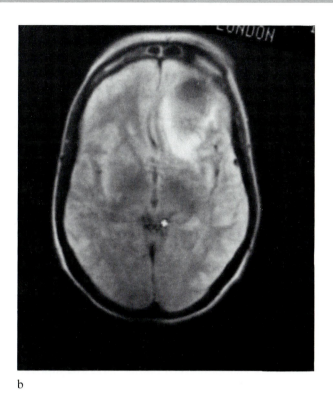

b

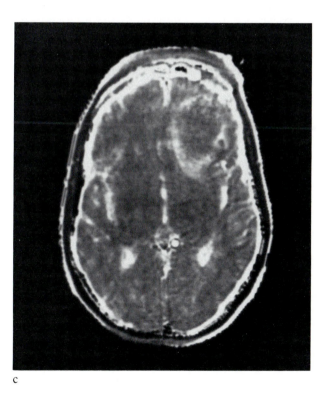

c

Figure 2.22

Meningioma: IR 1500/44/500
(**a**), SE 1500/80 (**b**), and T_2
map (**c**). The lesion is well
defined in (**a**). The T_2 map (**c**)
indicates that its T_2 shows little
or no increase.

3

Flow phenomena

William G Bradley

Few aspects of magnetic resonance (MR) imaging are as potentially confusing as the effect of motion on the MR image. While the MR image is anatomically similar to the image produced by CT, the MR appearance of flowing blood has no correlate in CT. Flowing blood can appear bright or dark, depending on the velocity and direction of flow.[1–12] To a first approximation, rapidly flowing blood appears dark ('flow void') and slowly flowing blood appears bright. This phenomenon is illustrated in Figure 3.1. This appearance is markedly influenced by factors related to the imaging sequence and to the MR imager itself. The signal from flowing blood depends on the position of the slice relative to the rest of the multislice imaging volume.[1] It depends on the repetition time TR, the echo-delay time TE, the echo number, and the slice thickness. In fast scanning techniques with short repetition times, gradient echoes, and flip angles less than 90°, flow has a different appearance than on standard 90°/180° spin-echo images.[13,14] The principles which affect the appearance of flowing blood also affect the appearance of flowing cerebrospinal fluid (CSF). Examples of CSF flow phenomena are given at the end of the chapter.

There are three independent factors which result in decreased signal intensity from flowing blood: high velocity,[1] turbulence,[10] and odd-echo dephasing.[15,16] These lead to the 'flow void',[7] or signal loss due to rapid flow, (shown in Figures 3.2 and 3.3) which permits normal arteries (Figure 3.3), aneurysms (Figure 3.2) and arteriovenous malformations (Figure 3.4) to be identified. There are also three independent factors which result in increased signal intensity: flow-related enhancement (FRE),[1] even-echo rephasing,[12] and diastolic pseudogating.[1] These phenomena result in signal gain which can be mistaken for intraluminal

pathology. Although these phenomena are independent and will be described separately, in practice they are almost always found in various combinations.

The causes of increased and decreased intensity can be considered under four separate categories: time-of-flight effects, phase effects, turbulence, and stagnation. Time-of-flight effects can cause signal loss at high velocity or signal gain at lower velocities for blood first entering the imaging volume, that is, FRE. Phase effects lead to signal loss on the first spin echo (odd-echo dephasing), however, under certain conditions this loss can be reversed on the second and subsequent even echoes (even-echo rephasing). Turbulence is actually random motion of fluid elements[17] and always causes irreversible signal loss.[10] Stagnation results in signal intensity due to the T_1, T_2, and proton density of unclotted blood and, therefore, has a greater dependence on TR and TE than when it is flowing rapidly. Stagnation can be due to a positional slowing of flow or to diastolic acquisition, either by intentional cardiac gating or by chance synchronization of the cardiac and MR cycles, that is, diastolic pseudogating.[1]

Time-of-flight effects

Time-of-flight effects are due entirely to motion. At low velocity, time-of-flight effects can lead to increased intraluminal signal due to replacement of previously exposed spins by fresh, unsaturated protons.[1] This is most prominent on single-slice techniques and near the entry surface of multislice techniques. Since it is the only true flow-related cause of signal greater than that of unclotted blood, it has been called flow-related enhancement.[1]

At higher velocities, time-of-flight effects lead to decreased signal. As the velocity increases, some spins will not be in the slice for both the 90- and 180° pulses which are required to produce a traditional spin echo. As the velocity continues to increase, this cause of signal loss increases (high velocity signal loss).[1]

High-velocity signal loss

In order to produce a traditional spin echo, a group of protons must be exposed to both a 90° and a 180° RF pulse. In the multislice techniques used commonly today, these pulses are slice-selective, that is, only the protons in a well-defined slice are exposed to the RF pulses. High velocity signal loss (Figure 3.5) or time-of-flight loss occurs when protons do not remain within the selected slice long enough to acquire both the initial 90° pulse and the subsequent 180° pulse to produce a traditional spin-echo signal. More signal is lost for later echoes because of the longer time interval between the initial 90° pulse and the 180° pulse preceding the last echo. As shown in Figure 3.6, the magnitude of the high-velocity signal loss is a linear function of velocity v and reflects the relative proportions of two populations of protons: those which are within the slice for the appropriate RF pulses and those which are not.[10] The latter can be further divided into protons which flow into the upstream side of the slice (not having acquired the initial 90° pulse) and those which flow out of the slice prior to acquisition of the 180° pulse. The protons which return a signal are those which flow a minimum distance of zero (on the downstream edge of the slice) and a maximum distance of one slice thickness dz (on the upstream edge of the slice) during the interval TE/2 between the 90° and 180° pulses. This corresponds to a maximum velocity of dz/(TE/2). Thus v/ dz/(TE/2) = vTE/2dz is the fraction leaving the slice and 1-vTE/2dz is the fraction remaining in the slice. In Figure 3.6, theoretical MR signal intensity is plotted as a function of velocity v.

Flow-related enhancement

When evaluating flow effects, it is important to remember that blood can become magnetized anywhere within the bore of the magnet while imaging is only performed in the homogeneous region in the center of the magnet. Flow-related enhancement (FRE)[1] or 'entry phenomenon' results when flowing blood enters the first slice of a multislice imaging volume. In this situation, the partially saturated (that is, demagnetized) blood remaining from the previous sequence is replaced by fresh, unsaturated blood, as shown in Figure 3.7). The strong signal from unsaturated blood reflects its full magnetization. It thus returns a stronger signal than that from the adjacent stationary tissue which is still partially saturated (to a degree depending on its own T_1 relaxation time and the repetition time TR).

The signal elicited from the vessel in the entry slice of a multislice technique comes from two populations of protons: a strong signal arising from the unsaturated, fully magnetized, upstream (inflowing) protons and a weaker signal arising from the protons in the downstream portion of the voxel which were within the slice at the time of the previous excitation (and are thus still partially saturated). The intraluminal signal is greatest at the velocity v where all the blood in the slice dz is replaced in the interval TR between excitations.[1] This occurs at:

$$v = \mathrm{d}z/\mathrm{TR}$$

For example, if the slice thickness dz is 1 cm and the repetition time TR is 1 sec, this corresponds to a velocity of 1 cm/sec, which is typically seen in veins.[1]

Flow-related enhancement is seen routinely during clinical MR imaging. Figure 3.1 demonstrates FRE in the slowly flowing femoral veins while there is absence of signal from the adjacent rapidly flowing femoral arteries. Figure 3.8 shows the lowest slices of a multislice imaging volume (which are the first sections encountered by the blood flowing cephalad in the femoral veins). Once the inflowing protons are exposed to their first 90° RF pulse, they return a strong signal which we see as FRE (Figure 3.8a). Exposure to subsequent 90° pulses deeper within the imaging volume elicits a weaker signal (Figures 3.8b and c), the maximum strength of which depends on the interval between excitations and on the amount of recovery of longitudinal magnetization which has occurred (reflecting the T_1 of the unclotted blood).

When flow occurs at the velocity shown in the above equation, maximal FRE is noted for a single-slice technique or in the entry slice of a multislice technique. Flow-related enhancement is a relative (rather than an absolute) phenomenon, that is, it reflects the relative signal of the flowing protons compared to those which are stationary outside the vessel. Thus FRE depends on the limited longitudinal recovery of the adjacent stationary tissue. It is therefore more pronounced at shorter repetition times.[1] The effect is also greater for stationary tissues with longer T_1 relaxation times.[1] This is supported by the experimental data shown in Figure 3.9. The above equation indicates that maximal FRE for short repetition times occurs at higher velocities.[1] This is also confirmed by the experimental data in Figure 3.9. By using Equation 3.1 and varying the slice thickness and the TR in a single-slice technique, the appearance of FRE allows the velocity in a vessel to be estimated.[18]

As the velocity increases above dz/TR, FRE can be seen in deeper slices, as illustrated in Figures 3.8 and 3.10–3.12.[10] Unsaturated protons project several slices into the imaging volume in a parabolic laminar flow profile, shown in Figure 3.11. Seen in three dimensions, this appears as a cone. Slicing across the cone produces a central high-intensity dot in the center of the vessel which enlarges to fill the entire lumen as one approaches the entry surface. This pattern of decreasing high-intensity circles is demonstrated in Figure 3.12 in the right common carotid artery. The subject in this case is a 30-year-old MR technologist. Were she an 80-year-old with a right hemispheric infarct, one might well question the presence of intraluminal pathology, and expose the patient to an unnecessary, invasive examination such as an arteriogram.

In order to understand the mechanism of FRE for slices deep to the entry slice, one must be familiar with a few details of the multislice imaging technique. 90° pulses for a given slice are separated by the repetition time interval TR. For the imaging volume as a whole, however, 90° pulses are applied more frequently, being separated by the interval between excitation of successive slices. If n slices are acquired during an interval TR, then the interval between excitations at successive levels is (TR/n). Excitation generally occurs for consecutive slices (that is, 1,2,3,...n) although odd-even excitation (1,3,5,...,2,4,6,...n) is also used. (For purposes of further discussion, we will only consider consecutive slice excitation hereafter.) As illustrated in Figure 3.13, the succession of 90° pulses appears as a slice excitation wave (SEW) moving through the imaging volume at a velocity v_0 of one slice thickness dz during the interval TR/n, that is

$$v_0 = \mathrm{d}z/(\mathrm{TR}/n)$$

For example, if consecutive, contiguous 1 cm slices are excited at intervals of 0.1 sec, then the SEW velocity is 10 cm/sec.

Intraluminal signal intensity depends on whether flow is in the direction of the SEW, that is, 'co-current', or against it, that is, 'countercurrent'.[19] As shown in the flow phantom experiments in Figure 3.14, signal intensity is much greater for flow countercurrent to the SEW than for co-current flow. This is true at both low and high velocity. This effect is also demonstrated in Figure 3.15 for central drainage of cortical veins into the superior sagittal sinus. Assuming the slices are numbered in the order they are acquired, this flow pattern will lead to co-current flow (at low slice numbers) and to countercurrent flow (at higher slice numbers) for multislice sagittal acquisition.

The explanation for the differences in co-current and countercurrent FRE is shown in Figures 3.16 and 3.17. These differences depend on the time available for recovery of longitudinal relaxation during the time between excitations. When less time is available for recovery of a significant fraction of the protons in the slice, signal intensity is relatively decreased. As shown in Figure 3.16, co-current flow results in some of the protons in the immediate upstream slice flowing into the slice to be excited. These protons have only had time TR/n to recover magnetization and thus return a relatively weak signal. As the velocity approaches v_0, all the protons in the slice were just excited by a 90° pulse as the SEW passed through the upstream slice. At lower velocities, the percentage of protons remaining from the previous passage of the SEW increases. These protons have had a longer period of time (TR) to recover and thus return a stronger signal. As the velocity approaches zero, all the protons have had time TR to recover—which, of course, is the same time available for the stationary protons around the vessel. The actual signal intensity at a particular velocity depends on the relative proportions of these two populations and whether the velocity is closer to zero or to v_0.

For countercurrent flow, less saturated downstream protons can flow back into the slice to be excited during the time interval TR/n. As shown in Figure 3.17, this motion produces gaps of less saturated protons which are exactly the same size as the overlap zones for co-current flow. These less saturated protons have had more time to recover magnetization since their last exposure to a 90° pulse and, therefore, they return a stronger signal. Exactly how unsaturated these protons are depends on whether there is an odd or even number of slices. As v approaches v_0, the width of the gap approaches the width of the slice. For an odd number of slices, the gap contains fresh, unsaturated protons which demonstrate true FRE. For an even number of slices, the gap contains protons which have had time 2TR to recover and thus return a stronger signal than for co-current flow where a shorter interval TR/n is available. The effect depends, of course, on the absolute T_1 of the flowing fluid and is also modified by dephasing effects and time-of-flight losses. Regardless, the intensity of protons flowing countercurrent to the SEW is always greater than those flowing in the same direction except for the entry slices.

Flow-related enhancement on fast scanning techniques

Fast scanning methods utilize gradient reversal to produce a gradient or field echo. In contrast to the traditional spin-echo, gradient-echo techniques do not utilize a 180° pulse. In a spin-echo image, flow perpendicular to the imaging plane causes signal loss due to flow during the interval between the 90- and the 180° pulses and on the basis of dephasing due to flow through the slice-selecting gradients. With fast scanning techniques, such as FLASH and GRASS which utilize gradient echoes, time-of-flight losses are decreased since there is no 180° pulse.[13,14] Thus FRE due to the entrance of fresh spins even at arterial velocities is unopposed by the factors which result in signal loss for a traditional spin echo. For this reason, FRE is much more prominent on FLASH and GRASS images. Figure 3.18 shows FRE in GRASS imaging. In addition, fast scanning techniques are often single slice (so every slice is an entry slice).

Reversible phase effects

Flow phenomena can be arranged in a hierarchy. Time-of-flight effects, for example, can be modified by phase effects. The above discussion of time-of-flight effects ignores phase effects and, thus, assumes that coherence is maintained by the spins in the voxel during flow. Phase effects can be separated into those which are reversible and those which are not. Reversible phase effects (odd-echo dephasing and even-echo rephasing) are similar to the partial rephasing resulting from the 180° pulse in a traditional spin echo. Irreversible phase effects (turbulence) are similar to the dephasing which results from randomly fluctuating internal fields which lead to irreversible T_2 decay.

Odd-echo dephasing

Laminar flow along a magnetic field gradient produces dephasing and therefore signal loss on the first and other odd echoes.[12,15,16] Dephasing results when all the protons in the voxel do not move at the same velocity through a magnetic field gradient and thus precess at different frequencies and accumulate different amounts of phase. To the extent that they are out of phase at the time of the spin echo, signal is lost. If laminar flow is steady and continues until a second echo is acquired, the dephasing seen on the first echo can be reconstituted on the second echo (see even-echo rephasing[12] below). When multiple echoes are acquired in an echo train,[20] all the odd echoes will have decreased signal intensity (due to dephasing) while the even echoes will have increased intensity signal (due to rephasing). To understand the dephasing-rephasing phenomenon seen in laminar flow, we must review the mechanism of traditional spin-echo formation.

Figure 3.19 is a schematic of the Carr Purcell Meiboom Gill spin-echo sequence.[20,21] Consider a hypothetical, microscopic group of protons which travel as a group and all experience essentially the same magnetic field. Since they remain in phase, they are called 'isochromats'.[8,12,21,22] Following the 90° pulse, isochromats begin to get out of phase due to magnetic field non-uniformities. Isochromats in a slightly stronger part of the field precess at a higher frequency and tend to get ahead of those in weaker parts of the magnetic field, that is, they 'accumulate more phase'. This results in flaring of the magnetization vectors in the rotating reference frame shown in Figure 3.19. The longer the time following the 90° pulse, the greater the relative phase accumulation by the more rapidly precessing protons.

Following a 180° rotation about the y-axis, dephased isochromats are flipped so that those which led now lag. Since they remain in a slightly stronger part of the magnetic field, however, they continue to precess at the higher frequency and eventually catch up with their more slowly precessing counterparts to generate a spin echo.[21]

The same phenomenon can be demonstrated by the spin-phase graph.[8] As shown in Figure 3.20, isochromats in a stronger part of the field gain phase until the 180° pulse. At this time, their phase is reversed and they suddenly lose exactly the amount of phase they had just gained. They continue to gain or lose phase at the same rate and regain coherence with their more slowly precessing counterparts at the time of the spin echo. At this time, there is no difference in phase angle between isochromats in different parts of the voxel. If the isochromats are allowed to dephase again after the first spin echo, they can be rephased again by a second 180° pulse, producing a second spin echo. Similarly, repeated 180° pulses produce multiple spin echoes in an echo train.

The phase graph can be used for the study of different types of flow. Two types of gradients across the voxel determine the degree of dephasing which will occur with flow: the magnetic field gradient and the velocity gradient.[15,16] The strength of the magnetic field gradient encountered depends on the direction of flow. The component of flow into the weaker slice-selecting gradient experiences less dephasing than that into the stronger readout gradient. (The phase-encoding gradient varies from zero to the full strength of the readout gradient so dephasing-rephasing will be less than that due to flow into the readout gradient.) The velocity gradient across the vessel is zero both in the no-flow situation and in idealizing plug flow.[17] In laminar flow, the velocity gradient across the vessel (and thus across each voxel spanning the vessel) increases as the velocity increases.[17]

Figure 3.21 demonstrates the change in phase angle (relative to that of protons in the main magnetic field) along the leading edge (stronger field) and lagging edge (weaker field) of the voxel.[12] When there is a magnetic field gradient but no flow, phase gain (or loss) relative to the mean field changes linearly with time. Flow into a gradient increases the rate of phase gain which then becomes quadratic in time (that is, phase is gained in proportion to $(time)^2$). The more rapid the flow, the greater the phase gain.

Figure 3.22 is a spin-phase graph for plug flow during a double-echo sequence. While protons on the leading edge of the voxel (in the stronger field) gain phase more rapidly than those on the lagging edge, the incremental quadratic phase gain is the same at all positions within the voxel because the velocity is the same at all positions across the voxel in plug flow. Although the isochromats do not return to a zero phase angle at the time of the first echo, they do all acquire the same positive phase angle, thus coherence is totally re-established. (With magnitude-reconstruction techniques, the phase angle per se does not influence signal intensity since real and imaginary components are added together.)

In laminar flow the situation is somewhat different, as shown in Figure 3.23. The spin-phase graph has three groupings of three curves each.[12] The major groupings reflect the magnetic field gradient (from front to back) across the voxel. Those acquiring phase most rapidly have the highest velocity in the center of the vessel. The three curves within each major grouping reflect radial position across the vessel. At the time of the first echo, the phase curves do not cross at one point as they did in plug flow but rather spread out, criss-crossing over an area. This represents dephasing or loss of coherence at the time of the first echo which results in signal loss.

Even-echo rephasing

As shown in Figure 3.23, the phase curves which had previously spread out (losing coherence at the time of the first echo) continue on to cross at a point (re-establishing coherence) at the time of the second echo.[12] This rephasing phenomenon reconstitutes the signal which had been lost at the time of the first echo in a manner analogous to the rephasing of an FID as a spin echo. As has been shown mathematically,[12] the rephasing only occurs for a flow of constant velocity into a linear gradient. Thus, when there are higher order terms for either flow (that is, acceleration or jerk)

or the field gradient, complete even-echo rephasing will not occur.

Even-echo rephasing results in higher signal intensity for even echoes compared to the preceding odd echoes.[12] This can be demonstrated using a flow phantom, shown in Figure 3.24, and in routine clinical imaging, as in Figures 3.3 and 3.25. This is primarily seen for 'symmetric echoes', that is, those where the TE of the second echo is twice that of the first. It is much reduced (or totally absent) for asymmetric echoes, for example, combinations such as TE 20 and 70 msec, unless the gradients are symmetric. It is also reduced when motion artifact suppression techniques are used. Although it is much weaker, even-echo rephasing can also be seen to an extent in turbulent flow,[10] and can be demonstrated mathematically if one assumes a Gaussian distribution to the random component of motion.[23,24] However, even-echo rephasing is much more prominent in laminar than in turbulent flow due to the random motion in the latter.

Figures 3.26–3.30 demonstrate use of the even-echo rephasing phenomenon in clinically relevant situations. A giant intracranial aneurysm is shown in Figure 3.26.[25] In comparing first- and second-echo images, the only region of signal gain (due to even-echo rephasing) is seen to be the patent lumen on the contrast-enhanced CT. Figure 3.27 shows even-echo rephasing in the right internal carotid artery due to slow flow; Figure 3.28 shows the same phenomenon in the basilar artery in a patient with brainstem infarcts. Even-echo rephasing is noted deep in the frontal lobe in Figure 3.29 in a patient with a venous angioma. Figure 3.30 shows two patients, both of whom have malignant external otitis. One of the severe complications of this chronic osteomyelitis of the temporal bone is thrombosis of the adjacent dural sinus. In Figure 3.30a and b, the sigmoid sinus is thrombosed and no even-echo rephasing is seen. In Figure 3.30c and d, even-echo rephasing is clearly demonstrated, documenting at least partial patency of that sigmoid sinus. Since many patients with suspected dural sinus thrombosis are hypercoagulable, the use of hypertonic contrast material for CT or angiography may aggravate the problem. MRI has been advocated in the evaluation of such patients, based on the sensitivity of even-echo rephasing to flow.[26]

The dephasing/rephasing seen on the first and second echo can only be produced by flowing isochromats. Thus when even-echo rephasing is seen, it is evidence of flow.[12] Usually, the relative signal increase on the second-echo image is apparent merely by inspection of the two images. In subtler cases where very slow flow must be distinguished from thrombosis, however, it may be necessary to compare the intensities using a cursor to define a region of interest on the computer monitor, as shown in Figure 3.31. Attempts to calculate a T_2 relaxation time in this situation may indicate prolonged or apparently negative T_2 values,[27,28] as illustrated in Figure 3.32.

Irreversible phase effects (turbulence)

'High velocity' and 'turbulence' are not equivalent terms. Turbulence is present when randomly fluctuating velocity components are found in both the axial and non-axial directions,[10] shown in Figure 3.33. This random motion produces dephasing and thus signal loss.

The velocity profile, that is, the variation in velocity across the vessel, is flatter for turbulent or 'plug' flow than for laminar flow, where the velocity profile is parabolic. As shown in Figure 3.34, several flow regions can be defined for flow rates in transition between laminar flow and turbulent flow in a tube.[10] Fully developed turbulence is present in the core. Laminar flow is present in a thin sublayer at the boundary of the tube. In between, there is a buffer zone separating the turbulent core from the laminar sublayer. Curiously, the magnitude of the random fluctuating velocity components, that is, the intensity of turbulence, is greatest in this buffer zone.[10]

As an approximation, onset of turbulence can be predicted using the Reynolds number Re which is defined:[10,17]

$$Re = \frac{density \times velocity \times tube\ diameter}{viscosity}$$

For Reynolds numbers less than 2100, laminar flow is generally present; for Reynolds numbers greater than 2100, turbulent flow is present. Laminar flow can be maintained at high velocity in small diameter tubes.[17] On the other hand, as Figure 3.35 demonstrates, turbulence can occur at low velocity in larger diameter tubes. It should be emphasized that this is a gross approximation, only applying to steady flow in smooth-walled tubes which do not branch.[10,17] Endothelial roughening due to atherosclerosis, vascular branching, and the acceleration and deceleration which accompany pulsatile flow all contribute to turbulent or 'disturbed' flow in arteries at lower velocities than predicted by the Reyonds number, as indicated in Figure 3.36.

Regions of laminar flow may be seen in association with otherwise turbulent flow. Laminar flow is seen within large-scale recirculation zones (eddies) downstream from a partial vascular obstruction.[10,29] If a double-echo technique is used, high signal may be seen in the eddies on the second-echo image due to even-echo rephasing, shown in Figure 3.37.

Stagnation

As flow decreases, approaching stagnation, the intraluminal intensity approaches that due to the intermediate (approximately 900 msec) T_1 and long T_2 (approximately 150 msec) of unclotted blood, as in Figure 3.38. Flow may be effectively stagnant during the majority of the spin-echo acquisitions whenever there is diastolic acquisition or if there is extended breathholding, particularly by a marginally claustrophobic patient. This may increase signal intensity in any vein affected by such respiratory maneuvers, that is, those within the head and neck as well as those in the abdomen.

Very slow flow

Flow in the jugular vein can be slowed significantly merely by positioning in the RF head coil. Figure 3.39 demonstrates high-signal intensity on the first-echo image in an interior slice due to positional slowing of drainage through the left jugular vein. The accompanying CT and angiogram show no evidence of pathology, that is, there is no glomus jugulare tumor. Slow drainage through the left jugular vein is noted when the patient is placed in the Townes position for the angiogram. The patient was in a similar position in the RF head coil at the time of the MR study, resulting in slow flow and high signal in the jugular bulb on that side.

Diastolic pseudogating

The high-signal intensity resulting from stagnation (shown in Figures 3.38 and 3.39) can also be seen in arteries under certain conditions.[1] Whereas venous flow is irregular, reflecting respiration and intermittent Valsalva maneuvers, arterial flow is as regular as the heartbeat. Over the period of one cardiac cycle, flow is alternately rapid (during systole) and slow or absent (during diastole). When MR image acquisition is intentionally gated to the R wave of the EKG, higher intraluminal signal is observed in arteries during diastole than during systole.

It is possible for the cardiac and MR cycles to become synchronized without intentional cardiac gating.[1] For example, if the heart rate is 60, a cardiac cycle is initiated every second. Should the TR of the MR imager also be set to 1.0 sec, the cardiac and MR cycles may remain in phase for the 2 to 8-minute acquisition (depending on the number of excitations and phase-encoded projections). Using a double-echo technique, 10 or so slices would typically be acquired during a 1.0 sec TR interval. At a heart rate of 60, approximately 30 per cent of the cardiac cycle is spent in systole and 70 per cent in diastole. Thus one would expect 3 of the 10 slices to show the flow void and 7 of the 10 slices to show higher signal due to the relatively slower flow. This is demonstrated in Figure 3.40. In this flow phantom, the 'heart rate' of the blood flow pump was set to 40 such that a new cardiac cycle began every 1.5 sec. The TR of the imager was also set to 1.5 sec, allowing 15 slices to be acquired sequentially. The resultant plot of signal intensity I (relative to a stagnant standard I_o) demonstrates high signal at the entry level (due to FRE) and a central peak due to diastolic acquisition. When this occurs by chance, it is called 'diastolic pseudogating',[1] and is demonstrated clinically in Figure 3.41.

The maximum signal due to diastolic pseudogating alone should not exceed that expected for stagnant, unclotted blood (for example, Figures 3.38 and 3.39). Whenever signal higher than this is seen, it reflects the additional presence of a separate flow phenomenon such as FRE. This is noted both on the phantom experiment in Figure 3.40 and in Figure 3.12 where diastolic pseudogating allowed the multislice FRE to be visualized. Whenever diastolic pseudogating is observed within an artery, the high signal can be potentially mistaken for thrombus or tumor. In such cases, the study should be repeated with intentional cardiac gating, positioning the patient such that the slice in question is in the interior of the imaging volume (rather than near an entry surface). If high signal is still seen on slices acquired during cardiac systole, then a lesion is likely to be present.

Combined flow phenomena

The flow phenomena discussed above often occur in combination. As the velocity increases from zero, FRE initially increases in the slices near the entry surface. At $v = dz/TR$, it is maximal in the first slice. As the velocity continues to increase, FRE will be noted in deeper slices, however, signal intensity may begin to decrease in the first slice due to offsetting time-of-flight losses and dephasing (Figure 3.9). First-echo dephasing increases as the velocity increases due to steepening of the parabolic velocity profile and decreasing intravoxel coherence. This tendency towards signal loss will partially decrease the signal gain which would have resulted from FRE. If a symmetric second-echo image is acquired and laminar flow continues at the same velocity until the second TE, then even-echo rephasing will reconstitute the signal loss which had occurred due to dephasing. However, signal loss due to time-of-flight effects will increase on the second-echo image because there is now three times as much

time available for outflow of spins prior to exposure to the second 180° pulse. The signal on the second echo will thus reflect offsetting influences: signal gain due to even-echo rephasing and signal loss due to increasing time-of-flight effects. For comparable velocities and vascular diameters, decreasing the slice thickness will increase the time-of-flight losses, decreasing signal intensity. As the vascular diameter decreases for a given velocity, the laminar parabolic profile will steepen, increasing the dephasing-rephasing effects.

When the signal intensity in a vein or dural sinus is particularly prominent on the second-echo image, associated FRE may be present. Even-echo rephasing should only restore signal which was lost on the first echo. Therefore, if the intensity on a second-echo image is greater than that expected on the basis of the T_1 and T_2 times of stagnant blood, associated FRE should be suspected (Figure 3.40). Since FRE may be masked by dephasing on the first-echo image, its influence may not be apparent until the second echo.

CSF flow

The flow phenomena which influence the intensity of flowing blood also affect the appearance of flowing CSF.[30-8] CSF motion reflects slow flow due to the circulation of CSF and more rapid flow due to superimposed cardiac pulsations.[30] The slow flow is due to the production of CSF by the choroid plexus inside the ventricles at a rate of approximately 500 cc/day. CSF flows through the aqueduct, out the foramina of Luschka and Magendie, through the basal cisterns, and eventually over the convexities where it is absorbed by the arachnoid villi. Superimposed on this slow steady flow of CSF is a more rapid to-and-fro motion due to transmitted cardiac pulsations.[30,39] These pulsations arise from the general expansion of the cerebral hemispheres during systole,[39] as well as from the systolic expansion of the choroid plexi[40] and the large arteries at the base of the brain. This to-and-fro motion of CSF occurs throughout the ventricles and basal cisterns but it is most obvious through the narrowest portion of the ventricular system, that is, the aqueduct, illustrated in Figure 3.42. Pulsatile flow can also be observed in the spinal subarachnoid space.[41] Since this flow originates at the foramen magnum, it is more prominent in the cervical subarachnoid space and decreases as one progresses towards the lumbar region.[33] The pulsatile motion of the CSF in the brain and spine can produce the same flow phenomena as noted above for blood. CSF flow phenomena, however, generally reflect slower flow rates and the much longer T_1 and T_2 of CSF.

Signal loss is most often seen in the aqueduct of Sylvius ('aqueductal flow void'),[30,34] shown in Figure 3.43. Since the velocity increases as the cross-sectional area decreases (for a constant volumetric flow rate), time-of-flight losses and first-echo dephasing are greatest in the aqueduct. This tends to be more pronounced on thinner slices and on more T_2-weighted images, both of which increase the influence of time-of-flight losses. Sections acquired through the upper fourth ventricle show signal loss which may reflect turbulence due to the venturi (nozzle) effect from the expanding jet of CSF,[42] illustrated in Figure 3.42. Occasionally, signal loss can also be observed in the lateral and third ventricles, particularly near the foramen of Monro, shown in Figure 3.43. Clinical conditions which decrease the flow of CSF through the aqueduct decrease the degree of signal loss.[32] This is particularly obvious for cases of aqueductal stenosis or other causes of aqueductal obstruction, as in Figure 3.44.

Clinical conditions which increase the pulsatile velocity of CSF through the aqueduct increase the magnitude of the flow void.[30,43] Because the cranium has a fixed volume, the systolic inflow of arterial blood must be countered by outflow of other non-compressible fluids such as venous blood or CSF. (A similar statement can be made for the supratentorial compartment which is defined inferiorly by the rigid tentorium.) There is a phase lag for venous outflow due to its passage through the capillary system, therefore, CSF must be vented from the supratentorial space (or calvarium) simultaneously with arterial inflow to avoid a pressure rise. CSF is vented from the supratentorial compartment mainly through the subarachnoid space (perimesencephalic cistern) and through the aqueduct. When the subarachnoid pathway is blocked, for example, by tumor, flow through the aqueduct increases,[44] as demonstrated in Figure 3.45.

Since marked signal loss is noted in all patients with a patent aqueduct on heavily T_2-weighted images, less heavily T_2-weighted images (for example, SE 2000/30) may be necessary to differentiate high- and low-flow states. The aqueductal flow void sign is particularly prominent in patients with chronic communicating hydrocephalus,[30] illustrated in Figure 3.46, including normal pressure hydrocephalus (NPH), shown in Figure 3.47. In this condition, flow of CSF through the aqueduct has been shown to be six to eight times normal[43] (Figure 3.48), and to decrease following successful ventricular shunting (Figure 3.49). On mildly T_2-weighted images, the most marked signal loss is seen in patients with NPH and the lowest degree of signal loss in patients with acute communicating hydrocephalus and atrophy,[30] as shown in Figure 3.50. The pulsatile flow of CSF through the aqueduct reflects many factors, among them the aqueductal diameter,[44] the resistance to outflow through cortical veins,[44] the ventricular surface area,[30] and the compliance of the ventricles[30] and the surrounding tissues. An increase in the diameter of the aqueduct (for example, due to communicating hydrocephalus) has the greatest effect on aqueductal flow since resistance decreases as the fourth power of the radius.[44] Decreased compliance due to stiff ventricles per se or resulting from periventricular gliosis or sclerosis of cortical veins (which are unable to vent venous blood adequately during diastole) may also contribute to the increased pulsatile motion of CSF through the aqueduct. Signal loss can also occur due to the radial to-and-fro motion of CSF around the basilar artery. On thin T_2-weighted images, the signal loss can lead to the misdiagnosis of basilar artery aneurysm,[45] as demonstrated in Figure 3.51.

High-signal intensity due to FRE may be noted in the basal cisterns, shown in Figure 3.52, and the ventricles, shown in Figure 3.53, particularly on slices near the entry surface of the imaging volume.[36] Such increased signal can be potentially mistaken for an arachnoid cyst (Figure 3.52), a tumor (Figure 3.53), a lipoma (Figure 3.54), or even subacute hemorrhage (Figure 3.55), depending on the signal intensity. When high-signal intensity is observed in an entry slice, the study should be repeated, repositioning the patient so that the slice in question is in the middle of the imaging volume, as in Figure 3.54 and 3.55. When symmetric double echoes are acquired, even-echo rephasing can be observed, particularly near the entry surface, as in Figures 3.53 and 3.54.

While we have not documented diastolic pseudogating in the context of flowing CSF, it can certainly occur. Figure 3.56 demonstrates increased signal within the third ventricle on an image acquired during diastole. Images acquired later in the cardiac cycle during the more rapid, systolic flow period show the usual signal loss. Hence synchronization of the cardiac and MR cycles could result in a 'pseudomass' within the third ventricle in Figure 3.56.

References

1 BRADLEY WG, WALUCH V, Blood flow: magnetic resonance imaging, *Radiology* (1985) **154**:443–50.

2 CROOKS L, SHELDON P, KAUFMAN L et al, Quantification of obstructions in vessels by nuclear magnetic resonance, *IEEE Trans Nucl Sci* (1982) **NS-29**:1181.

3 CROOKS LE, MILLS CM, DAVIS PL et al, Visualization of cerebral and vascular abnormalities by NMR imaging. The effects of imaging parameters on contrast, *Radiology* (1982) **144**:843–52.

4 MILLS CM, BRANT-ZAWADZKI M, CROOKS LE et al, Nuclear magnetic resonance: principles of blood flow imaging, *AJNR* (1983) **4**:1161–6.

5   MORAN P, A flow velocity zeugmatographic interlace for NMR imaging in humans, *Magn Reson Imaging* (1982) **1**:197–203.

6   SINGER JR, CROOKS LE, Nuclear magnetic resonance blood flow measurements in the human brain, *Science* (1983) **221**:654–6.

7   GEORGE CR, JACOBS G, MACINTYRE WJ et al, Nuclear magnetic resonance whole-body imager operating at 3.5 kgauss, *Radiology* (1982) **143**:169–74.

8   SINGER JR, NMR diffusion and flow measurements and an introduction to spin phase graphing, *Phys E Sci Instrum* (1978) **11**:281–9.

9   AXEL L, Blood flow effects in magnetic resonance imaging, *AJR* (1984) **143**:1157–66.

10 BRADLEY WG, WALUCH V, LAI KS et al, The appearance of rapidly flowing blood on magnetic resonance images, *AJR* (1984) **143**:1167–74.

11 KAUFMAN L, CROOKS L, SHELDON P et al, The MR signal intensity patterns obtained from continuous and pulsatile flow models, *Radiology* (1984) **151**:421–8.

12 WALUCH V, BRADLEY WG, NMR even echo rephasing in slow laminar flow, *J Comput Assist Tomogr* (1984) **8**:594–8.

13 HAASE A, MATTHAEI D, HANICKE W et al, FLASH imaging: rapid NMR imaging using low flip-angle pulses, *J Magn Reson* (1986) **67**:258–6.

14 FRAHM J, HAASE A, MATTHAEI D, Rapid three-dimensional MR imaging using the FLASH technique, *J Comput Assist Tomogr* (1986) **10**:363–8.

15 VALK PE, HALE JD, CROOKS LE et al, MRI of blood flow: correlation of image appearance with spin-echo shift and signal intensity, *AJR* (1981) **146**:931–9.

16 VON SCHULTHESS GK, HIGGINS GB, Blood flow imaging with MR: spin-phase phenomena, *Radiology* (1985) **157**:687–95.

17 BIRD RB, STEWART WE, LIGHTFOOT EN, *Transport phenomena*, (Wiley: New York 1960) 153–8.

18 KUCHARCZYK W, KELLY WM, DAVIS DO et al, Intracranial lesions: flow-related enhancement of MR images using time-of-flight effects, *Radiology* (1986) **161**:767–72.

19 BRADLEY WG, OTTO RJ, KLEIN BD et al, Comparison of co-current and countercurrent flow-related enhancement, *Radiology* (1987) **165**(P):365.

20 CARR HY, PURCELL EM, Effects of diffusion on free precession in nuclear magnetic resonance experiments, *Phys Rev* (1954) **94**:630–8.

21 HAHN EL, Spin echoes, *Phys Rev* (1958) **80**:580–94.

22 HAHN EL, Detection of sea-water motion by nuclear precession, *J Geophys Res* (1960) **65**:776–7.

23 DEGENNES PG, Theory of spin echoes in a turbulent field, *Phys Lett* (1960) **29A**:20–1.

24 DEVILLE G, LANDESMAN A, Experiences d'echos de spins dans un liquide en ecoulement, *J Physique* (1971) **32**:67–72.

25 ALVAREZ O, HYMAN RA, Even echo MR rephasing in the diagnosis of giant intracranial aneurysm, *J Comput Assist Tomogr* (1986) **10**(4):699–701.

26 MCMURDO SK Jr, BRANT-ZAWADZKI M, BRADLEY WG et al, Fural sinus thrombosis: study using intermediate field strength MR imaging, *Radiology* (1986) **161**:83.

27 HRICAK H, AMPARO E, FISHER MR et al, Abdominal venous system: assessment using MR, *Radiology* (1985) **156**:415–22.

28 KUCHARCZYK W, BRANT-ZAWADZKI M, LEMME-PLAGHOS L et al, MR technology: effect of even-echo rephasing on calculated T_2 values and T_2 images, *Radiology* (1985) **157**:95–101.

29 MOTOMIYA M, KARINO T, Flow patterns in the human carotid artery bifurcation, *Stroke* (1984) **15**:50–6.

30 BRADLEY WG, KORTMAN KE, BURGOYNE B, Flowing cerebrospinal fluid in normal and hydrocephalic states: appearance on MR images, *Radiology* (1986) **159**:611–16.

31 SHERMAN JL, CITRIN CM, Magnetic resonance demonstration of normal CSF flow, *AJNR* (1986) **7**:3–6.

32 SHERMAN JL, CITRIN CM, BOWEN BJ et al, MR demonstration of altered cerebrospinal fluid flow by obstructive lesions, *AJNR* (1986) **7**:571–9.

33 SHERMAN JL, CITRIN CM, GANGAROSA RE et al, The MR appearance of CSF pulsations in the spinal canal, *AJNR* (1986) **7**:879–84.

34 CITRIN CM, SHERMAN JL, GANGAROSA RE et al, Physiology of the CSF flow-void sign: modification by cardiac gating, *AJNR* (1986) **7**: 1021–4.

35 BERGSTRAND G, BERGSTROM M, NORDELL B et al, Cardiac gated MR imaging of cerebrospinal fluid flow, *J Comput Assist Tomogr* (1985) **9**:1003–6.

36 ENZMANN DR, RUBIN JB, DELAPAZ R et al, Cerebrospinal fluid pulsation: benefits and pitfalls in MR imaging, *Radiology* (1986) **161**:773–8.

37 RUBIN JB, ENZMANN DR, Harmonic modulation of proton MR precessional phase by pulsatile motion: origin of spinal CSF flow phenomenon, *AJNR* (1987) **8**:307–18.

38 RUBIN JB, ENZMANN DR, Imaging of spinal CSF pulsation by 2DFT magnetic resonance: significance during clinical imaging, *AJNR* (1987) **8**:297–306.

39 DUBOULAY GH, Pulsatile movements in the CSF pathways, *Br J Radiol* (1966) **39**:255–62.

40 BERING EA Jr, Choroid plexus and arterial pulsations of cerebrospinal fluid: demonstration of the choroid plexuses as a cerebrospinal fluid pump, *Arch Neurol Psychiatr* (1955) **73**:165–72.

41 LANE B, KRICHEFF II, Cerebrospinal fluid pulsations at myelography: a videodensitometric study, *Radiology* (1974) **110**:579–87.

42 WHITE DN, WILSON KC, CURRY GR et al, The limitation of pulsatile flow through the aqueduct of Sylvius as a cause of hydrocephalus, *J Neurol Sci* (1979) **42**:11–51.

43 BRADLEY WG, FEINBERG D, OPENSHAW KL et al, Comparison of MR cardiac-gated aqueductal flow velocity measurement in healthy individuals and in patients with hydrocephalus, *Radiology* (1986) **194**:(P)161.

44 BRADLEY WG, WHITTEMORE AR, JINKINS JR et al, CSF flow patterns in hydrocephalus: correlation of clinical and phantom studies using MRI, *Radiology* (1987) **165**(P):78.

45 BURT TB, MR of CSF flow phenomenon mimicking basilar artery aneurysm, *AJNR* (1987) **8**(1):55–8.

46 Figures reproduced from Bradley WG, Blood and CSF flow phenomena in magnetic resonance imaging. In Stark DD, Bradley WG, eds. *Magnetic resonance imaging*. (Mosby and Co: St Louis 1988) Chapter 7.

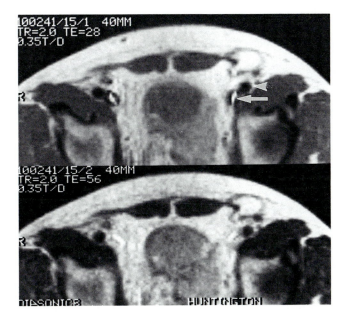

Figure 3.1

Flow-related enhancement and high-velocity signal loss in a patient with carcinoma of the bladder. Increased signal in slowly flowing femoral veins (arrow) is due to unsaturated protons entering section. Absence of signal from the adjacent femoral arteries (arrowhead) reflects loss of signal due to turbulence, dephasing, and time-of-flight losses (SE 2000/28).[1]

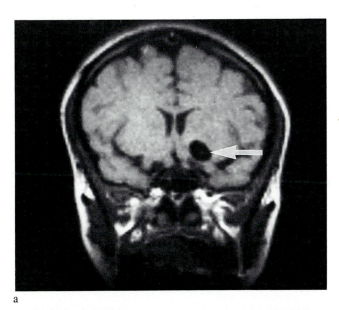

a

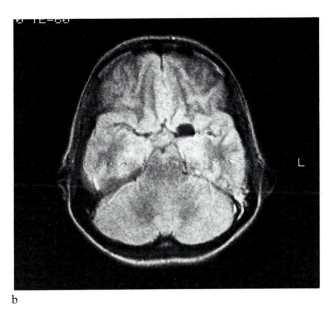

b

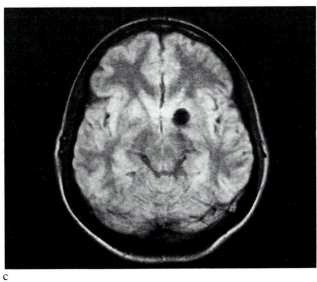

c

Figure 3.2

Left middle cerebral artery aneurysm. Flow void is found within 2 cm (arrow) due to turbulence, dephasing, and time-of-flight losses.
(**a**) Coronal section (SE 500/40).
(**b**) Axial section through base of aneurysm (SE 2000/60).
(**c**) Higher axial section through dome (SE 2000/30).[46]

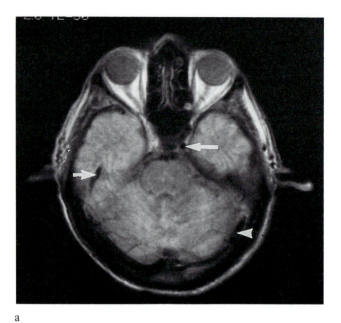 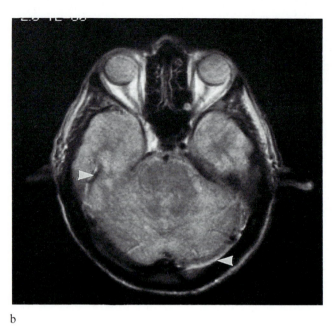

a   b

Figure 3.3

Arterial flow void. Normal
signal loss due to rapid arterial
flow in patent left carotid artery
(arrow). (Thrombosed right
carotid artery does not have
flow void.) Note also first echo
dephasing (arrowheads) and
even echo rephasing in veins
and left transverse sinus. (**a**) SE
2000/30. (**b**) SE 2000/60.

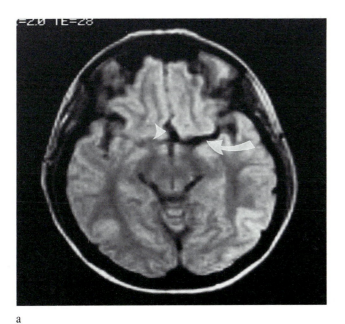

a

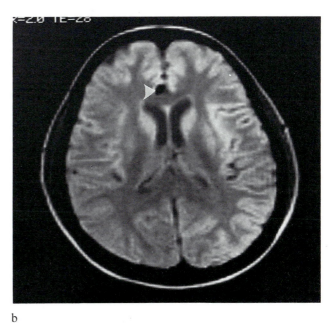

b

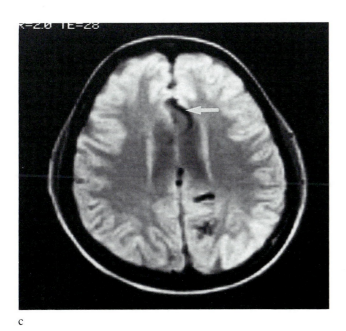

c

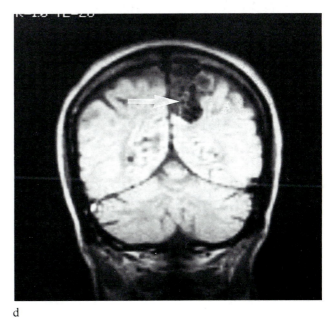

d

Figure 3.4

Arteriovenous malformation (AVM). Signal loss is noted in AVM due to time-of-flight losses, turbulence, and dephasing (SE 2000/28). (a) Axial section through Circle of Willis showing enlarged left middle cerebral (curved arrow) and anterior cerebral (arrowhead) arteries supplying AVM (SE 2000/28). (b) Axial section through lateral ventricles showing enlarged anterior cerebral artery (arrowhead) (SE 2000/28). (c) Axial section through lateral ventricular roofs showing enlarged anterior cerebral artery (arrow) and other abnormal vessels comprising AVM (SE 2000/28). (d) Coronal section demonstrating flow void associated with AVM (arrow) (SE 1000/28).

Time =   t   t + ½ TE
       (90° pulse ▨)   (180° pulse ▧)

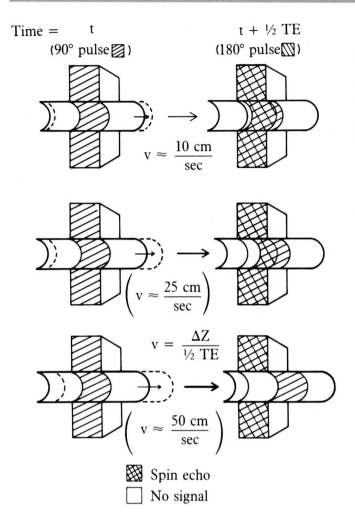

$$v \approx \frac{10 \text{ cm}}{\text{sec}}$$

$$\left(v \approx \frac{25 \text{ cm}}{\text{sec}} \right)$$

$$v = \frac{\Delta Z}{½ \text{ TE}}$$

$$\left(v \approx \frac{50 \text{ cm}}{\text{sec}} \right)$$

▨ Spin echo
▢ No signal

Figure 3.5

High-velocity (time-of-flight) signal loss. Protons must acquire both a 90° pulse and a 180° pulse to emit spin echo (crosshatch). Protons that acquire a 90° pulse and then leave section prior to acquiring 180° pulse emit no signal. Protons flowing into the section following selective 90° pulse also emit no signal.[1]

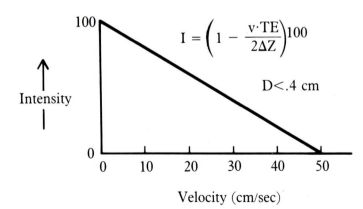

$$I = \left(1 - \frac{v \cdot TE}{2 \Delta Z} \right) 100$$

D < .4 cm

Intensity

Velocity (cm/sec)

Figure 3.6

High-velocity signal loss. Predicted intraluminal intensity (*I*) is plotted as function of velocity *v* for tubes less than 0.4 cm in diameter (*D*). This illustrates linear relationship predicted between signal intensity and velocity, slice thickness, and echo-delay time TE (ignoring dephasing effects). (This curve is based on a TE of 28 msec and a slice thickness of 7 mm.)[10]

Time =   t   t. + TR

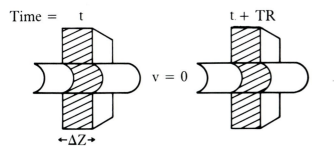

$$v = 0$$

←ΔZ→

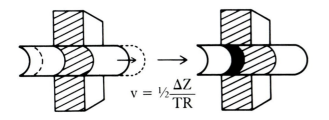

$$v = \tfrac{1}{2}\frac{\Delta Z}{TR}$$

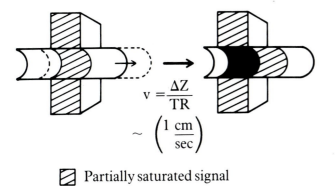

$$v = \frac{\Delta Z}{TR}$$

$$\sim \left(1\,\frac{cm}{sec}\right)$$

▨ Partially saturated signal
■ Unsaturated (maximum) signal

Figure 3.7

Flow-related enhancement. Under conditions of slow flow, unsaturated protons enter section with full magnetization and emit stronger signal than protons in adjacent, partially saturated, stationary tissue. Maximum effect occurs when velocity equals section thickness divided by TR.[1]

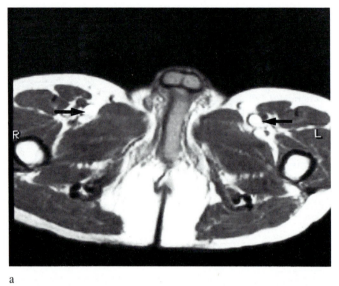

a

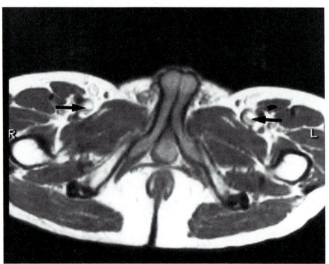

b

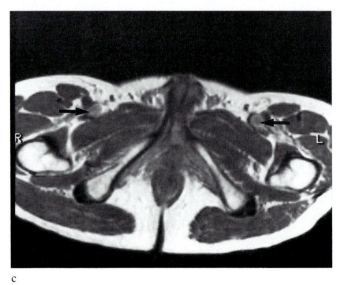

c

Figure 3.8

Flow-related enhancement. The first three slices encountered by inflowing venous blood in the femoral veins (arrows) are shown in **a-c**. Note the progressive decrease in signal intensity on deeper slices (SE 1000/30).[46]

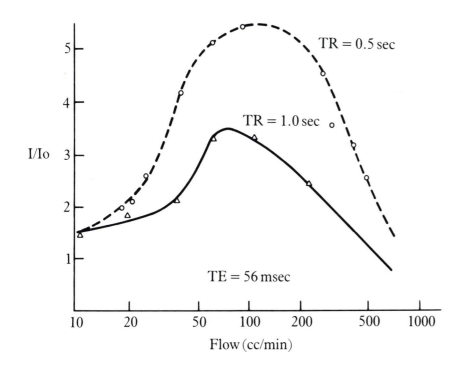

Figure 3.9

Flow-related enhancement and high-velocity signal loss in flow phantom. Intraluminal signal I is initially increased (relative to stationary signal I_0) due to unsaturated protons entering section. Effect is best seen at low velocity and is accentuated at short TR. Signal is lost as velocity is increased due to offsetting time-of-flight losses and dephasing.[1]

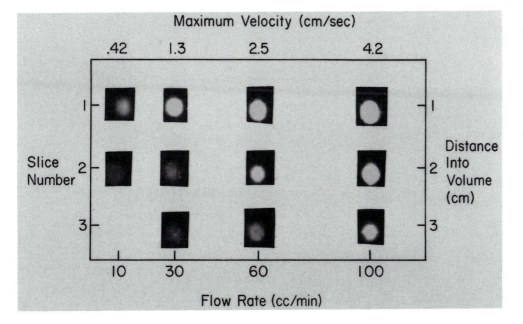

Figure 3.10

Multislice flow-related enhancement. Signal intensities demonstrated as function of volumetric flow rate, calculated maximum velocity, and distance into volume. Highest intensity is seen on entry slice (number 1) with decreasing signal (and decreasing cross-sectional area) noted on deeper slices (SE 500/28).[10]

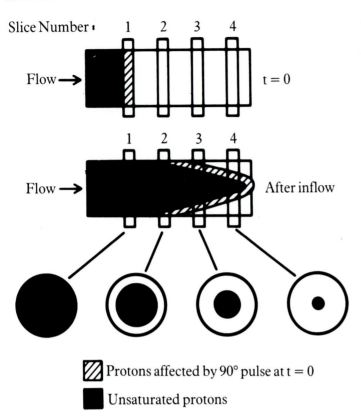

Slice Number   1   2   3   4

Flow →   t = 0

Flow →   After inflow

⧄ Protons affected by 90° pulse at t = 0

■ Unsaturated protons

Figure 3.11

Multislice flow-related enhancement. Parabolic laminar flow profile projects several slices into imaging volume. In three dimensions the high-signal inflowing protons form a cone. Cross-sections of laminar profile result in decreasing cross-sectional area for central zone of high-intensity, unsaturated protons deeper in imaging volume.[10]

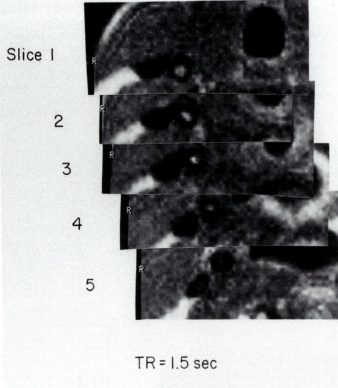

Slice I

2

3

4

5

TR = 1.5 sec

TE = 28 msec

Figure 3.12

Multislice flow-related enhancement in right common carotid artery (SE 1500/28, non-gated). Decreasing intraluminal signal is noted for slices deeper in imaging volume.[10]

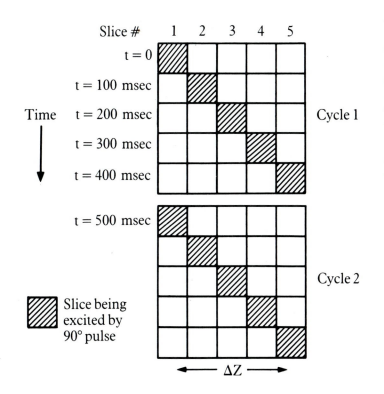

Time

t = 0
t = 100 msec
t = 200 msec
t = 300 msec
t = 400 msec

Cycle 1

t = 500 msec

Cycle 2

Slice being excited by 90° pulse

ΔZ

Figure 3.13

Slice excitation wave (SEW). Cyclic excitation of consecutive slices is indicated by crosshatching on two 500 msec cycles over two repetition periods. For a slice thickness of 1 cm, the SEW in this example moves at a velocity of 1 cm/100 msec or 10 cm/sec.[46]

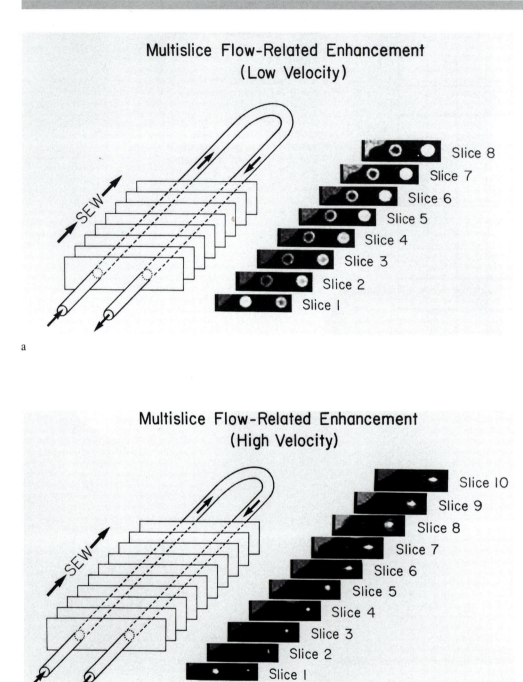

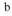

Figure 3.14

Comparison of co-current and
countercurrent flow-related
enhancement. (**a**) At low
velocity (1 cm/sec), note deeper
penetration into imaging
volume of unsaturated protons
for flow countercurrent to slice
excitation wave (SEW). (**b**) At
high velocity (10 cm/sec), high
signal is only noted in the
center of the stream.
(Dephasing effects lead to loss
of signal in the region of
greatest shear, that is, steepest
velocity gradient, towards the
periphery.)[46]

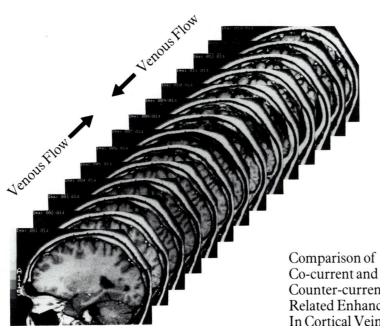

Comparison of
Co-current and
Counter-current Flow
Related Enhancement
In Cortical Veins

Figure 3.15

Clinical comparison of co-current and countercurrent flow-related enhancement (FRE). Cortical veins drain centrally into superior sagittal sinus from both sides of head. Deeper penetration of FRE is noted for flow countercurrent to SEW compared to co-current flow.[46]

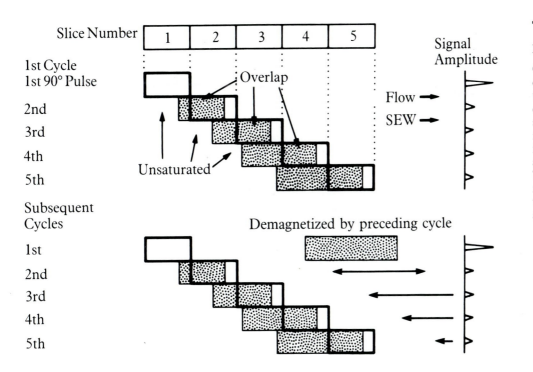

Figure 3.16

Co-current flow-related enhancement. When flow is in the same direction as the slice excitation wave (SEW), protons saturated or depolarized recently (time interval TR/n) flow into next slice to be excited and thus return a weak signal. The percentage of this 'overlap' zone approaches 100 as the velocity of the blood approaches that of the SEW.

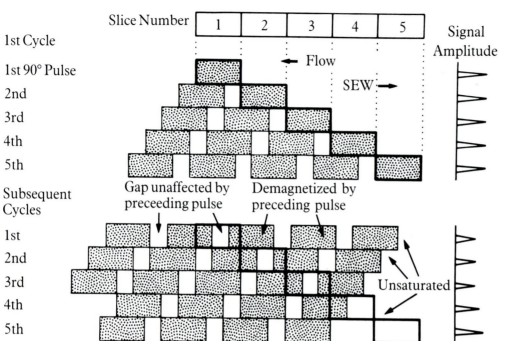

Slice Number

1st Cycle

1st 90° Pulse

2nd

3rd

4th

5th

← Flow

SEW →

Signal
Amplitude

Subsequent
Cycles

1st

2nd

3rd

4th

5th

Gap unaffected by
preceeding pulse

Demagnetized by
preceeding pulse

Unsaturated

Figure 3.17

Countercurrent flow-related
enhancement. When flow is
countercurrent to the slice
excitation wave (SEW),
protons which have had at least time
2TR to recover flow into the
slice to be excited. The size of
this 'gap' approaches that of the
slice as the velocity approaches
that of the SEW. The stronger
signal from the protons flowing
countercurrent (versus co-
current) to the SEW is due to
the longer time available for
longitudinal recovery.

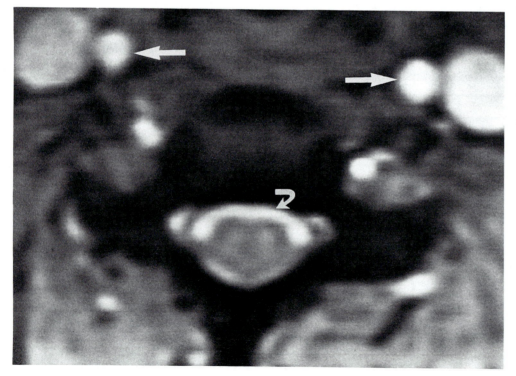

Figure 3.18

Flow-related enhancement in
GRASS imaging. Note high
signal from inflowing blood
(straight arrows) and CSF
(curved arrow) due to single
(entry) slice and short TR.

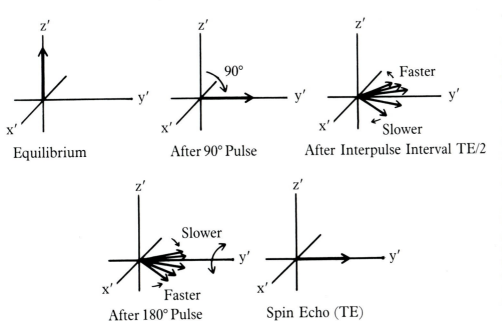

Figure 3.19

Carr Purcell Meiboom Gill (CPMG) spin echo. In rotating reference frame, magnetization (solid arrow) is rotated into x'y'-plane by 90° radiofrequency (RF) pulse. Dephasing causes flaring of the magnetization as some protons precess faster and some slower than average (due to relatively stronger and weaker local magnetic fields). After interpulse interval TE/2, 180° pulse is applied that causes rotation about y'-axis and flared magnetization vectors begin to rephase. At TE rephasing is complete and coherent spin echo is emitted.[1]

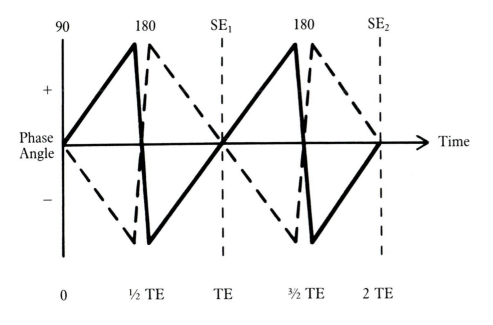

Figure 3.20

Spin-phase graph. Phase is either lost or gained relative to average precessional frequency by protons in weaker and stronger parts of the magnetic field. Sign of phase is reversed by each 180° pulse, at 1/2TE and 3/2TE. Coherence is re-established at the time of each spin echo (SE$_1$ and SE$_2$).[1]

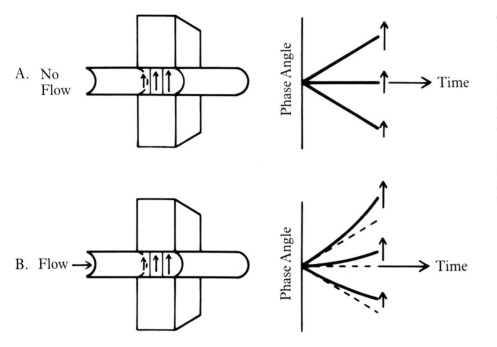

Figure 3.21

Accelerated phase gain due to flow into an increasing magnetic field. When a gradient is present without flow (above), rephasing occurs as it would in any other non-uniform magnetic field. When blood flows into an increasing magnetic field (below), phase is gained more rapidly (that is, quadratically in time).[1]

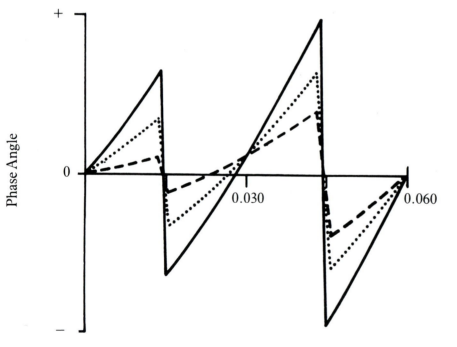

Figure 3.22

Computer simulation of plug flow. Phase angle of isochromats in stronger half of field is plotted as a function of time (spin echoes occur at 0.030 and 0.060 sec). Positive phase angle at time of first spin echo is due to quadratic phase gain. Complete rephasing occurs for both echoes.[1]

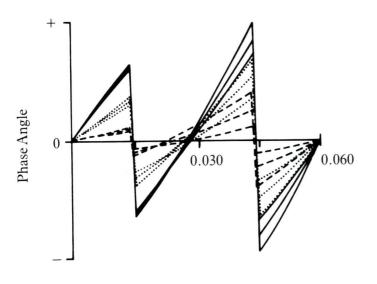

Time in Seconds

Figure 3.23

Computer simulation of laminar flow. Phase angles of isochromats at different positions in voxel field are plotted as a function of time with spin echoes occurring at 0.030 and 0.060 sec. Three groups of three curves each are shown. Within each group the isochromats that gain phase most rapidly are in the center of the stream at the highest velocity. The group with solid lines is at the leading edge of the voxel where the magnetic field is strongest, while the dashed line corresponds to spins on the lagging edge of the voxel where the field is weaker.[1]

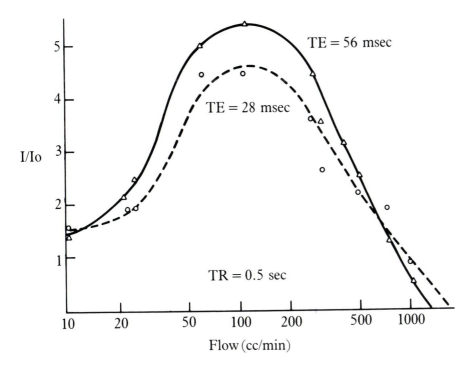

Flow (cc/min)

Figure 3.24

Even-echo rephasing in flow phantom. Second echo is more intense than the first in slow laminar flow. This is due to rephasing effects that arise from constant flow into the linear gradient. (I = intraluminal signal; I_0 = stationary signal.)[1]

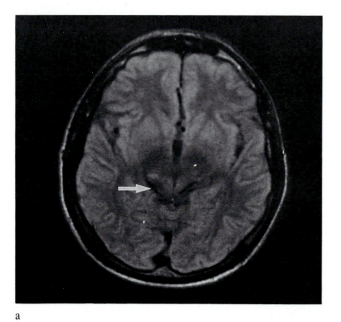

a

Figure 3.25

Even-echo rephasing in the
basal veins of Rosenthal.
(**a**) First-echo dephasing
produces signal void (arrow) on
SE 2000/30 image. (**b**) Even-
echo rephasing (arrow)
produces strong signal on
second echo (SE 2000/60).

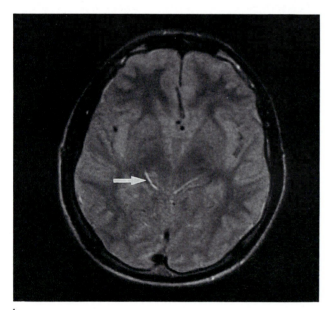

b

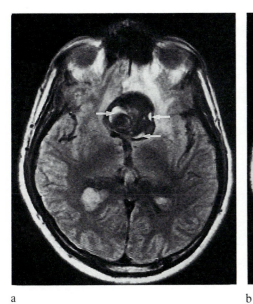 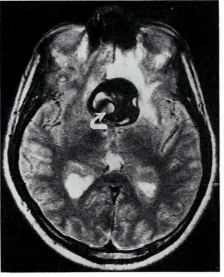 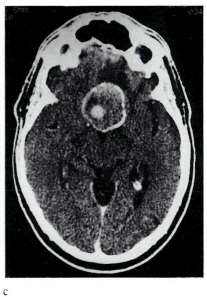

a   b   c

Figure 3.26

Giant intracranial aneurysm.
(**a**) First-echo image shows
several areas of high signal due
to extracellular methemoglobin
in mural thrombus (arrows)
(SE 2000/30). (**b**) On second-
echo image (SE 2000/60), signal
increase is only seen in patent
lumen (curved arrow),
reflecting even-echo rephasing.
(**c**) Position of patent lumen
confirmed on contrast-
enhanced CT.[46]

Figure 3.27

Even-echo rephasing in slow
arterial flow. (**a**) First-echo
image demonstrates apparently
normal flow void (arrow) in the
right internal carotid artery (SE
2000/30). (**b**) Second-echo
image demonstrates even-echo
rephasing (arrow), suggesting
slow flow (SE 2000/60). Duplex
doppler examination (not
shown) confirmed the presence
of a high-grade stenosis and
slow flow.

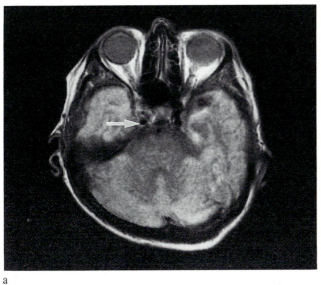 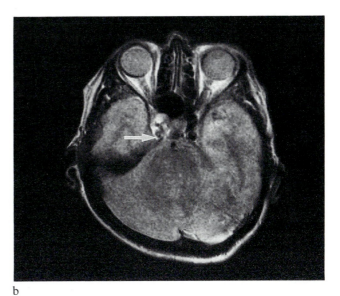

a   b

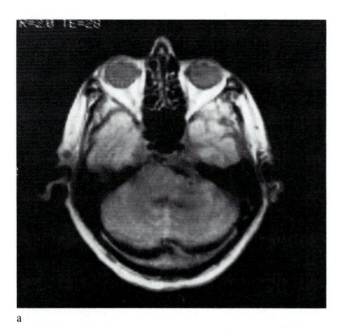

a

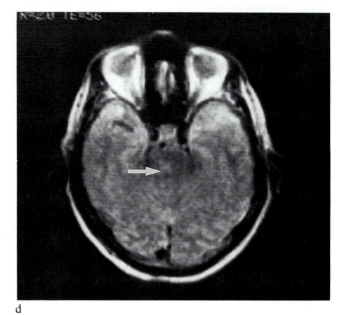

b

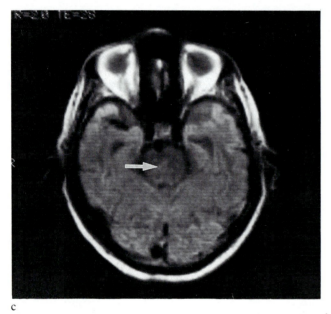

c

d

Figure 3.28

Even-echo rephasing in slow
arterial flow. (**a**) First-echo
image at the level of the pons
(SE 2000/28). (**b**) Second echo
image demonstrates even-echo
rephasing in the basilar artery
(arrow) suggesting slow flow
(SE 2000/56). (**c–d**) Higher
section through pontine
isthmus demonstrates
brainstem infarct (arrow) (SE
2000/28 and 56). Subsequent
angiogram (not shown)
demonstrated high-grade
stenosis of the vertebral arterial
origins.

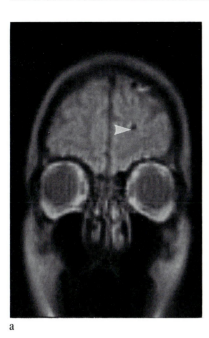
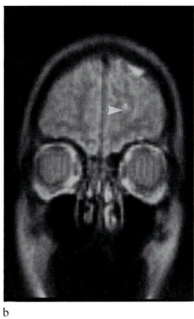
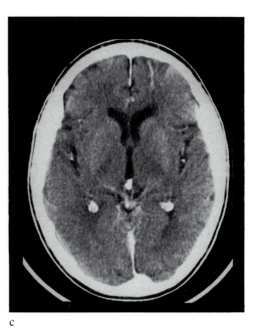

a   b   c

Figure 3.29

Venous angioma. (**a**) First-echo image shows flow void (arrowhead) in location atypical for normal vein (SE 2000/28). (**b**) Second-echo image shows even-echo rephasing (arrowhead) suggesting slow flow in an abnormal medullary vein or venous angioma (SE 2000/56). (**c**) Contrast-enhanced CT confirms presence of vascular abnormality.

Figure 3.30

Dural sinus thrombosis and patency. (**a–b**) First- and second-echo images (SE 2000/28 and 56) in patient with malignant external otitis and documented sigmoid sinus thrombosis (arrow). No even-echo rephasing is seen. (**c–d**) SE 2000/28 and 56 acquired in another patient with malignant external otitis but in whom the sigmoid sinus demonstrates even-echo rephasing (arrow), indicating patency.[46]

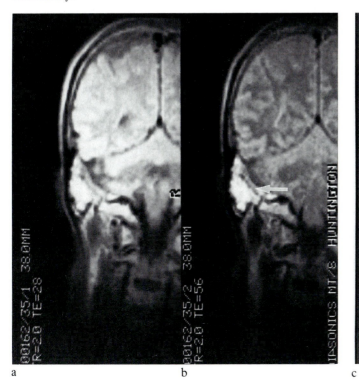

a   b

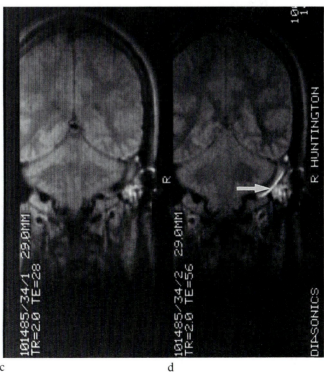

c   d

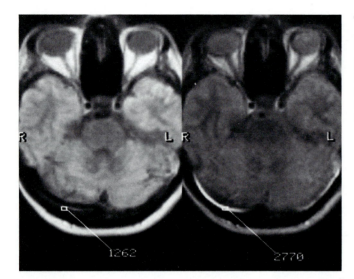

Figure 3.31

Even-echo rephasing. Documentation of absolute signal increase in transverse sinus indicated by computer cursor (SE 2000/28 and 56).

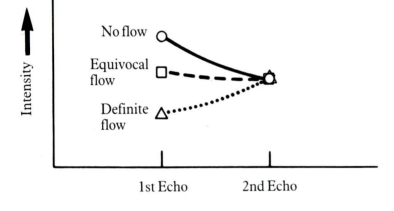

Figure 3.32

Change in measured T_2 relaxation time as a function of flow. When the intensity of the second echo is greater than the first, an apparently negative T_2 relaxation time results due to flow (first-echo dephasing and even-echo rephasing). When very slow flow is present, the T_2 will appear to be prolonged (rather than negative) and flow cannot be said unequivocally to be present.[46]

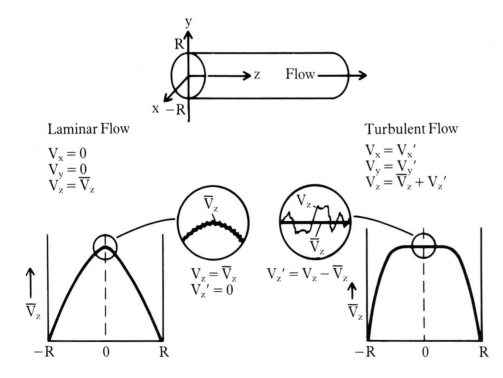

Figure 3.33

Comparison of laminar and turbulent flow. For flow in tube of radius R in axial (z) direction, velocity components in non-axial direction (v_x and v_y) are zero during laminar flow. Actual velocity in axial direction (v_z) is equal to time-smoothed mean ($\bar{v}_z$). In turbulent flow, fluctuating velocity components are present (indicated by superscript primes, for example, v_x').[10]

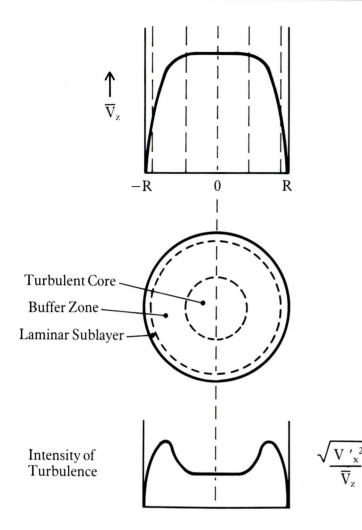

Figure 3.34

Transitional flow in tube of radius R. Top, lateral view: flattened flow profile of time-smooth mean velocity ($\bar{v}_z$) is shown. Middle, axial view: turbulent core, buffer zone, and laminar sublayer are demonstrated. Bottom, lateral projection: intensity of turbulence is plotted as function of radial position. Magnitude of fluctuating velocity component, $v_x'^2/\bar{v}_z$ (that is, intensity of turbulence), is greatest in transitional (buffer) zone.[10]

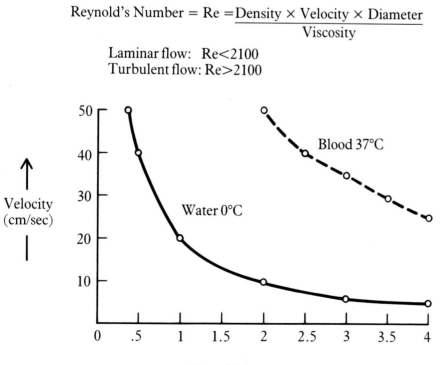

$$\text{Reynold's Number} = \text{Re} = \frac{\text{Density} \times \text{Velocity} \times \text{Diameter}}{\text{Viscosity}}$$

Laminar flow: Re<2100
Turbulent flow: Re>2100

Figure 3.35

Reynold's relationship. Using the Reynold's number, the onset of turbulence can be predicted as a function of velocity, vascular diameter, density, and viscosity. Turbulence occurs sooner at higher velocity, larger vascular diameter, and lower viscosity (for example, water versus blood).

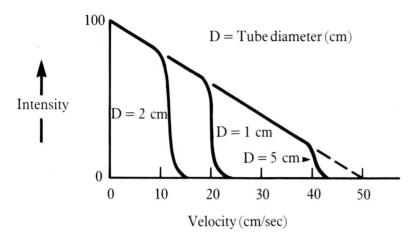

Figure 3.36

Effect of turbulence on high-velocity signal loss. In addition to time-of-flight losses shown by limiting diagonal curve, there is signal loss due to turbulence. Notice that turbulence (and therefore signal loss) occurs at lower velocities for larger diameter vessels while laminar flow is maintained at higher velocities for smaller diameter vessels.[46]

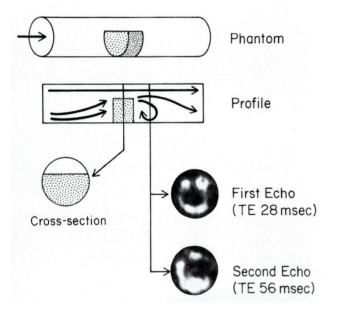

Figure 3.37

Even-echo rephasing downstream from obstruction in turbulent flow. Plastic (Lucite) phantom is shown schematically, as are flow patterns in lateral projection. Actual axial MR images 1 cm downstream from obstruction are shown, demonstrating even-echo rephasing in eddy. TR = 500 msec.[10]

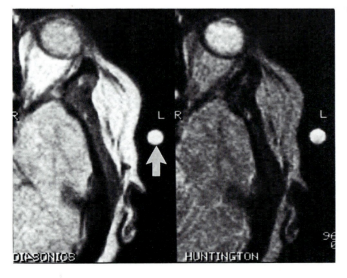

Figure 3.38

Intensity of stagnant blood. Intensity of unclotted blood within heparinized tube (arrow) is demonstrated on SE 3000/40 and 80 images. The high-signal intensity reflects the relatively long T_2 (approximately 150 msec) of unclotted blood.[46]

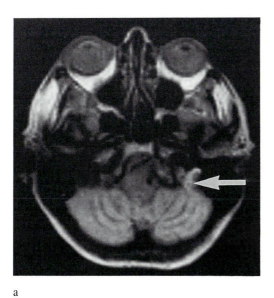

a

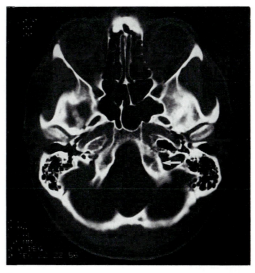

b

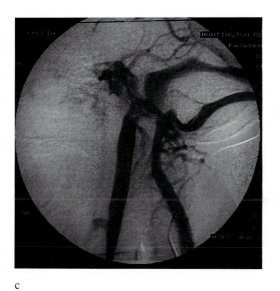

c

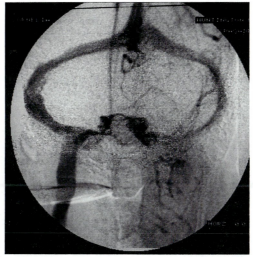

d

Figure 3.39

Positional slowing of drainage through left jugular vein.
(a) High-signal intensity (arrow) noted within left jugular bulb in first-echo image (SE 2000/28) on non-entry slice. In view of the clinical presentation (left-sided tinnitis), glomus jugulare tumor was suspected. (b) CT with bone windows demonstrates enlarged jugular bulb with normal cortication (arrow) and no evidence of bone destruction to suggest a glomus tumor. (c) Off-lateral angiogram demonstrates high-riding left jugular bulb.
(d) Slight flexing of neck for Townes view results in marked slowing of drainage through the left jugular system. The patient was in a similar position at the time of MR imaging. The high-signal intensity noted in (a) is thus attributed to positional slowing of venous drainage on the left side.

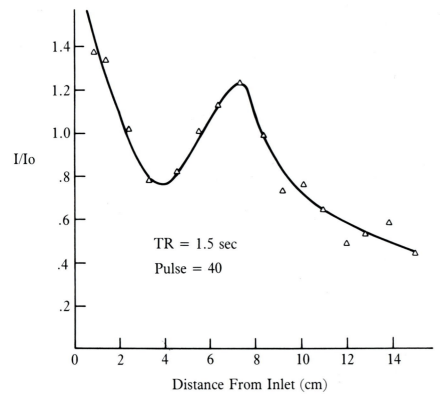

I/Io

TR = 1.5 sec

Pulse = 40

Distance From Inlet (cm)

Figure 3.40

Intensity profile in gated pulsatile flow (flow phantom). Ratio of flowing to stationary water (I/I_0) is plotted as a function of distance from the entry surface during a 15-slice acquisition. Increased intensity near the inlet is due to flow-related enhancement. Central peak is due to acquisition during slower diastolic flow.[1]

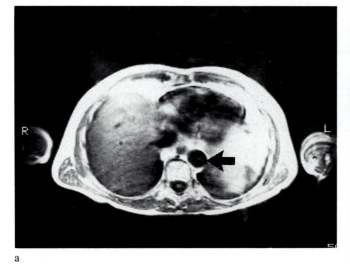

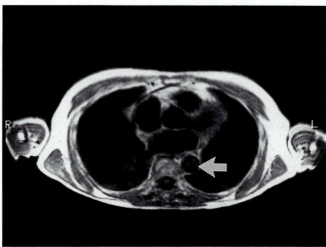

a   b

Figure 3.41

Diastolic pseudogating. In patient with heart rate of 60 and MR repetition time TR of 1.0 sec, chance synchronization of the cardiac and MR cycles results in relatively increased signal intensity in the descending aorta (arrow) during relatively slow flow. (**a**) Systole. (**b**) Diastole delay after R wave noted for each section.[46]

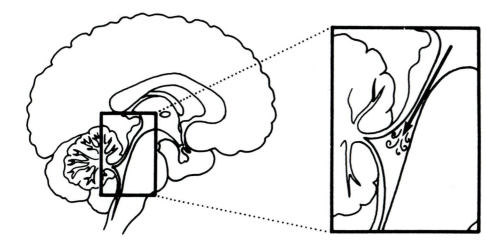

Figure 3.42

CSF flow through aqueduct and upper fourth ventricle. The velocity of CSF pulsating through the aqueduct is higher than elsewhere in the ventricular system due to the smaller cross-sectional area. As the CSF stream expands into the upper fourth ventricle, turbulence occurs due to a venturi effect.[46]

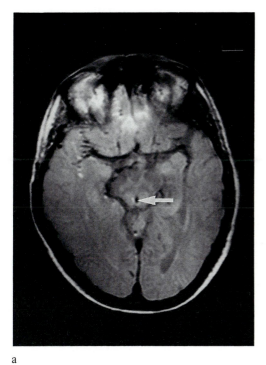

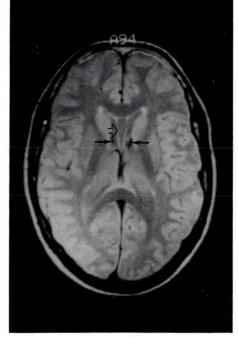

a   b

Figure 3.43

Normal CSF flow voids.
(a) Signal loss due to normal to-and-fro motion of CSF through aqueduct (arrow) (SE 2000/30).
(b) CSF flow voids (arrows) noted at foramen of Monro in another patient with incidental cavum septum pellucidum (open arrow).

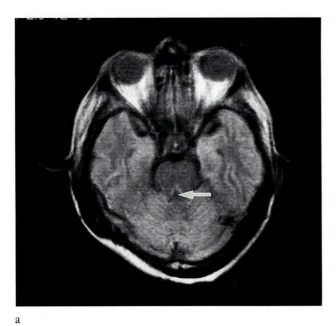

a

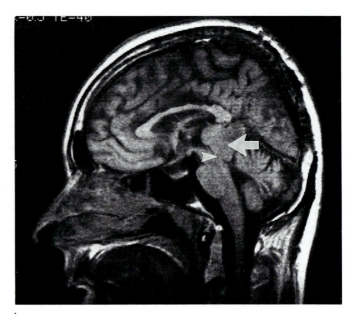

b

Figure 3.44

Aqueductal stenosis due to
tectal tumor. (**a**) Absent
aqueductal flow void (arrow)
(SE 2000/30). (**b**) Tectal tumor
(arrow) compresses aqueduct
(arrowhead), slowing CSF flow
(SE 500/40).

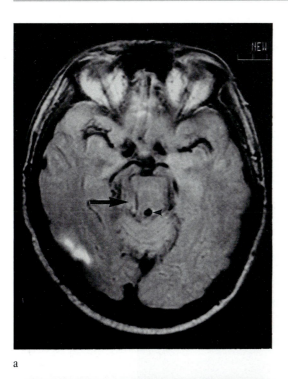

a

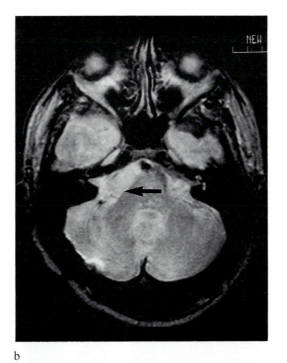

b

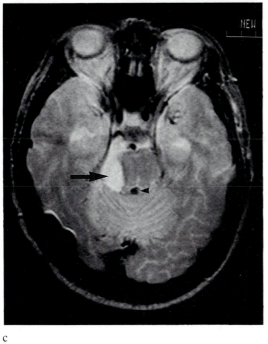

c

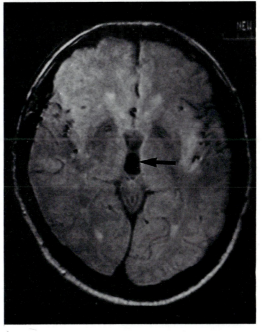

d

Figure 3.45

Hyperdynamic CSF flow state due to obstructed extraventricular pathways. (**a**) Axial section through posterior fossa demonstrating meningioma in right cerebellopontine angle cistern (arrow) (SE 2500/30). (**b**) Axial section showing meningioma (arrow) in right perimesencephalic cistern, displacing pontine isthmus and obstructing extraventricular flow of CSF. Note marked signal void in aqueduct (arrowhead) due to secondary increase in intraventricular CSF flow (SE 2500/30). (**c**) Second echo through same level as (**b**) (SE 2500/60). (**d**) CSF flow void in third ventricle (SE 2500/30).

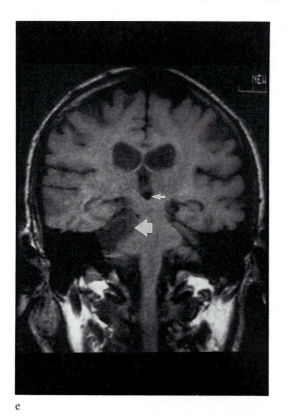

e

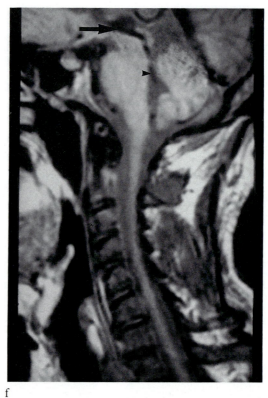

f

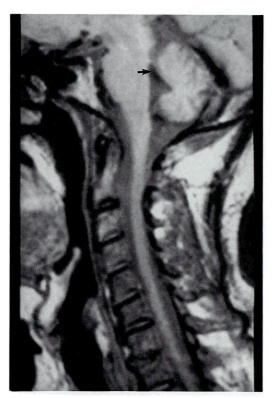

g

Figure 3.45 *continued*

(**e**) Coronal section
demonstrating transtentorial
meningioma (arrow) and CSF
flow void in third ventricle
(arrowhead) (SE 600/20).
(**f–g**) Sagittal sections
demonstrating CSF flow void in
third (arrow) and fourth
(arrowhead) ventricles (SE 600/20).

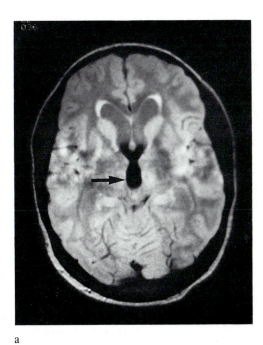

a

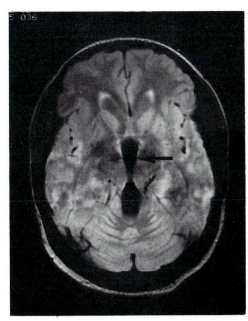

b

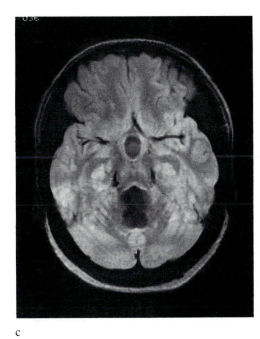

c

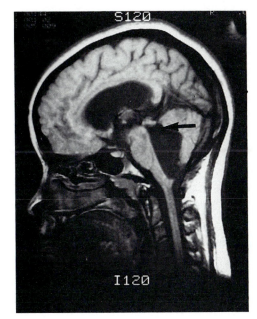

d

Figure 3.46

Hyperdynamic CSF flow in chronic communicating hydrocephalus. (**a**) Axial section through foramen of Monro demonstrating marked flow void (arrow) (SE 2500/30). (**b**) Axial section through aqueduct and upper fourth ventricle (SE 2500/30). (**c**) Axial section through fourth ventricle (SE 2500/30). (**d**) Midline sagittal section showing CSF flow void (arrow).[46]

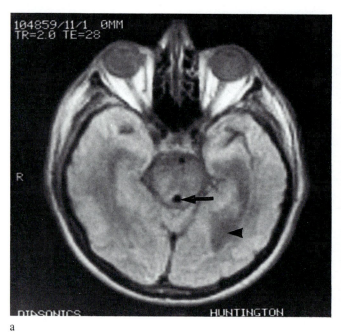
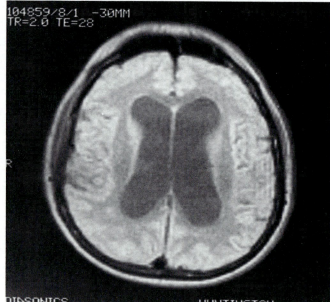

a   b

Figure 3.47

Hyperdynamic CSF flow in
patient with clinical NPH.
Greater signal loss is noted in
aqueduct (arrow) than in lateral
ventricles (arrowhead) because
of hyperdynamic flow of CSF.
(**a**) Section through aqueduct
(SE 2000/28). (**b**) Section
through lateral ventricles.[30]

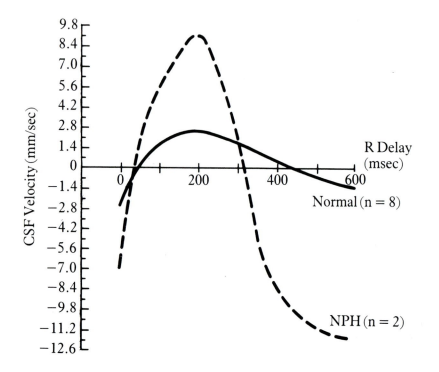

Figure 3.48

Aqueductal CSF velocity. CSF
velocity through the aqueduct
is measured as a function of the
cardiac cycle using the 'velocity
density imaging' technique.
Average CSF velocity is
demonstrated in eight normal
volunteers. In two patients with
untreated normal pressure
hydrocephalus (NPH), the CSF
velocities are seen to be six to
eight times normal. (Although
relative velocities should be
accurate, absolute velocities
may be low due to errors from
higher-order motion terms,
such as acceleration.)[46]

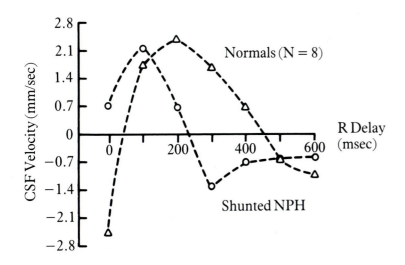

Figure 3.49

CSF velocity profile in treated normal pressure hydrocephalus (NPH). Following successful shunting, CSF velocity has returned to normal, although the peaks occur earlier than in normals.

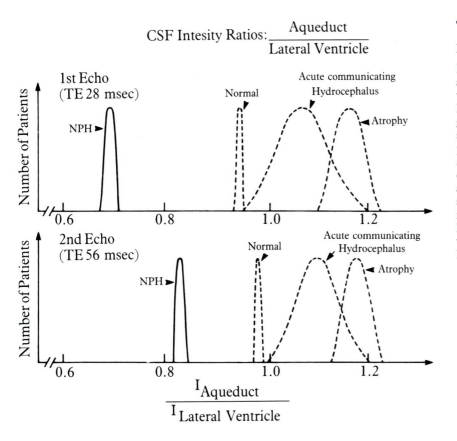

Figure 3.50

Ratio of CSF intensity in aqueduct compared to lateral ventricles in healthy and hydrocephalic patients. The greatest relative aqueductal signal loss is noted in normal pressure hydrocephalus (NPH) and the least is noted in acute communicating hydrocephalus and atrophy. While aqueductal signal loss can also be observed in healthy individuals, this is less marked than in patients with chronic communicating hydrocephalus (NPH).[30]

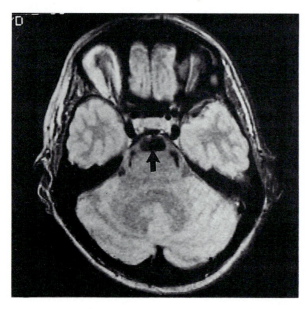

a

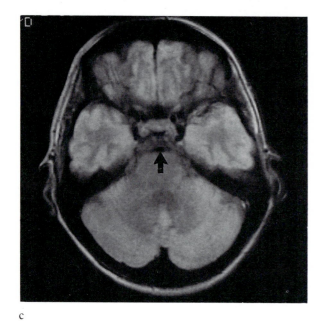

b

c

Figure 3.51

Pseudoaneurysm of the basilar artery. (**a**) 2.5 mm thick SE 2000/50 image of the basilar artery demonstrating prominent flow void suggesting aneurysm (arrow). (**b**) Even-echo rephasing on second-echo image (SE 2000/100) partially restores signal loss. (**c**) 1 cm thick section (SE 2000/30) at the same level demonstrates normal diameter basilar artery (arrow). The signal loss in (**a**) reflects dephasing radial due to motion of the CSF around the pulsating basilar artery.[46] The dephasing is increased with the use of stronger gradients (for thinner slices) and longer echo delay times TE.

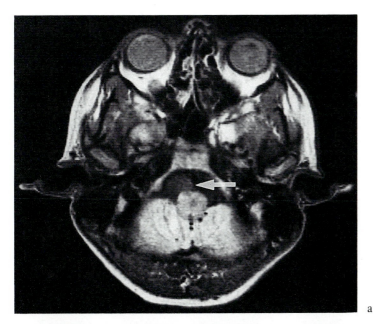

a

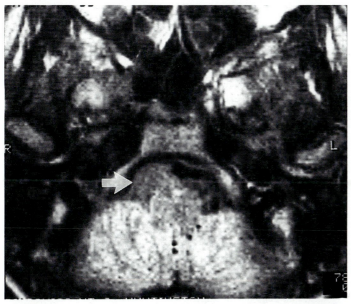

b

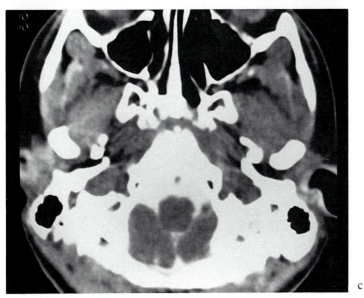

c

Figure 3.52

Pseudomass in (**a**) First-echo image (SE 2000/40) demonstrates well marginated intermediate intensity 'mass' in the right medullary cistern which was suspected of being an arachnoid cyst. (**b**) On the enlarged second-echo image (SE 2000/80), the 'mass' has CSF intensity (arrow). The vertebral arteries are both in the left of midline. (**c**) Metrizamide CT study is normal. The high-signal intensity in the right medullary cistern thus represents flow-related enhancement due to the to-and-fro motion of CSF through the foramen magnum. The dephasing due to the radial motion of CSF surrounding the vertebral arteries in the left medullary cistern leads to local signal loss.[46]

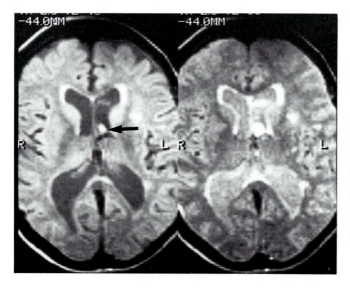

Figure 3.53

Pseudomass near the foramen of Monro. High-signal CSF near the foramen of Monro (arrow) reflects retrograde CSF flow entering the first slice of the imaging volume. This could be potentially mistaken for colloid cyst or subependymoma (SE 2000/40). Second-echo image (SE 2000/80) demonstrates increase in apparent size and intensity of lesion due to even-echo rephasing.

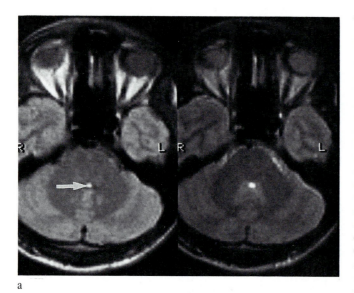

a

b

Figure 3.54

Pseudomass in fourth ventricle. (**a**) High-signal intensity (arrow) in fourth ventricle could be potentially mistaken for lipoma, dermoid, or other fatty mass. Since this is the lowest slice of the multislice imaging volume, this represents flow-related enhancement due to inflowing CSF (SE 2000/40). Even-echo rephasing further increases intensity of mass on second-echo image (SE 2000/80). (**b**) Comparable section through another acquisition several slices in from the entry surface shows no evidence of high-signal intensity in fourth ventricle, confirming suspicion of flow artifact (SE 2000/40 and 80).[46]

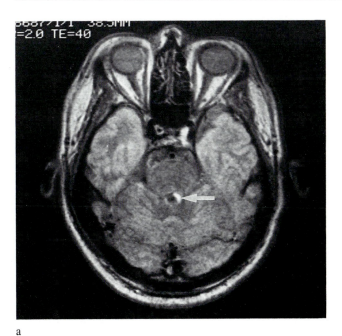

a

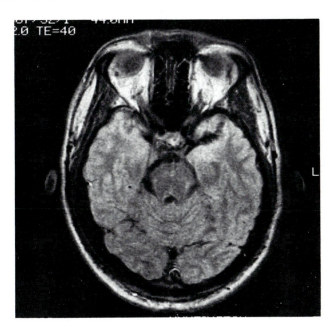

b

Figure 3.55

Pseudo-subacute hemorrhage due to flow-related enhancement. (**a**) High-signal intensity noted in left periaqueductal region (arrow). In this patient with acute onset of brainstem symptoms, this was originally suspected to be for subacute hemorrhage (SE 2000/40). (**b**) On repeat section through same level as (**a**) (now several slices in from entry surface), there is no evidence of high-signal intensity. The high signal noted in (**a**) (the lowest slice in the imaging volume) represents flow-related enhancement due to the pulsatile motion of CSF back and forth through the aqueduct.

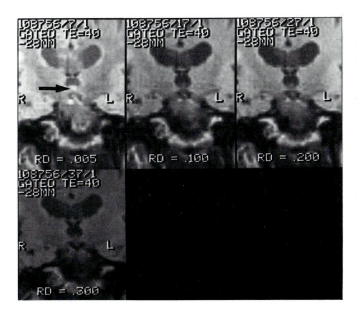

Figure 3.56

Diastolic pseudogating as a potential cause of increased CSF signal intensity. Four gated images are shown with variable delay from the R wave of the EKG ('RD' is R delay in seconds). Note increased signal in third ventricle (arrow) during mechanical diastole which is not seen (arrow) in systole. Similar signal can be seen when there is chance synchronization of cardiac and MR cycles, that is, diastolic 'pseudogating'.[46]

4
Tumors

Graeme Bydder

Introduction

Magnetic resonance imaging (MRI) of central nervous system tumors has evolved rapidly since the first publication on the subject in 1980.[1] In the initial phases of MRI, marked changes were observed in tumors as a consequence of their differences in T_1 and T_2 compared with brain, but the spatial resolution of MRI was limited. As a result, the principal area of advantage for MRI was in the posterior fossa where the quality of CT images was frequently degraded by the presence of artifact from bone.[2,3] With improvements in technology MRI then began to compete with X-ray computed tomography (CT) in the supratentorial compartment. The development of gadolinium-DTPA (Gd-DTPA) for clinical use in 1983 overcame the principal disadvantage of MRI.[4-6] With this agent in use, meningiomas were much better demonstrated and it became much easier to distinguish macroscopic tumor from edema. In the years that have followed, the quality of MR images has continued to improve and new techniques have been introduced to increase the sensitivity of MRI to associated hemorrhage and improve the speed of the examination. Three-dimensional techniques have also been developed and provide a method for visualizing tumors in any plane.

In this chapter a classification of tumors is described, followed by an outline of the typical MRI features of tumors. Individual tumor types are then discussed.

Tumor classification

According to the need, a variety of tumor classifications can be used. These can be based on clinical or radiological criteria, as well as pathological considerations. The scheme used in this chapter was developed by Russell and Rubenstein at the Armed Forces Institute of Pathology,[7] and is summarized in Table 4.1. The scheme subdivides tumors by tissue type and by region, with some overlap between the two groups.

Typical MRI features of intracranial tumors

The MRI features of tumors can be divided from center to periphery into tumor mass, edema, mass effect, hydrocephalus, and distant effects.

The proton density of the tumor mass may be increased or decreased. In general, there is some increase with malignant tumors, although a decrease is seen with some benign tumors and in regions of dense calcification.

The fact that the T_1 and T_2 of the tumor mass are generally increased was first described by Damadian in 1971,[8] but exceptions to this pattern were recognized even at this early stage. It has been recognized that there may be a wide spread of T_1 and T_2 values even within a single histological classification and that there is overlap between different pathological groupings.[9,10] Since the tumor mass may contain calcification and cysts as well as hemorrhagic and necrotic areas, it is not surprising that single characteristic values of T_1 and T_2 have not been found. In addition, some gliomas show areas of variable malignancy and there may be differences within a tumor between viable, well vascularized, well oxygenated cells at the rim, and cells at the center which have an inadequate blood supply.

Table 4.1 Tumor classification.

I   Tumors of neuroglial cells
     1   Astrocytoma
     2   Glioblastoma multiforme
     3   Oligodendroglioma
     4   Ependymoma

II   Tumors of neuronal cells or primitive, bipotential precursors
     1   Medulloblastoma
     2   Neuroblastoma
     3   Ganglioneuroma/ganglioglioma

III   Tumors of the cranial nerves
     1   Schwannoma
     2   Neuroma
     3   Neurinoma

IV   Tumors of mesodermal origin
     1   Meningioma/meningiosarcoma

V   Tumors of the reticuloendothelial system
     1   Primary lymphoma
     2   Metastatic lymphoma

VI   Tumors of blood vessels
     1   Hemangioblastoma
     2   Cavernous hemangioma

VII   Tumors of choroid plexus and related structures
     1   Choroid plexus papilloma/carcinoma
     2   Intraventricular meningioma
     3   Colloid cyst

VIII   Tumors of pineal origin
     1   Germ cell tumors
        (a)   Germinoma
        (b)   Teratoma,
        (c)   Choriocarcinoma/embryonal carcinoma
     2   Pineal cell tumors
        (a)   Pineocytoma
        (b)   Pineoblastoma
     3   Other pineal tumors

IX   Tumors of maldevelopment
     1   Epidermoid cyst
     2   Dermoid cyst
     3   Teratoma
     4   Craniopharyngioma
     5   Hamartoma
     6   Neurofibromatosis

X   Local tumors
     1   Pituitary tumors
        (a)   Macroadenoma
        (b)   Microadenoma
     2   Chordoma
     3   Chondroma/chondrosarcoma
     4   Glomus tumor

XI   Metastatic tumors

Peritumoral edema produces an increase in T_1 and T_2, and since this is the same basic change as that usually produced by the tumor mass it may be difficult to detect the margin between the two pathological processes. It is known from X-ray CT stereotactic biopsy studies that malignant cells often extend beyond the apparent rim of tumor on CT, and similar difficulties in the definition of the margin between tumor and edema might reasonably be expected with MRI. By using a wider variety of sequences and intravenous Gd-DTPA, definition of the margin between the bulk of the tumor and surrounding edema has improved, as illustrated in Figure 4.1, but difficulties remain at the microscopic level.

Mass effects are generally better displayed with T_1-weighted sequences than with spin-echo (SE) sequences. The advantage of MRI in comparison with X-ray CT is most marked in regions where the CT is degraded by the presence of artifact or partial-volume effects from bone. This includes the apex of the skull, the posterior fossa, and the skull base. In addition, mass effects may be better demonstrated in particular cases by direct sagittal or coronal imaging.

Hydrocephalus is well demonstrated with MRI. The sagittal plane is useful to show the region of the aqueduct. In addition, periventricular edema can be demonstrated without confusion with partial-volume effects between brain and CSF by the use of appropriate SE sequence.

There are often some remote effects associated with tumors, including periventricular changes not associated with hydrocephalus and changes in the properties of CSF (decreased T_1 and T_2) attributable to increased protein content.

With the use of Gd-DTPA, dural and meningeal enhancement may be observed. These features may also be present with X-ray CT, but are easily obscured by the presence of the adjacent skull.

Tumors of neuroglial cells

Astrocytomas

Astrocytomas are conventionally classified into grades I to IV. Grade III and grade IV astrocytomas can be considered independently under the term 'glioblastoma multiforme'. Astrocytomas make up 35 per cent of all primary intracranial tumors. They occur most frequently in children and young adults. The site of occurrence varies with age; childhood tumors are most frequently located in the posterior fossa, whereas those in adults are more often supratentorial in location. Grades I and II tumors are typically slow growing. These tumors may differentiate with time and undergo frank malignant transformation.

Supratentorial astrocytomas are typically solid and infiltrating, and produce relatively little edema and mass effect. On MR examination, these lesions appear as conspicuous, high-intensity abnormalities on T_2-weighted images, and as less conspicuous low-intensity abnormalities on T_1-weighted images, and hence reflect prolongation of T_2 and T_1 relaxation times, respectively, as shown in Figure 4.2. T_1 prolongation is typically less than that seen with grades III and IV tumors. In the absence of conspicuous signal-intensity abnormalities, loss of the normal distinction between gray and white matter may indicate the presence of tumor.

Cystic lesions occur most frequently in the posterior fossa and are often termed 'juvenile astrocytomas'. Cystic supratentorial lesions are less common. When compared to solid tumors, the cystic lesions are better defined with smoother borders. The intensity of cyst fluid varies with its protein and iron content, but is usually greater than that of CSF on conventional T_1- and mildly to moderately T_2-weighted sequences. This reflects the influence of hydration-layer water, which causes significant T_1-shortening and minimal T_2-shortening.

In both solid and cystic lesions, calcification is frequent and identifiable on CT in up to 30 per cent of cases. Magnetic resonance imaging is relatively insensitive to calcification.[11] Very large and/or dense areas of calcification are demonstrated as foci of decreased signal intensity.

Grade I and II tumor enhancement is typically less pronounced than in higher-grade lesions.

Intratumoral hemorrhage is infrequent in lower-grade lesions, but when it occurs it may dominate the clinical presentation and obscure the underlying tumor.[12]

Glioblastoma multiforme

These tumors represent more than 60 per cent of all gliomas. They occur most commonly in middle age, and there is a 3:2 male preponderance. The lesions grow rapidly and carry a poor prognosis. Presenting symptoms may reflect involvement of local structures or a generalized increase in intracranial pressure. The tumors are most frequently supratentorial in location and may extend across the midline through central white matter structures such as the corpus callosum (the 'butterfly glioma', illustrated in Figure 4.3). On T_2-weighted MR images, these tumors appear as irregular, high-intensity lesions with moderate to marked surrounding edema. Signal heterogeneity may reflect necrosis, cyst formation, and/or calcification or hemorrhage; the latter is shown in Figure 4.4. The central tumor may often be distinguished from surrounding edema by the latter's shorter T_1 and longer T_2 relaxation times. Thus tumor usually appears less intense than edema on both T_1- and T_2-weighted

images. As Figure 4.5 shows, the distinction between tumor and edema can be demonstrated more consistently by administration of Gd-DTPA.

The incidence of multicentric glioblastoma is estimated to be between 2 and 5 per cent of all gliomas. The majority of these multicentric tumors are small satellite lesions adjacent to a large central tumor. Less frequently, multiple lesions may be widely separated and occasionally occur in opposite hemispheres. Tumors apparently discontinuous on CT examination may be connected by 'microscopic' extensions, and this continuity may be more apparent on MRI than on CT.

The optic nerve is another site where gliomas are seen, and such a tumor is shown in Figure 4.6.

Oligodendrogliomas

Oligodendrogliomas represent 5 to 7 per cent of all primary intracranial gliomas. They occur most frequently in adults. Typically slow-growing, they produce chronic focal symptoms, most often seizures, and may reach a large size prior to detection. There is predilection for frontal lobe involvement. Like other low-grade, solid neoplasms, these tumors appear as focal areas of increased signal intensity on T_2-weighted images, with relatively little edema or mass effect. Large and extensive calcifications, readily apparent on CT examination, may be relatively inconspicuous on the MR study. Small intratumoral cysts may result in foci of relatively decreased signal intensity on T_1-weighted and mild to moderately T_2-weighted images.

Ependymomas

Ependymomas represent 5 to 6 per cent of all primary intracranial gliomas. They are often located about the lateral and third ventricles. In adults, fourth ventricular involvement is more typical, illustrated in Figure 4.7. They appear as well-defined, hyperintense lesions on T_2-weighted MR images. On T_1-weighted sagittal sections, the lesions may invaginate into the fourth ventricle, indicating their ependymal origin. Despite the low histologic grade of these lesions, their periventricular location may result in seeding of tumor via CSF pathways, resulting in a poor prognosis.

Tumors of neuronal cells or primitive bipotential precursors

Medulloblastoma

Medulloblastomas occur exclusively within the posterior fossa. They occur mainly in children, although adults can be susceptible. Tumors generally occur in the midline and arise from the anterior medullary velum. The tumor is highly cellular and locally invasive. Extension into the fourth ventricle and vermis is common, with deformity and obstruction of the aqueduct. Hydrocephalus is common and metastatic seeding along CSF pathways occurs frequently. T_1 and T_2 are typically increased. Gadolinium-DTPA is useful in demonstrating seeding of the tumor.

Neuroblastomas

Primary intracranial neuroblastomas are now reclassified under the heading of primitive neuroectodermal tumors. These are rare tumors of childhood. Calvarial or skull-base metastases from primary lesions of the thorax or abdomen are more common. Primary lesions occur most frequently in the cerebral hemispheres. Calcification, cysts, and intratumoral hemorrhage are non-specific features.

Ganglioneuromas/gangliogliomas

These uncommon tumors are composed of abnormal neural and glial cell elements. Occurring most often in children and young adults, they may affect any intracranial site, but there is a predilection for involvement of the temporal lobe or structures about the third ventricle. The tumors are slow-growing and symptoms are most often related to focal irritation. The lesions are predominantly solid and are manifested by areas of increased signal intensity on T_1-weighted MR images. Multiple small tumoral cysts may be seen and are reflected as foci of relatively decreased signal intensity on T_1- and mildly T_2-weighted images and increased intensity on heavily T_2-weighted images. Focal calcification is a characteristic feature on CT, but is typically inconspicuous on MRI.

Tumors of the cranial nerves

Schwannomas, neuromas, and neurinomas are typically well-defined, rounded lesions, which are often hyperintense on T_2-weighted MR images. Specific diagnosis relies on the demonstration of an extra-axial mass at a characteristic location, such as the internal auditory canal (acoustic neuroma)[13,14] (Figures 4.8–4.10), the jugular fossa (ninth nerve neuroma) (Figure 4.11), or Meckel's cave (trigeminal neuroma) (Figure 4.12).

Eighth nerve (acoustic) tumors represent more than 90 per cent of all neuromas. Trigeminal neuromas typically appear as rounded or bilobulated masses, expanding into the cavernous sinus and extending over the superior aspect of the petrous apex into the superior cerebellopontine angle cistern. Denervation of the affected muscles of mastication may produce a unilateral decrease in bulk and increase in signal intensity due to increased fat deposition.

Tumors of mesodermal origin

Meningiomas

Meningiomas represent 13 to 18 per cent of all intracranial neoplasms and most often affect middle-aged and elderly adults. Females are preferentially affected by a 2:1 ratio. Multiple meningiomas may be seen in patients with neurofibromatosis. These lesions are most often located along meningeal surfaces in the parasagittal region, lateral convexity, the falx, the sphenoid ridge, the olfactory groove (Figure 4.13), cerebellopontine angle (Figure 4.14), the petrous ridge, and the tentorium, in order of descending frequency. Rarely, intraventricular meningiomas may arise from meningeal rests in the choroid plexus. Meningiomas are typically slow-growing lesions. Grossly, they appear well-defined and globular or lobulated, less often assuming an en plaque configuration, shown in Figure 4.15. Erosion and/or hyperostosis of adjacent bony structures is a characteristic finding on plain films or CT, but may be difficult to appreciate on MRI. Histologically, these tumors are composed of firm, fibrous tissue, occasionally divided by denser septae. Calcification may be both diffuse (psammomatous) or focal (amorphous and globular).

As previously described, meningiomas appear as isointense or hyperdense masses on CT, with varying degrees of surrounding edema and intense, homogeneous enhancement. Several studies have indicated the relative insensitivity of MRI in the depiction of these lesions,[15,16] in part reflecting limitations in the image quality of prototype systems. Signal intensity of these lesions may vary significantly. Many meningiomas are similar to gray matter in signal intensity over a wide range of imaging parameters. Heavily calcified lesions appear hypointense on both T_1- and T_2-weighted images, whereas other tumors appear hypointense on T_1-weighted images and hyperintense on T_2-weighted images. In general, the T_2 relaxation time is less prolonged than that of gliomas. Accurate diagnosis relies on demonstration of extra-axial mass effect, manifested as displacement of adjacent brain parenchyma and superficial vessels. Meningiomas are often separated from adjacent brain by a low-intensity capsule. This lack of capsular signal may be related to dense fibrous tissue or displaced vessels. The internal matrix of these lesions is typically uniformly granular or speckled. Occasionally, intratumoral septations may yield a pathognomonic, spoke-wheel appearance. Reactive edema appears hyperintense on T_2-weighted images and may mask an underlying isointense tumor. Focal calcifications and bony changes are readily demonstrable by CT but are poorly depicted by MRI. These lesions enhance intensely following intravenous administration of Gd-DTPA.[17,18]

Meningiosarcomas cannot be differentiated from their benign counterparts in most cases. This diagnosis is typically made on the basis of clinical and/or histologic criteria. Poorly defined tumor margins, marked heterogeneity, and/or prominent edema are indicative of tumor aggressiveness.

A significant proportion of meningiomas show only a slight increase in T_1 over white matter and a T_2 within the normal range for brain. The use of highly T_2-dependent sequences therefore produces little soft tissue contrast. With medium TI inversion recovery (IR) sequences, the slight difference between tumor and white matter may be sufficient to define the lesion. In addition, the greater anatomical detail available with IR images helps in identification of mass effects. When Gd-DTPA is used, meningiomas are usually enhanced and this enhancement is maximal with the medium TI IR sequence. Since highly T_2-dependent sequences are normally used for the detection of pathology in the brain (IR sequences are generally used much less frequently) there is a possibility of missing meningiomas. On the other hand, if IR sequences are used routinely for screening purposes the time of examination must be increased.

Magnetic resonance imaging has potential advantages over CT in the demonstration of lesions adjacent to the convexity of the skull at the base of the brain and in the posterior fossa. Meningioma-en-plaque and dural involvement may be better demonstrated, although calcification is not.

It is also possible that measurement of T_1 and T_2 may provide a guide to tumor consistency and therefore surgical approach. Softer tumors tend to have a longer T_1 and T_2 than harder tumors.

Although results obtained with MRI in meningioma have improved, some doubt remains about the exact way in which an examination sensitive for meningioma should be integrated into routine practice. Since the symptoms of meningioma are not specific there is often no particular indication to perform an examination specifically designed to detect this tumor. Missing a meningioma may not be important if it is a small incidental finding in the region of the falx, but the same sized tumor in the optic canal or in the foramen magnum may be highly significant. These issues are not yet fully resolved but the need to detect meningiomas in screening examinations may affect the choice of sequences, the length of time of screening examinations, and the extent to which Gd-DTPA is used in routine practice.

Tumors of the reticuloendothelial system

Primary lymphomas

Primary lymphoma is also referred to as 'microglioma' and 'reticulum cell sarcoma'. It is relatively rare, representing approximately 1 per cent of all intracranial neoplasms. Typically, primary CNS lymphomas are limited to the brain but are occasionally associated with occult or subsequently demonstrated extracranial disease. Primary lymphoma most often affects males in the fifth and sixth decades and frequently occurs in immunosuppressed patients, such as those with acquired immune deficiency syndrome (AIDS). The tumor affects both brain parenchyma and meninges and is often multicentric in location. Midline or paramedian structures are preferentially affected. The tumors are typically infiltrating and are associated with relatively little mass effect or edema. As with other parenchymal neoplastic processes, tumors are most conspicuously demonstrated as high-intensity abnormalities on T_2-weighted images, as in Figure 4.16.

Metastatic lymphomas

Metastatic involvement of the brain by systemic lymphoma may have an appearance similar to that of primary lymphoma, but typically there is a greater incidence of leptomeningeal involvement. In other cases, intracranial spread of systemic lymphoma mimics metastatic carcinoma.

Tumors of blood-vessel origin

Hemangioblastomas

Hemangioblastomas usually present in the third and fourth decades, occasionally in association with polycythemia. Hemorrhage may lead to an abrupt presentation. Patients with Hippel-Landau disease may have associated tumors in multiple locations.

Hemangioblastomas are usually irregular and often occur with cysts and an associated mural nodule. They are highly vascular.

The T_1 and T_2 of these tumors are prolonged, as shown in Figure 4.17. Cystic components may be recognized, as well as serpiginous areas of altered signal intensity due to the vascular changes.

Cavernous angiomas

Cavernous angioma is a form of vascular malformation rather than a true neoplasm, but may mimic a tumor in its clinical presentation and appearance on CT or MRI. Cavernous angiomas are usually subcortical in location and occur most frequently in the temporal lobe. On MR examination, they appear as well-defined, rounded lesions, hyperintense on T_2-weighted images, with lesion heterogeneity related to calcification and a relatively complex matrix. They may contain foci of hemorrhage with resultant intensity variations dependent on the age of the hemorrhage. Mild mass effect may be noted with acute or subacute hemorrhagic lesions. More usually, the lack of mass effect or change on serial examinations suggests this diagnosis.

Tumors of the choroid plexus and related structures

Choroid plexus papillomas/carcinomas

These lesions represent less than 1 per cent of all primary intracranial tumors, and the majority occur in patients in the first decade. Males are affected more often than females. Fifty per cent of these lesions are found within the fourth ventricle; lateral ventricular lesions are more common on the left side. On MR examination, papillomas appear as lobulated, somewhat heterogeneous lesions, hyperintense on T_2-weighted images, originating from the choroid plexus and expanding into the ventricle, as shown in Figure 4.18. Carcinomas are characterized by invasion of the adjacent brain parenchyma. Both papillomas and carcinomas may cause disproportionate ventricular enlargement, secondary to overproduction of CSF.

Intraventricular meningiomas

These rare lesions arise from meningeal rests in the choroid plexus and usually involve the lateral ventricle. As with meningiomas elsewhere, isointensity with gray matter over a broad range of pulsing parameters is a common MR feature.

Colloid cysts

Colloid cysts are relatively rare, benign tumors, which are usually located within the anterior third ventricle. They are thought to arise from either the vestigial paraphysis or diencephalic ependymal pouches. Classically, these lesions present in adults with symptoms of obstructive hydrocephalus, which is sometimes intermittent or related to variation in head position. Because of their critical location at the foramen of Monro, even lesions less than 1 cm in diameter may be symptomatic. Lesions measuring 3 cm or greater are occasionally seen. On MRI the signal intensity of these lesions is extremely variable, demonstrated in Figure 4.19.

Pineal region tumors

Current classification systems divide these lesions into those of germ cell origin (germinomas, teratomas, choriocarcinomas, and embryonal carcinomas), those of pineal cell origin (pineocytomas and pineoblastomas), metastases to the pineal gland, tumors of maldevelopment origin (epidermoids and dermoids), and tumors arising from adjacent structures (gliomas of the epithalamus, corpus callosum, and mid-brain tectum). Cross-sectional imaging is used to detect and localize the tumor and to demonstrate invasion of adjacent structures or spread via ependymal or CSF pathways. Figure 4.20 illustrates a pinealoma in a characteristic site.

Germ cell tumors

Germinomas

Pineal germinomas, also referred to as atypical teratomas, are the most common of the pineal tumors, representing more than 50 per cent of all primary pineal neoplasms. These lesions occur most often in the second and third decades and males are affected much more often than females. Germinomas may occur anywhere along the axis between the pineal gland and the hypothalamus, with more anterior lesions giving rise to the term 'ectopic pinealoma'. Multiple midline tumors are occasionally seen. As with other pineal region tumors, spread via ependymal or CSF pathways is not uncommon. These tumors are often radiosensitive. Demonstration of a pineal region tumor in a young male may warrant a trial of radiotherapy. If a decrease in tumor size is demonstrated, this may indicate the need for further cranial irradiation and possibly irradiation of the spinal axis as well.

On MR examination, these lesions are often best appreciated on sagittal sections. Tumors arising within the pineal cistern produce anteroinferior displacement and distortion of the midbrain tectum, often associated with a clinical presentation of limited upgaze (Parinaud's syndrome). 'Ectopic' lesions may be located anywhere between the pineal cistern and the suprasellar cistern. These lesions are hyperintense on T_2-weighted images and are frequently heterogeneous, reflecting focal calcification, hemorrhage, and/or cyst formation. Although some investigators have reported distinguishing features of various pineal region neoplasms on CT examination, in our experience, the signal-intensity pattern on MR is non-specific, and demographic data (patient age and sex) may take precedence in the determination of appropriate therapeutic intervention.

Teratomas

Pineal region teratomas also affect young males. Theoretically, these lesions would be expected to be the most heterogeneous of all pineal region tumors, as they reflect the inclusion of various germ cell elements.

Choriocarcinomas/embryonal carcinomas

Choriocarcinomas and embryonal cell carcinomas are rare and invasive lesions. On MR examination, they also appear hyperintense on T_2-weighted images with varying degrees of heterogeneity and involvement of adjacent structures.

Pineal cell tumors

Pineocytomas and pineoblastomas may affect patients of either sex at any age. A pineocytoma is the most common pineal region neoplasm in young females. On MR examination, pineocytomas appear as relatively well-defined, homogeneous lesions, whereas pineoblastomas typically appear more irregular and invasive.

Tumors of maldevelopmental origin

Epidermoid cysts

Epidermoid cysts represent 1 per cent of all intracranial neoplasms. Presumably present from birth, they typically remain asymptomatic until adulthood, with a peak incidence of clinical presentation in the fifth decade.

Epidermoid cysts result from inclusion of ectodermal elements during closure of the neural tube in the fifth week of fetal life. Early inclusion results in midline lesions; later inclusion results in increasing laterality. On gross examination, these lesions are well-defined, cystic structures with glistening, irregular, nodular surfaces and are thus appropriately termed 'pearly tumors'. The cyst is filled with waxy or flaky material composed of cholesterol crystals and keratinized debris. The most frequent location is in the cerebellopontine angle cistern, shown in Figure 4.21, with other common locations including the parasellar region, the fourth ventricle, and the pineal cistern.

On MR examination, these lesions appear heterogeneous and hyperintense on T_2-weighted images, reflecting the presence of proteinaceous debris within the tumor. Despite their cholesterol content, T_1-shortening is noted in the minority of lesions, presumably because the cholesterol is in the solid state. Typically, these tumors appear as extra-axial lesions extending along natural tissue planes and producing relatively little mass effect. A heterogeneous appearance on MR examination reflects the complexity of the internal matrix and is often seen in large lesions.

Dermoid cysts

These less common lesions result from inclusion of epithelial cells and skin appendages, such as hair follicles and sebaceous or sweat glands, during closure of the neural tube. They are more frequently located in the midline. Anterior lesions are often associated with a midline bone or skin defect. The contents of dermoid cysts are buttery in texture and the partially liquefied cholesterol produces T_1-shortening and resultant hyperintensity on T_1-weighted images. These lesions frequently contain punctate or rim-like calcification, but this is relatively inconspicuous on MR examination.

Teratomas

These lesions contain elements of all three germ cell lesions. As previously discussed, malignant or aggressive lesions (that is, teratoid tumors or atypical teratomas) are most frequently located in the pineal region. Benign teratomas are more often located about the third ventricle or sella. Teratomas have a heterogeneous appearance on MR examination, reflecting the contributions of the various germ cell elements.

Craniopharyngiomas

These lesions represent 3 per cent of all intracranial tumors and are among the more common intracranial neoplasms of childhood. There is a bimodal age distribution with tumors occurring most frequently in the first and second decades, followed by a second peak in the fifth decade. Originating from epithelial rests along the vestigial craniopharyngeal duct, they are usually suprasellar in location, although there is frequently an intrasellar component as well. Patients typically present with a hypothalamic or chiasmal syndrome.

Grossly, these lesions may be cystic, solid, or complex. The cysts may be rich in liquefied cholesterol or high in protein content, which will produce T_1-shortening and hyperintensity on T_1-weighted images, as in Figure 4.22. The T_1 relaxation time is mildly prolonged in solid lesions. The T_2 relaxation time is almost always prolonged, yielding hyperintensity on T_2-weighted images, although there are occasional exceptions.[19] Craniopharyngiomas often contain nodular or shell-like calcifications, which are almost always better demonstrated by CT than by MRI.

Hamartomas

Intracerebral hamartomas are unusual tumors which may be divided into two distinct categries: hypothalamic and multiple. Hypothalamic hamartomas are isolated lesions, which occur sporadically, usually in young males who present with precocious puberty. The lesions are conspicuously demonstrated on sagittal images. Magnetic resonance signal intensity may vary considerably. Foci of T_1-shortening may be observed in fat-containing lesions.

Multiple intracerebral hamartomas are associated with tuberous sclerosis. Histologically, superficial cortical lesions are associated with gliosis and cellular atypia. These lesions appear hyperintense on a T_2-weighted MR image. The subependymal hamartomas of tuberous sclerosis are typically more benign and often heavily calcified. They produce little, if any, alteration of MR signal intensity and are most often apparent only by virtue of their extension into CSF-containing ventricles. The hamartomas of tuberous sclerosis may degenerate into giant cell astrocytomas. Because they are usually located about the foramen of Monro, they produce obstructive hydrocephalus. These lesions appear hyperintense on T_2-weighted images and often produce significant focal mass effect and surrounding edema.

Neurofibromatosis

Neurofibromatosis (von Recklinghausen's disease) is included under the category of maldevelopment tumors, since the lesions associated with this disease appear to result from a congenital, generalized dysplasia rather than from differentiation and transformation of previously normal cell lines. Neurofibromatosis is typically classified into peripheral and central subcategories. The peripheral form is manifested by multiple, subcutaneous nerve sheath tumors; the central form is characterized by tumors arising from the brain parenchyma, ependyma, meninges, or nerve roots. The histology of central tumors varies greatly. Eighth nerve neuromas, convexity meningiomas, and low-grade optic gliomas are often seen. Less frequently, low-grade gliomas may be found elsewhere within the cerebral or cerebellar hemispheres and intraparenchymal hamartomas are also found in patients with this disorder.[20] The MR appearance of individual lesions is described elsewhere in this chapter.

Local tumors

Pituitary tumors

Pituitary adenomas represent up to 20 per cent of all intracranial neoplasms. Macroadenomas (those greater than 1 cm in diameter) often produce symptoms by virtue of local mass effect, typically a visual-field deficit related to compression of the suprajacent optic complex. Less frequently, tumor compression of normal pituitary tissue results in either hypopituitarism or increased prolactin production. Histologically, most macroadenomas have chromophobic staining characteristics. They are non-secreting tumors which may grow quite large before they are detected or produce clinical symptoms.

Macroadenomas are best demonstrated on thin-slice sagittal and coronal MR sections, as in Figure 4.23. On T_1-weighted images, these lesions are isointense to slightly hypointense, and extrasellar extension into the suprasellar cistern can be readily identified, often with 'waisting' as the tumor passes through the diaphragm sella. Lateral extension into the cavernous sinuses is easily diagnosed when the tumor encases the internal carotid artery. However, subtle invasion of the medial portion of the cavernous sinus can be difficult to distinguish from tumoral compression without true invasion. On T_2-weighted images, the tumors appear hyperintense, and compressive edema within adjacent brain parenchyma is more conspicuously demonstrated. Macroadenomas are usually homogeneous in signal intensity; but occasionally heterogeneity may indicate the presence of intratumoral necrosis, cyst formation, calcification, and/or hemorrhage.

Pituitary microadenomas are more common lesions than macroadenomas. They become symptomatic by virtue of overproduction of trophic hormones: prolactin, adrenocorticotrophic hormone (ACTH), or human growth hormone (HGH). Prolactin-secreting tumors are by far the most common functioning adenomas, primarily affecting young females and producing amenorrhea and galactorrhea. Tumors secreting ACTH and HGH produce the clinical syndromes of Cushing's disease and gigantism or acromegaly, respectively

Several investigators have described the efficacy of MRI in the evaluation of patients with microadenomas. The current sensitivity of MRI in the detection of these lesions is comparable to that of contrast-enhanced, direct coronal high-resolution CT.[20-2] Microadenomas are most apparent on thin-slice T_1-weighted sagittal and coronal MR sections, where they appear as isointense or hypointense foci relative to the normal gland, illustrated in Figure 4.24. Associated alterations in pituitary gland size and contour and infundibular displacement may be observed. However, subtle erosion of the bony sella is difficult to detect with MRI. Preliminary studies suggest that intravenous administration of Gd-DTPA may significantly increase the effectiveness of MRI in the evaluation of microadenomas.

Chordomas

These tumors arise from notochordal remnants and are most frequently located in the sacrum and clivus. Chordomas are rare lesions that usually occur in the sixth to eighth decades. Males are affected more frequently than females. The tumors produce focal bone destruction, often eroding through the clivus into adjacent structures such as the sphenoid sinus, the pituitary fossa, and the prepontine cistern. Clinical symptoms are most often related to compression of adjacent neural structures, classically the cranial nerves.

Chordomas are well demonstrated on T_1-weighted sagittal and coronal images. Clival involvement is manifested by replacement of normal high-intensity clival marrow. These tumors are irregularly margined and have a heterogeneous signal intensity. The latter feature may be related in part to intratumoral calcification. The appearance of a chordoma may be simulated by a metastatic carcinoma involving the clivus.

Chondromas/chondrosarcomas

These rare tumors originate from the dura and skull base and produce an extra-axial mass effect. Clinical symptoms relate to local bone destruction and compression and/or invasion of adjacent neural structures. On MR examination, both chondromas and chondrosarcomas are characterized by homogeneous or mottled, low-signal intensity, reflecting the proton density of their chondroid matrix.

Glomus tumors

Cranial glomus tumors involve the middle ear and/or the jugular fossa. Glomus jugulare tumors typically occur in adults from 30 to 80 years of age. They are highly vascular and locally invasive. They can grow into the posterior fossa through the jugular foramen, internal auditory meatus, or hypoglossal canal. Involvement of the middle ear is common as involvement of cranial nerves in the skull base. They are generally inhomogeneous with a prolonged T_2 and sometimes display vascular features.

Metastatic tumors

Metastatic lesions represent up to 40 per cent of all intracranial tumors. By virtue of its high sensitivity, MRI has proved effective in the diagnosis of these lesions. It may demonstrate small lesions not revealed by CT, particularly in the posterior fossa. More importantly, MRI may demonstrate two or more lesions when only one is shown by CT, significantly altering differential diagnostic considerations and therapeutic implications. Multiplicity is the hallmark of metastatic disease. An isolated metastasis cannot be reliably differentiated from either a primary brain tumor or an active inflammatory process, such as an abscess. Parenchymal metastases appear as high-intensity lesions on T_2-weighted images, usually with edema and mass effect. As with high-grade gliomas, central tumor can often be separated from high-intensity surrounding edema on heavily T_1- or T_2-weighted images, due to slight differences in T_1 and T_2 relaxation times. However, tumor enhancement with intravenous Gd-DTPA is a more reliable method of distinguishing tumor from edema, as demonstrated in Figure 4.25.

Meningeal metastases may be manifested as alteration of normal meningeal signal intensity and secondary subdural effusions or obstructive hydrocephalus.[23] Calvarial lesions are less apparent on MRI than on CT with appropriate window settings. Involvement of the diploic space and replacement of the normal fatty marrow results in decreased MR signal intensity. Skull-base lesions are well demonstrated by direct coronal and/or sagittal images and intracranial extensions can be readily assessed.

Non-neoplastic mass lesions

As with CT, the MR appearance of an intracranial neoplasm may be mimicked by a variety of non-neoplastic conditions, such as abscesses, cysts (Figure 4.26), and giant aneurysms. In the appropriate clinical setting, the patient's history and the results of other diagnostic tests may take precedence in the determination of the appropriate therapy.

References

1 HAWKES RC, HOLLAND GN, MOORE WS et al, Nuclear magnetic resonance tomography of the brain: a preliminary clinical assessment with demonstration of pathology, *J Comput Assist Tomogr* (1980) **4**:577–86.

2 MCGINNIS BD, BRADY TJ, NEW PFJ et al, Nuclear magnetic resonance (NMR) imaging of tumors in the posterior fossa, *J Comput Assist Tomogr* (1983) **7**:575–84.

3 RANDELL CP, COLLINS AG, YOUNG IR et al, Nuclear magnetic resonance imaging of posterior fossa tumors, *AJR* (1983) **141**:489–96; *AJNR* (1983) **4**:1027–34.

4 GRAIF M, BYDDER GM, STEINER RE et al, Contrast enhanced MR imaging of malignant brain tumors, *AJNR* (1985) **6**:855.

5 FELIX R, SCHORNER W, LANIADO M et al, Brain tumors: MR imaging with gadolinium-DPTA, *Radiology* (1985) **7**:97–104.

6 BRADLEY WG, BRANT-ZAWADZKI M, BRASCH RC et al, Initial clinical experience with Gd-DPTA in North America: MR contrast enhancement of brain tumors, *Radiology* (1985) **157**(P):125.

7 RUBENSTEIN LJ, *Tumors of the central nervous system*, (Armed Forces Institute of Pathology: Bethesda 1972).

8 DAMADIAN R, Tumor detection by nuclear magnetic resonance, *Science* (1971) **171**:1151–30.

9 ARAKI T, INOUYE T, SUZUKI H et al, Magnetic resonance imaging of brain tumors: measurement of T_1, *Radiology* (1984) **150**:95–8.

10 LEBAS JF, LEVIEL JL, DECORPS M et al, NMR relaxation times from serial stereotactic biopsies in human brain tumors, *J Comput Assist Tomogr* (1984) **8**: 1048–57.

11 TSURUDA JS, BRADLEY WG, MR detection of intracranial calcification, *AJNR* (1987) **8**: 1049–55.

12 ATLAS SW, GROSSMAN RI, GOMORI JM et al, Hemorrhagic intracranial malignant neoplasms: spin echo MR imaging, *Radiology* (1987) **164**:71–7.

13 NEW PFJ, BACHOW TB, WISMER GL et al, MR imaging of the acoustic nerves and small acoustic neuromas at 0.6T: prospective study, *AJR* (1985) **144**:1021–6.

14 CURATI WL, GRAIF M, KINGSLEY DPE et al, Acoustic neuromas: Gd-DTPA enhancement in MR imaging, *Radiology* (1986) **158**:447–51.

15 BRADLEY WG, WALUCH V, YADLEY RA et al, Comparison of CT and MR in 400 patients with suspected disease of the brain and cervical spinal cord, *Radiology* (1984) **152**:695–702.

16 ZIMMERMAN RD, FLEMING CA, SAINT-LOUIS LA et al, Magnetic resonance imaging of meningiomas, *AJNR* (1985) **6**:149–58.

17 BYDDER GM, KINGSLEY DPE, BROWN J et al, MR imaging of meningiomas including studies with and without gadolinium-DTPA, *J Comput Assist Tomogr* (1985) **9**:690–7.

18 SCHORNER W, LANIADO M, NIENDORF HP et al, Time dependent changes in image contrast in brain tumors after gadolinium-DPTA, *AJNR* (1986) **7**:1013–18.

19 PUSEY E, KORTMAN KE, FLANNIGAN BD et al, MR of craniopharyngiomas: tumor delineation and characterization, *AJNR* (1987) **8**:65–9.

20 HURST TW, NEWMAN SA, CAIL WS, Multifocal intracranial MR abnormalities in neurofibromatosis, *AJNR* (1988) **9**:293–6.

21 PECK WW, DILLON WP, NORMAN D et al, High resolution MR imaging of microadenomas at 1.5T: experience with Cushing disease, *AJNR* (1988) **9**:1085–9.

22 POJUNAS KW, DANIELS DL, WILLIAMS AL et al, MR imaging of prolactin secreting microadenomas, *AJNR* (1986) **7**:209–13.

23 DAVIS PC, FRIEDMAN NC, FRY SM et al, Leptomeningeal metastasis: MR imaging, *Radiology* (1987) **163**:449–54.

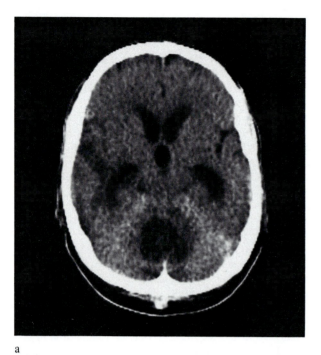

a

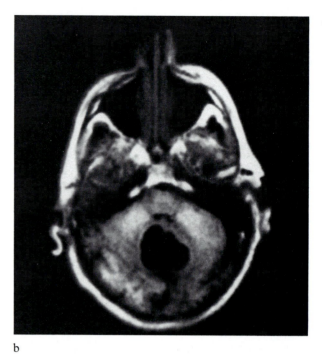

b

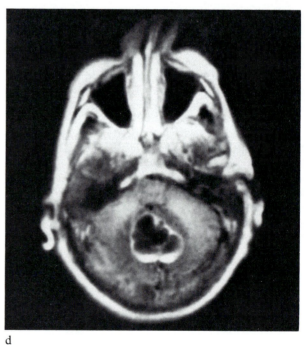

c

d

Figure 4.1

Metastatic carcinoma. X-ray
CT (**a**) and IR 1500/44/500 (**b**)
images before enhancement
compared with X-ray CT (**c**)
and IR 1500/44/500 (**d**) images
after enhancement. A ring of
enhancement is seen in (**c**) and
(**d**). The changes are more
readily seen with MRI.

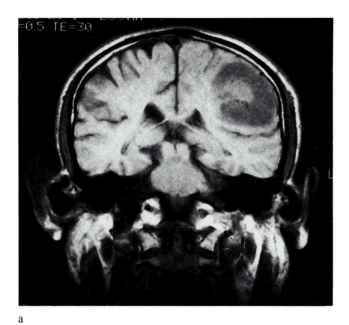
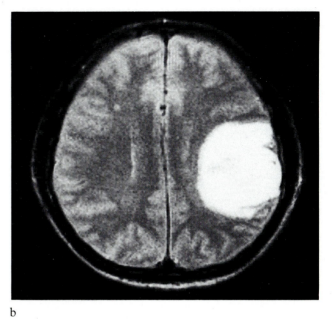

a

b

Figure 4.2

Astrocytoma grade II. Coronal
SE 500/30 (**a**) and SE 2000/60
(**b**) images. The tumor has a
prolonged T_1 and T_2 and there
is evidence of structure within
it.

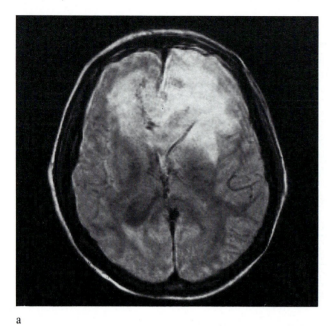

a

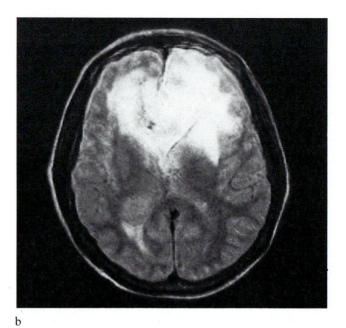

b

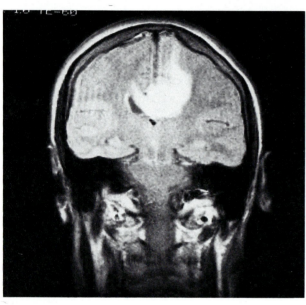

c

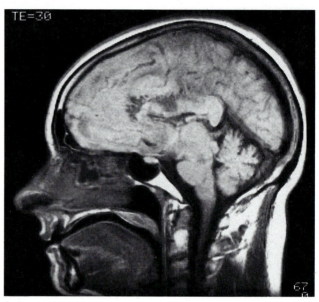

d

Figure 4.3

Butterfly glioma. SE 500/30 (**a**), SE 2000/60 (**b**), coronal SE 1000/60 (**c**), and sagittal SE 500/30 (**d**) images. The increased signal intensity in (**a–c**) extends across the midline.

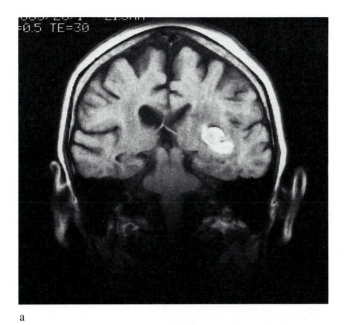

a

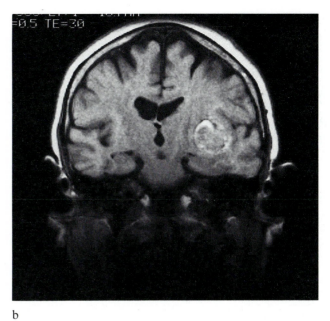

b

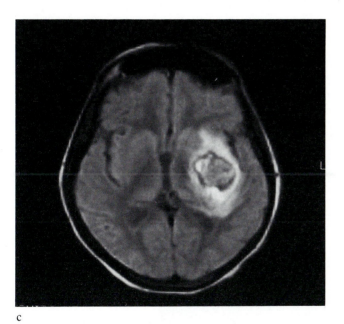

c

Figure 4.4

Hemorrhagic glioma. Coronal
SE 500/30 (**a**), coronal SE 500/
30 (**b**), and SE 2000/30 (**c**)
images. The tumor displays
high signal-intensity regions in
(**a**) and (**b**) but a low-intensity
margin with surrounding
edema in (**c**).

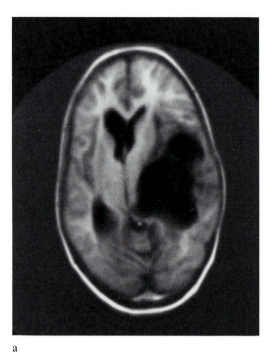

a

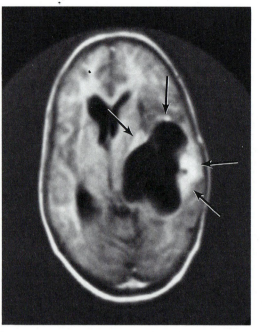

b

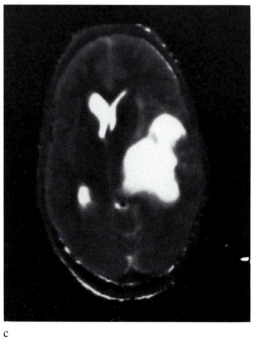

c

d

Figure 4.5

Astrocytoma grade III. IR
1500/44/500 images before (**a**)
and after (**b**) IV Gd-DTPA; T_1
maps before (**c**) and after (**d**)
Gd-DTPA. Areas of
enhancement are seen in (**b**)
(arrows). The T_1 value of the
cyst is lower after Gd-DTPA
(**d**) than before (**c**).

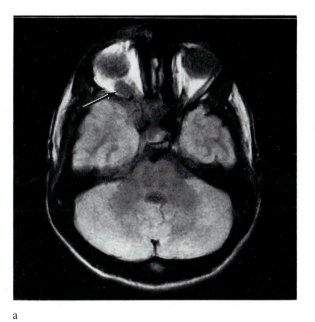

a

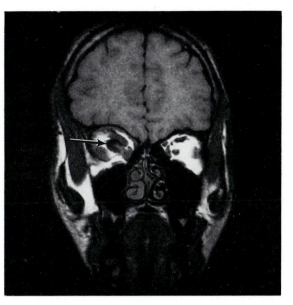

b

Figure 4.6

Optic nerve glioma. SE 2000/30
(**a**) and coronal SE 500/40 (**b**)
images. The tumor (arrows) has
a low-signal intensity on both
images.

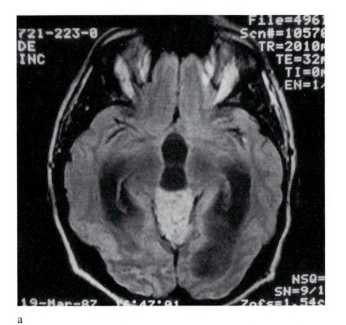

a

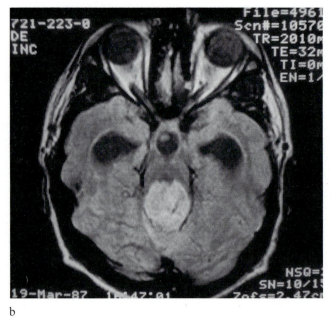

b

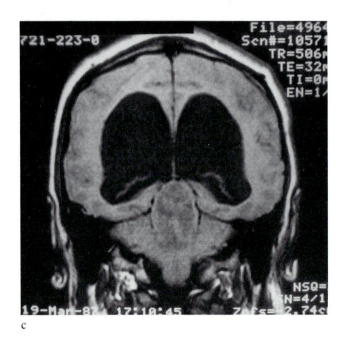

c

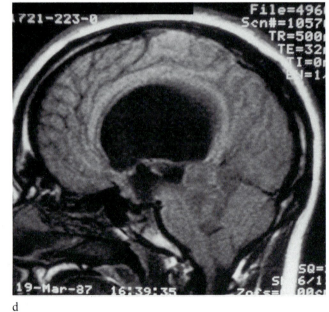

d

Figure 4.7

Ependymoma. SE 2010/32 (**a**),
SE 2000/32 (**b**), coronal SE 506/
32 (**c**), and sagittal SE 500/32
(**d**) images. The tumor is
occupying much of the fourth
ventricle and obstructing CSF
flow, producing
hydrocephalus. *(Courtesy of
Meredith A Weinstein MD,
Cleveland, Ohio)*

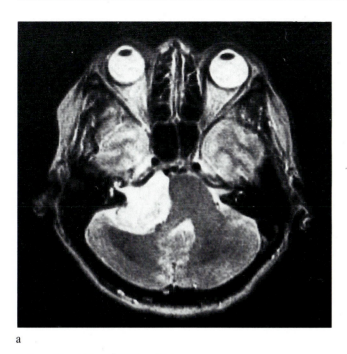

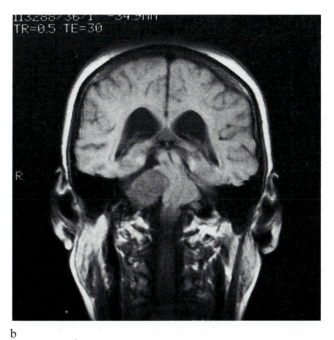

a

b

Figure 4.8

Acoustic neuroma. SE 3000/80
(**a**) and coronal SE 500/30 (**b**)
images. The tumor has a high-
signal intensity on (**a**) and a low
intensity on (**b**).

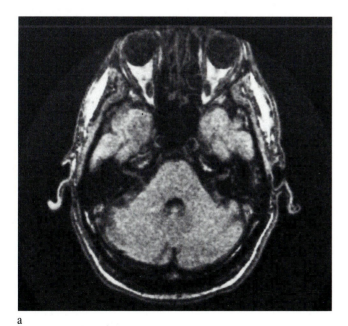

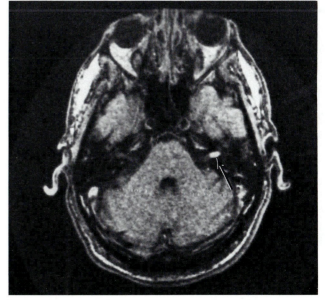

a

b

Figure 4.9

Intracanalicular acoustic
neuroma. PS 200/33 images
before (**a**) and after (**b**) IV Gd-
DTPA. The tumor displays
enhancement (arrow).

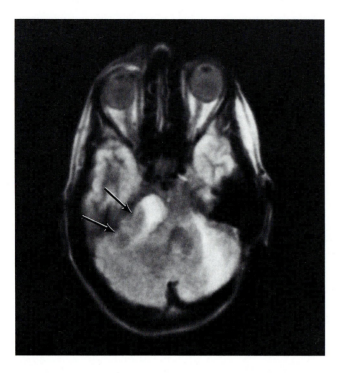

Figure 4.10

Cystic acoustic neuroma. SE 1580/80 image. The tumor has high- and low-signal intensity (arrows) components.

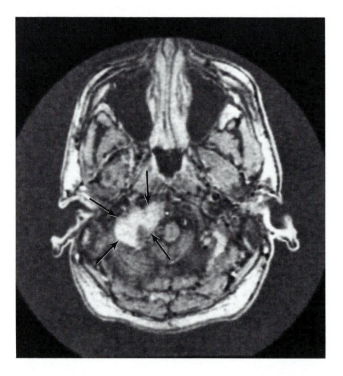

Figure 4.11

Glomus jugulare tumor. PS 300/33 image. The tumor is visualized at the base of the brain (arrows).

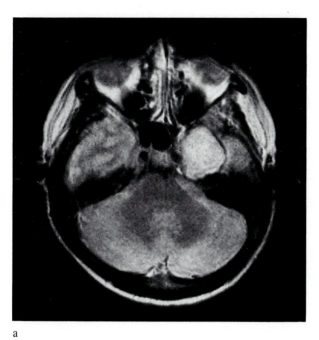

a

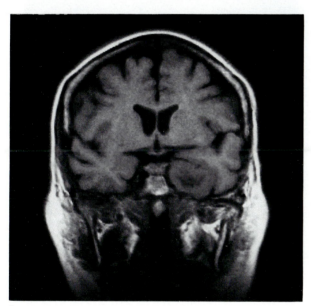

b

Figure 4.12

Trigeminal neuroma. SE 2000/
60 (**a**) and coronal SE 500/30
(**b**) images. The tumor is seen
in a parasellar location.

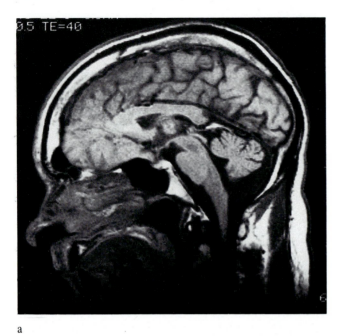

a

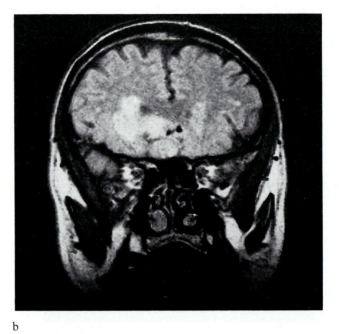

b

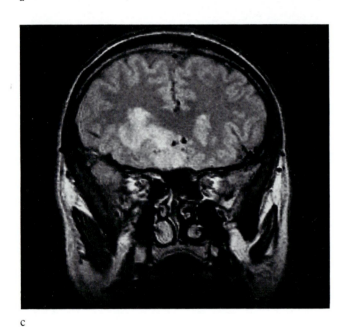

c

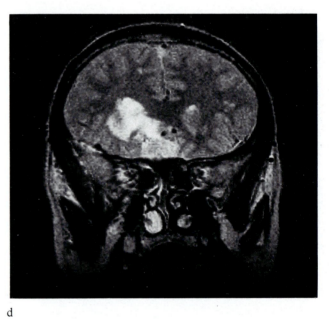

d

Figure 4.13

Meningioma of olfactory
groove. Sagittal SE 500/40 (**a**),
coronal SE 1000/40 (**b**), coronal
SE 1500/40 (**c**), and coronal SE
1500/80 (**d**) images. The tumor
shows low contrast compared
with brain and edema.

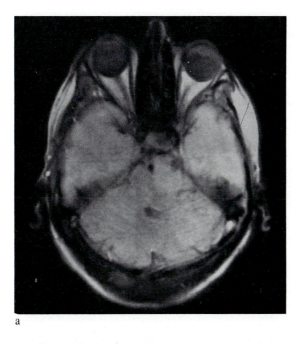

a

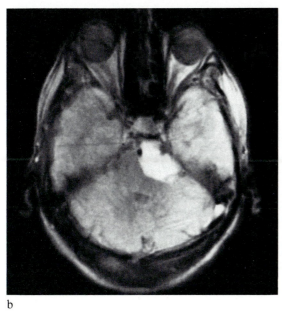

b

Figure 4.14

Cerebellopontine angle
meningioma. SE 200/33 images
before (**a**) and after (**b**) IV Gd-
DTPA. The tumor displays a
high level of enhancement.

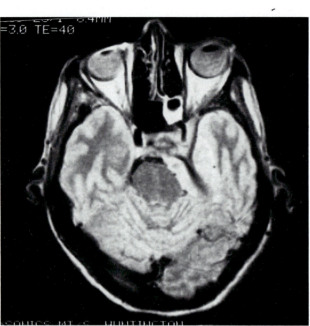

a

b

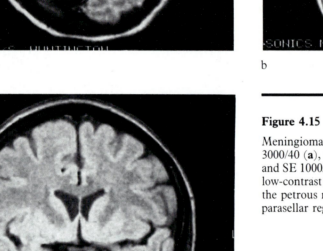

c

Figure 4.15

Meningioma-en-plaque. SE
3000/40 (**a**), SE 1000/40 (**b**),
and SE 1000/40 (**c**) images. The
low-contrast tumor is seen on
the petrous ridge and in the
parasellar region.

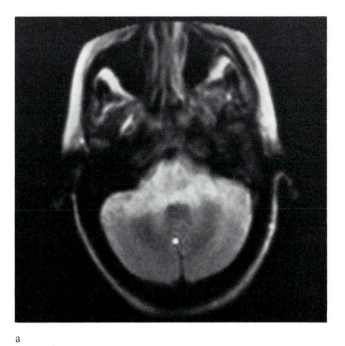

a

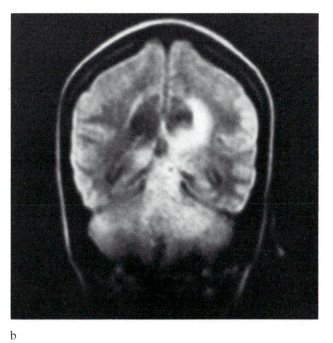

b

Figure 4.16

Primary lymphoma. SE 1580/80 (**a**), coronal SE 1580/80 (**b**), and sagittal SE 1580/80 (**c**) images. The tumor is spread widely within the brainstem and periventricular regions.

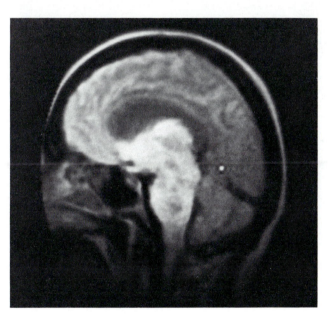

c

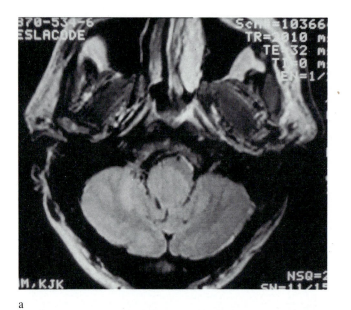

a

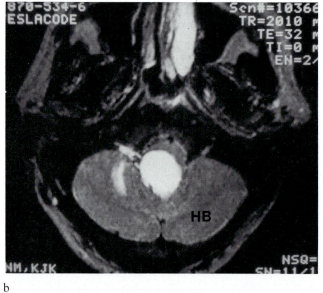

b

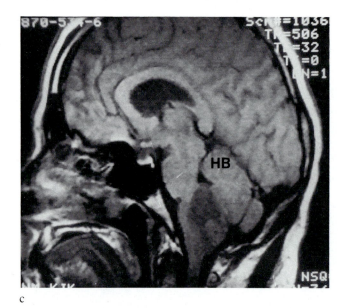

c

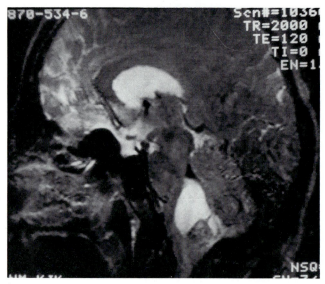

d

Figure 4.17

Hemangioblastoma. SE 506/32 (**a**), SE 2010/32 (**b**), sagittal SE 506/32 (**c**), and sagittal SE 2000/120 (**d**) images. The tumor is invading the fourth ventricle and expanding the brainstem.*(Courtesy of Meredith A Weinstein MD, Cleveland, Ohio)*

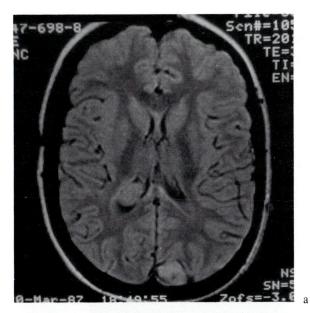

a

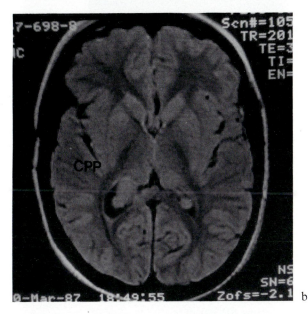

b

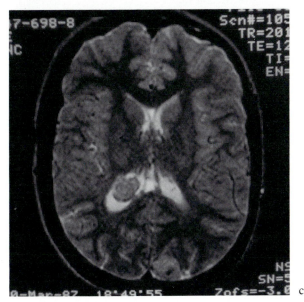

c

Figure 4.18

Papilloma of the choroid
plexus. SE 206/32 (**a**), SE 2010/
32 (**b**), and SE 2010/120 (**c**)
sequence. The tumor is seen in
the lateral ventricle. *(Courtesy of
Meredith A Weinstein MD,
Cleveland, Ohio)*

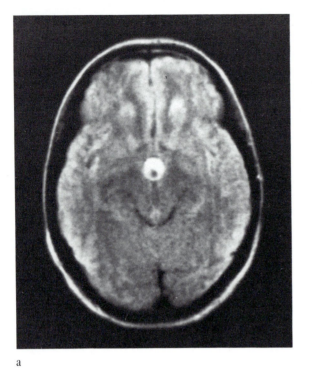

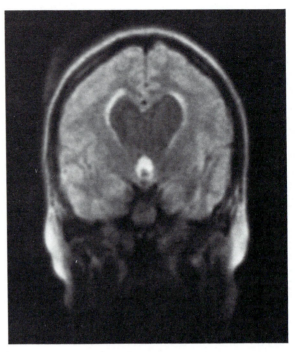

a   b

Figure 4.19

Colloid cyst. SE 1500/80 (**a**)
and coronal SE 1500/80 (**b**)
images. The cyst has a high-
signal intensity with a small
dark area within it.
Periventricular edema is noted.

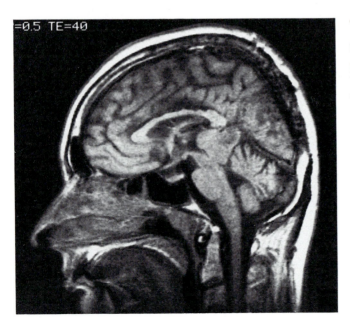

Figure 4.20

Pinealoma. Sagittal SE 500/40.
The tumor is seen in the
characteristic site.

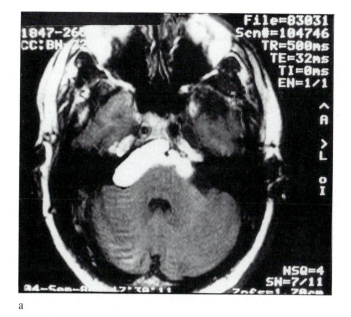

a

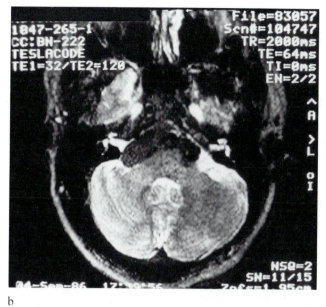

b

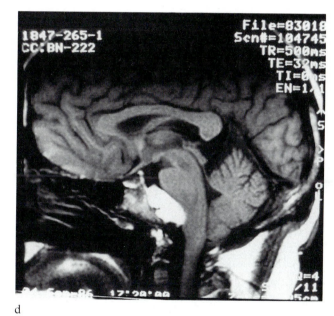

c   d

Figure 4.21

Epidermoid cyst. SE 500/32
(**a**), SE 2000/64 (**b**), coronal SE
500/32 (**c**), and sagittal SE 500/
32 (**d**) images. The tumor has a
short T_1 and T_2. *(Courtesy of
Meredith A Weinstein MD,
Cleveland, Ohio)*

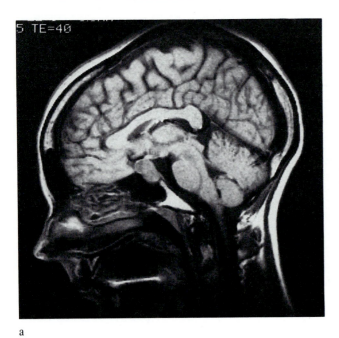

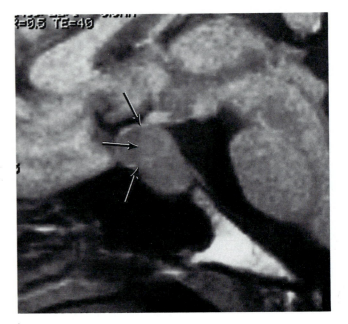

a

b

Figure 4.22

Craniopharyngioma. Sagittal
SE 500/40 (**a**) and enlarged
sagittal SE 500/40 (**b**) images. A
fluid level is seen within the
tumor on (**b**) (arrows).

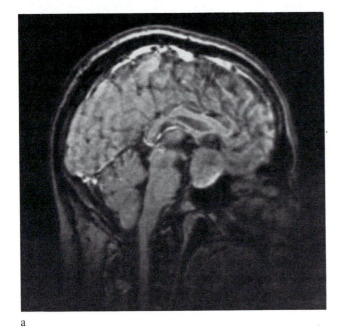

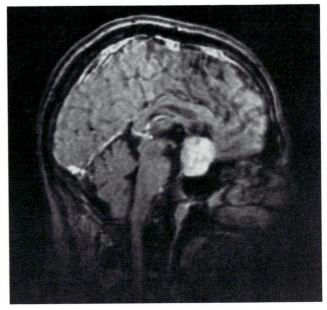

a

b

Figure 4.23

Pituitary macroadenoma. PS
300/33 sequence before (**a**) and
after (**b**) IV Gd-DTPA. The
tumor shows marked inferior
extension.

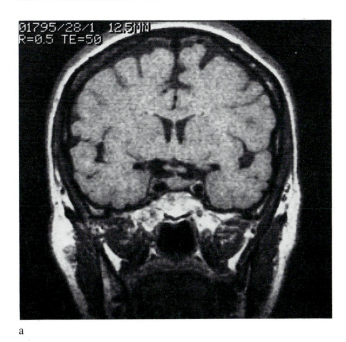

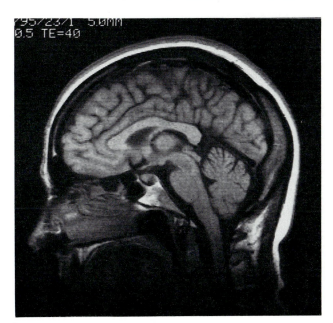

a

b

Figure 4.24

Pituitary microadenoma.
Coronal SE 500/80 (**a**) and
sagittal SE 500/40 (**b**). The
tumor displays an upward
convexity and deviates the
infundibulum.

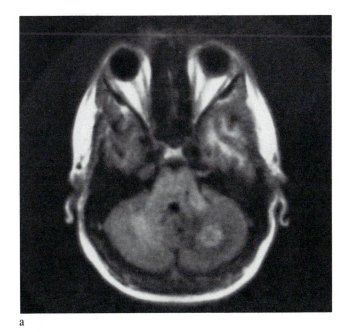

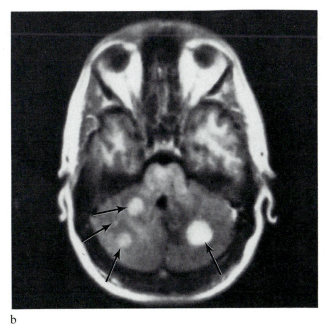

a

b

Figure 4.25

Malignant melanoma
metastases. IR 1500/44/500
images, before (**a**) and after (**b**)
IV Gd-DTPA. More metastases
are seen in (**b**) (arrows).

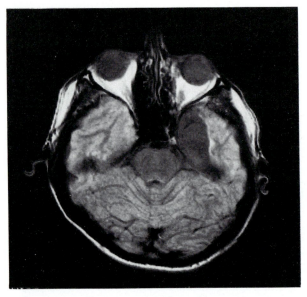

a

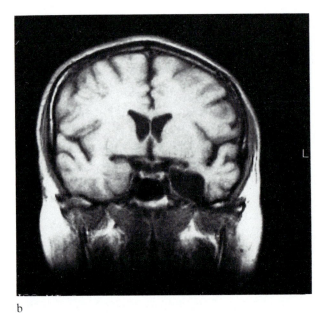

b

Figure 4.26

Arachnoid cyst. SE 2000/30 (**a**)
and coronal SE 500/30 (**b**) images.
The cyst is displacing the
adjacent temporal lobe.

5

Ischemia-infarction

William G Bradley

Stroke is the third leading cause of death in the USA, exceeded only by heart disease and cancer. Over 300 000 people are affected annually by cerebral ischemia.[1] Half of these will develop fixed neurologic deficits.[2] Symptoms in the other half will resolve without a fixed deficit. Resolution within 24 hours is called a transient ischemia attack (TIA); resolution within three days is generally known as a RIND (reversible ischemia neurologic deficit). Each time a stroke occurs, there is a 15 to 35 per cent chance of death.[2] When hemorrhage is present, the mortality figure rises to between 60 and 80 per cent.[2] As the elderly population increases in the future, stroke will become an even more important diagnostic and therapeutic problem.

'Stroke' is a non-specific term indicating an acute neurologic event. While arteriosclerosis is by far the leading cause of stroke, acute neurologic events can also result from hemorrhage secondary to rupture of an aneurysm or bleeding from an AVM. Less common causes of stroke include bleeding into metastatic or primary tumors or, even less commonly, subdural hematomas. Since arteriosclerotic strokes usually involve a known vascular distribution, they are generally distinguishable from strokes due to other causes by either CT or MRI.

The use of CT or MRI is indicated in the acute setting since subsequent treatment, such as anticoagulation or surgical decompression, may depend on the findings of hemorrhage and mass effect from the imaging study. Unfortunately, when an arteriosclerotic etiology of stroke has been determined, the degree of abnormality on MRI or CT may not correlate well with the degree of clinical impairment. According to its location, a relatively large lesion on MRI may be totally asymptomatic, minimally symptomatic, or quite symptomatic. This is certainly true for the correlation between MR findings and the degree of psychometric impairment in deep white matter infarction.[3] It is also true regarding the hemorrhage associated with stroke. While hemorrhage in the first several days post ictus is almost always symptomatic (due to reperfusion following embolization), petechial hemorrhage in the second week post ictus is rarely symptomatic.[1] Finally, clinical decisions regarding anticoagulation are currently based on the initial detection of hemorrhage by CT. How these clinical decisions will be modified by the MR detection of subtler levels of acute hemorrhage (using high-field or gradient-echo techniques) remains to be determined.

Pathophysiology

The pathophysiologic events comprising cerebral ischemia and infarction have been discussed in considerable detail by other authors.[1,2,4–10] Some—but certainly not all—of these events are visible by MRI. Additional events may only be apparent by MR spectroscopy.[11] As the word 'ischemia' implies, these events result from decreased blood supply to the brain. Since blood contains both oxygen and glucose, ischemia is to be differentiated from hypoxia or anoxia (decreased or absent oxygen) and hypoglycemia (decreased glucose), both of which can produce stroke-like symptoms. While anoxia and hypoglycemia tend to be global, that is, to involve the entire intracerebral circulation, ischemia can be *either* focal or global.

143

Symptoms associated with focal ischemia depend on the part of the brain involved. All global processes eventually lead to coma. In addition, focal lesions differ from global processes in their dependence on the time course of the occlusion. Slow, focal occlusion may not produce ischemic symptoms if there is time for development of collateral pathways. Such pathways are not available, of course, for global ischemia.

Following interruption of blood supply to the brain, oxidative phosphorylation ceases.[6] As anaerobic pathways attempt to maintain cellular metabolism, lactic acid is formed and ATP levels fall. Since ATP is required to power the sodium/potassium pump, it too begins to fail. As a result, sodium begins to enter the cell and potassium begins to leave. The influx of sodium is matched by an influx of water during the first few hours,[1] and the cell swells. At this point, the cell becomes non-functional and the patient may become symptomatic, depending on the location of the lesion.[6] The additional cellular water is known as 'cytotoxic edema' (Figure 5.1a), in contrast to the more common 'vasogenic edema' (Figure 5.1b), produced by blood-brain barrier breakdown.[5] Ischemic or cytotoxic edema is reversible. While function is lost, structure has been maintained.[6] Thus, if the blood supply to the cell is re-established, function can be restored.

Several groups have investigated the MR features of cytotoxic edema in an attempt to distinguish reversible from irreversible damage.[8-10] The usual animal model for cytotoxic edema is triethyl tin (TET) intoxication.[5] While this produces cellular swelling, it also causes vesicles to appear in the myelin sheaths.[9] The ultrafiltrate in these vesicles is essentially pure water, which has longer T_1 and T_2 times than the more proteinaceous vasogenic edema.[8-10] Using the TET model of cytotoxic edema, therefore, a 'fast' and 'slow' relaxing compartment can be found (compared to the single 'fast' compartment model of vasogenic edema).[8-10] However, the myelin vesicles which lead to the long relaxation times in the slow compartment may be an artifact of the TET model and may not be related to clinical ischemia per se. Thus fitting the decay curves with one or two exponentials to determine the number of compartments has not been found to be useful clinically to distinguish cytotoxic from vasogenic edema.

There have been two anecdotal reports of cytotoxic edema suggested by MRI in the clinical setting. In one case, the cortex adjacent to an AVM was hyperintense prior to embolization and returned to normal intensity after embolization,[12] as illustrated in Figure 5.2. This was interpreted as ischemia due to a vascular steal phenomenon from the high flow AVM. In another report, two patients with lupus cerebritis had focal hyperintensity in the cortex which returned to normal after steroid treatment.[13] In general, it is difficult to distinguish between cytotoxic and vasogenic edema by MRI as they tend to be intermixed,[6] and both demonstrate high signal on T_2-weighted images.

If the ischemia persists, proteins in the electron-transport chain become reduced and catalyze the formation of free radicals.[6] These pathologically-produced free radicals attack the fatty acid moieties (for example, arachadonic acid) on the phospholipids in the cellular membranes and those of organelles such as mitochondria. Their breakdown leads to accumulation of free fatty acids.[6] These add to the osmolarity of the ischemic region, drawing in more water. As the mass effect increases, the microcirculation becomes more compromised, increasing the ischemia.

Continued ischemia and acidosis first destroy the mitochondria and then the cytoplasmic membranes. Loss of vascular endothelial integrity follows, which leads to breakdown in the blood-brain barrier and accumulation of vasogenic edema. When the defects in the blood-brain barrier are large enough, the infarct will be enhanced with iodinated contrast on CT or gadolinium-DTPA on MRI.[1]

If perfusion to the ischemic, hyperosmotic tissues is re-established via the normal vessels (for example, by breakup of an embolus) or via collaterals, the edema can worsen significantly. The mass effect can lead to further compromise in the microcirculation, extending the infarction into the penumbra of less damaged tissue surrounding the central lesion and separating it from the normal brain at the periphery.[1] Reperfusion can also increase tissue damage by subjecting the friable ischemic endothelium to arterial pressures, leading to gross vascular disruption and hemorrhage. This is thought to be the mechanism responsible for hemorrhagic infarction (Figure 5.3) in the setting of embolic stroke following breakup of the embolism.[2]

If perfusion is not re-established, the infarct remains 'bland' by CT criteria during the first week. During the second week, asymptomatic petechial hemorrhage (Figure 5.4) has been noted in 42 per cent of previously bland infarcts by CT.[14] Grossly, during the first two weeks, the vasogenic edema (and concomitant mass effect) increases and then plateaus. During the third week, the mass effect begins to resolve (Figures 5.4f and g).

During the 'subacute phase', which begins several days to a week post ictus, 'luxury perfusion' is noted, producing enhancement in a typical gyral pattern, as shown in Figure 5.5. This is probably due to neovascular capillary proliferation,[4] with formation of an incomplete blood-brain barrier. Loss of autoregulation in leptomeningeal collaterals has also been suggested as a mechanism for luxury perfusion.[2] Such enhancement can be seen up to 8 to 10 weeks post ictus. If it persists beyond this time, a neoplasm should be suspected.

In the 'chronic phase' the loss of brain substance

becomes evident. Microscopically, there is a general loss of cellular elements and demyelination. Since myelin is hydrophobic, this allows an increase in the water content of the damaged tissue. Small cystic spaces appear between the remaining cellular elements, replacing a portion of the normal parenchyma. Pathologically the brain softens; this is called 'encephalomalacia'.[1,2] As the repair continues, there is continued loss of brain substance, enlargement of the overlying subarachnoid space, and eventually confluence of some of the small cystic spaces into larger cysts. On CT, the encephalomalacic brain appears hypodense. On moderately T_2-weighted MRI, two zones can be seen: a zone of hyperintensity adjacent to the normal brain and a more peripheral region of CSF intensity, as shown in Figure 5.6. The hyperintensity on moderately T_2-weighted MRI appears to correlate with the small cystic spaces seen microscopically and thus has been called 'microcystic encephalomalacia',[15] or 'gliosis'. The larger cystic spaces which appear CSF-like on moderately T_2-weighted MR images are called 'macroscopic encephalomalacia'.[15] Since the macrocystic encephalomalacia has the same signal intensity as CSF, it can be difficult to separate it from the overlying enlarged subarachnoid space. It has been postulated that the amount of microcystic encephalomalacia reflects the degree of mass effect present at the time of the acute infarct.[15] A similar pattern of central microcystic encephalomalacia and peripheral macrocystic encephalomalacia can be seen after surgery, as illustrated in Figure 5.7, or following trauma.

The different MR characteristics of microcystic and macrocystic encephalomalacia are due to the different environments of water in the brain. The many small cysts in the microcystic form provide a large surface area which attracts the water molecules in hydration layers. As discussed in Chapter 1, this hydration-layer environment has a shorter T_1 than CSF, which tends to increase its signal intensity.[16] In the macrocystic form, water is predominately in the bulk phase, and this explains its similarity in appearance to CSF.

Large vessel disease

The carotid bifurcation is the most common site of atherosclerotic disease leading to cerebral infarction.[2] There are three ways by which disease of the carotid bulb can lead to intracranial symptoms.[2] The first is occlusion due to plaque formation; however, unilateral disease is usually asymptomatic due to crossover flow at the Circle of Willis. On the other hand, carotid disease tends to be bilateral. Thus when flow through both carotid arteries falls below the threshold necessary for normal metabolic activity, symptoms will

occur. A second mechanism for stroke in the setting of carotid disease is embolization of small thrombi formed on the surface of an ulcerated plaque. A third (less common) mechanism is embolization of the plaque material itself.[2]

Thrombi from the cervical carotid artery or, less commonly, the intracranial carotid siphon generally flow into the middle cerebral distribution.[2] This produces infarction in the temporal, posterior and lateral frontal, and lateral parietal lobes, shown in Figures 5.8 and 5.9. Emboli to the anterior cerebral artery involve medial portions of the frontal and parietal lobes adjacent to the falx (Figure 5.10). Total occlusion (Figure 5.11) or very slow flow (Figure 5.12) in the internal carotid artery without sufficient crossover flow through the circle of Willis leads to infarction in both the anterior and middle cerebral arterial distributions (Figures 5.6 and 5.13).

The posterior cerebral circulation is less commonly involved by embolic disease than the anterior circulation, since the posterior cerebral arteries are normally supplied by the vertebrobasilar system which tends to have less arteriosclerosis.[2] Infarcts of the occipital lobes (Figure 5.14), brainstem (Figures 5.15 and 5.16), and cerebellum (Figures 5.15 and 5.17) are more commonly due to arteriosclerotic narrowing of local small arteries or extracranial emboli from ulcerated plaques in the subclavian artery, aortic arch or from thrombi originating in the heart.[2] Brain stem infarcts (Figure 5.18) are often seen in hypertensive patients with subcortical arteriosclerotic encephalopathy and deep white matter infarcts.[17] Both brain stem infarcts[18] and deep white matter infarcts[3] are better seen by MRI than CT due to the relative insensitivity of the older modality in the posterior fossa and periventricular region, respectively. While MRI is more sensitive than CT in lesion detection in these locations, correlation with clinical findings is poor.[3,18] Other brainstem lesions without mass effect, such as infiltrating gliomas and central pontine myelinolysis (Figure 5.19), can potentially be confused with brainstem infarcts.

On MRI, the typical bland infarct is characteristically hypointense on T_1-weighted images and hyperintense on T_2-weighted images, relative to normal brain, as illustrated in Figure 5.4. These changes reflect T_1 and T_2 prolongation due to increased water content. The T_1 and T_2 prolongation can be seen within the first hour after vascular occlusion in experimental animals.[1] Lack of a normal flow void (Figure 5.11) in the occluded vessel may be visualized by MRI and help determine the level of obstruction. When flow is slow but not totally obstructed, even-echo rephasing (see Chapter 3) may be seen in arteries if a symmetric second echo is acquired (Figures 5.12 and 5.16).

Mass effect from acute infarction increases over the first week, plateaus during the second week, and begins to resolve by the third week. On heavily T_2-weighted images at high field, interstitial hemorrhage can often be seen during the second week, as in Figure 5.4. This does not depend on whether or not the patient has been anticoagulated and does not correlate with worsening of symptoms. When present, frank hemorrhage generally occurs within the first several days and definitely does correlate with clinical worsening. Hemorrhagic infarcts (Figure 5.3) are generally due to embolic disease with subsequent breakup of the embolus and reperfusion of the ischemic region. The appearance of hemorrhage is described in detail in Chapter 7. Following hemorrhagic infarction, local hemosiderin deposition is noted which may persist forever, as depicted in Figure 5.3. If the hemorrhage breaks into the ventricular system, the patient may be left with a porencephalic cyst, shown in Figure 5.8.

Global ischemia generally results from high-grade stenoses of the carotid arteries. Cardiac arrythmias and hypotension can also be causative in their own right or can add to otherwise subclinical stenoses. As the perfusion pressure drops below the autoregulatory threshold, the blood supply to the brain becomes linearly dependent on systolic blood pressure. As the blood pressure continues to drop, the areas of the brain which are at the distal ends of a given vascular supply, or those between two vascular territories, begin to experience ischemia first. These 'watershed' infarcts are located in the periventricular region (Figure 5.18) between the deep medullary circulation (for example, the lenticulostriate and thalamoperforator arteries) and the superficial cortical circulation (such as the middle cerebral artery). In the chronic setting, this mechanism may be responsible for deep white matter infarction (see below). Infarcts can also be noted in the watershed regions between the major vascular territories, as in Figure 5.20, due to selective decrease in the blood supply to two neighbouring vessels and their corresponding vascular territories.

In adults, the gray matter has a higher metabolism than the white and is, therefore, more susceptible to acute cessation of blood supply.[1,2] Thus, adult infarcts are characterized by combined cortical and subcortical involvement in a wedge-shaped vascular distribution, as shown in Figures 5.6, 5.9 and 5.17. In young children, the white matter is hypermetabolic relative to gray matter due to the extensive myelination taking place.[1] Thus, global ischemia in children involves the periventricular white matter for two reasons: the watershed configuration of the vascular supply and the relative hypermetabolism of the white matter. The resulting periventricular leukomalacia (Figure 5.21) reflects the sensitivity of this region to ischemia. Thalamic iron deposition (Figure 5.21) has been noted in such children following severe ischemic anoxic events, such as cardiopulmonary arrest, drowning, or umbilical cord compression during delivery.[19]

Infarction secondary to subarachnoid hemorrhage may be multifocal due to spasm in multiple vessels. While MRI lacks the spatial resolution to demonstrate the vascular spasm per se, it easily shows the resulting infarcts. Although MRI is generally less sensitive than CT in the detection of subarachnoid hemorrhage, it may demonstrate the lesion responsible for the hemorrhage, for example, aneurysm or AVM, and may demonstrate a subarachnoid thrombus near the site of origin of the bleeding. (Chapter 7 covers this topic in more detail.)

Infarction can occur secondary to meningitis, particularly the basilar, granulomatous forms. The resulting infarcts may be cortical or deep within the white matter due to lenticulostriate involvement. A similar distribution of infarcts can be seen in leptomeningeal carcinomatosis.

Infarction can result from trauma. Contusions generally occur adjacent to fixed, bony structures. Thus the finding of gliosis in the inferior frontal lobes suggests prior trauma, as in Figure 5.22. Shearing injury to the white matter results from rotatory trauma to the brain. Axonal shearing injury can produce a pattern similar to deep white matter infarction. Shearing injuries tend to involve long white matter tracts, including the entire corona radiata from the vertex to the hypothalamus shown in Figure 5.23. They can be relatively limited (Figure 5.23) or more severe (Figures 5.24 and 5.25), involving large portions of the periventricular white matter. The most severe injuries occur at the corticomedullary junction, illustrated in Figure 5.26, simulating subcortical infarcts. These have the worst prognosis.

Infarction can occur secondary to other lesions in the brain which have significant mass effect. When the brain herniates against the free edge of the falx or the tentorium, vascular compression may lead to infarction in the distribution of the particular vessel. Subfalcine herniation, for example, may catch the anterior cerebral artery between the falx and the medial edge of the herniating frontal lobe, leading to infarction of the ipsilateral anterior cerebral distribution. Temporal lobe mass effect may catch the posterior cerebral artery between the mesial aspect of the temporal lobe and the free edge of the tentorium at the incisura, leading to infarction of the ipsilateral occipital lobe.

Small vessel disease

Arteriosclerosis of the small perforating vessels leads to lacunar infarcts ('lacunes', Figure 5.27) in the deep gray structures, that is, the basal ganglia. These are often found in the setting of hypertension. When they involve the posterior limb of the adjacent internal capsule, a predictable symptom complex develops. Lacunes at the genu of the internal capsule lead to contralateral facial palsy. Lesions from the genu to the midportion of the posterior limb lead to contralateral hemiparesis involving the upper body and legs. Lesions of the posterior half of the posterior limb produce contralateral hemisensory deficits. Lacunes of the subthalamic nucleus may produce hemiballismus.[20] Hypertensive arteriosclerosis of the lenticulostriate and thalamoperforator arteries may be associated with hemorrhage due to rupture of small Charcot-Bouchard aneurysms (Figure 5.28).

Lesions of the medium-sized perforating vessels can also produce deep white matter infarction, shown in Figures 5.18 and 5.29. These vessels are particularly prone to arteriosclerosis. They also have a long parenchymal course[21] and are, therefore, among the first vessels to be affected when the general perfusion of the brain is decreased with advancing age.[22,23]

There has been substantial controversy regarding the etiology of the high-intensity lesions which are found so ubiquitously in the elderly population in the periventricular white matter and centrum semiovale.[21-30] Some investigators have suggested that these lesions are enlarged perivascular spaces and this may well be true at the vertex (Figure 5.30) or adjacent to the anterior commissure (Figure 5.31). These tend to be round or oval and are always well-marginated. They represent enlarged Virchow-Robin spaces (which are extensions of the subarachnoid space). When severe, they produce a state known as 'état criblé', shown in Figure 5.32.[25] Others have suggested that periventricular demyelination without associated infarction can lead to the observed abnormalities.[26]

In a recent report, MRI–histopathologic correlation was obtained in 14 elderly cadaver brains.[27] Using MRI to guide the subsequent histopathologic evaluation, the larger, irregular bright spots in the periventricular region and centrum semiovale were found to represent small central infarcts with surrounding reactive astrocytes.[27] When immunostained against glial fibrillary acidic protein (GFAP), IgG, and albumin, these reactive astrocytes were seen to align with the myelin sheaths in a pattern known as 'isomorphic gliosis'.[27,31] They were found over a much larger volume than the central cavity of the infarct, generally extending outward in the direction of the flow of edema at the time of blood-brain barrier breakdown. In fact, it is hypothesized that the astrocytes become reactive, taking up the serum proteins at the time of acute infarction and blood-brain barrier breakdown.[32] The general lack of correlation between the size and extent of the abnormalities on MRI and degree of psychometric impairment[3] may be due to the fact that most of the abnormality on MRI is still functional brain in the zones of isomorphic gliosis surrounding the central non-functional infarct cavity. In addition, correlation is poor because these small non-functional areas in the center of the MR abnormality may not involve tracts which are symptomatic when destroyed.

Deep white matter infarction is aggravated following radiation therapy to the brain.[33] This presumably reflects the additive effects of subclinical arteriosclerosis and radiation vasculitis of the long penetrating vessels with resulting watershed infarction downstream, illustrated in Figure 5.33. When patients who have received whole brain irradiation are compared with age-matched controls, the incidence of deep white matter infarction increases markedly with age.[33]

The small vessels of the brain may also be involved by autoimmune or infectious vasculitis leading to small cortical infarcts in their distribution. Systemic lupus erythematosus (SLE) is the most common cause of autoimmune vasculitis in the brain (Figure 5.34), and can also produce a pattern of central patchy hyperintensity similar to that of multiple sclerosis (MS), as shown in Figure 5.35. This pattern has been called 'lupus sclerosis'. When an MS pattern is found in combination with small cortical infarcts, the possibility of a vasculitis should be considered.

Focal deep white matter abnormalities have also been noted in patients with common or classic migraine, demonstrated in Figure 5.36. In a recent series of 18 patients with migraine, 50 per cent had abnormalities which appeared like deep white matter infarcts on their MR scans.[34] These patients did not have complicated or 'hemiplegic' migraine, nor did they have neurologic deficits at the time of MR examination. The abnormalities were deep within the white matter, without a particular propensity for the occipital lobes. These were presumably due to small infarcts secondary to vascular spasm from the migraine; however, this etiology is speculative at this time. Regardless of the pathophysiology, the presence of migraine headaches should be questioned in patients presenting with a pattern similar to deep white matter infarction or MS.

Venous disease

Infarction can result from venous obstruction as well as from arterial occlusion.[2] Following venous obstruction, edema accumulates upstream leading to compromise of the microcirculation and so-called 'venous infarcts', which are shown in Figure 5.37. These tend to be hemorrhagic.[2] Infarction is more often produced by thrombosis of individual cortical veins rather than dural sinuses, since alternative collateral pathways of venous drainage can develop in the latter circumstance. Nevertheless, the finding of multiple hemorrhagic infarcts should prompt a search for thrombus in the dural sinuses (Figure 5.37c) or in the veins draining the area of abnormality.

References

1 BRANT-ZAWADZKI M, Ischemia. In: Stark DD, Bradley WG, eds. *Magnetic resonance imaging.* (CV Mosby and Co: St Louis 1988) 299–315.

2 HORTON JA, Cerebral infarction. In: Latchaw RE, ed. *Computed tomography of the head, neck, and spine.* (Year Book Medical Publishers: Chicago 1985) 101–15.

3 BRANT-ZAWADZKI M, FEIN G, VAN DYKE C et al, Magnetic resonance of the aging brain: patchy white matter lesions and dementia, *AJNR* (1985) **6**(5):675–82.

4 GOLDBERG HI, Stroke. In: Lee SH, Rao KCVG, eds. *Cranial computed tomography.* (McGraw-Hill: New York 1967) Chapter 15.

5 KLATZO I, SEITELBERGER F, eds, *Brain edema,* (Springer: New York 1967).

6 SHALLER CA, JACQUES S, SHELDEN CH, The pathophysiology of stroke: a review with molecular considerations, *Surg Neurol* (1980) **14**:433–43.

7 GARCIA JH, Experimental ischemic stroke: a review, *Stroke* (1984) **15**(1):5–14.

8 NARUSE S, HORIKAWA Y, TANAKA C et al, Proton nuclear magnetic resonance studies on brain edema, *J Neurosurg* (1982) **56**:747–52.

9 GO KG, EDZES HT, Water in brain edema—observations by the pulsed nuclear magnetic resonance technique, *Arch Neurol* (1975) **32**:462–5.

10 BAKAY L, KURLAND RJ, PARRISH RG et al, Nuclear magnetic resonance studies in normal and edematous brain tissue, *Exp Brain Res* (1975) **23**:241–8.

11 BRANT-ZAWADZKI M, WEINSEIN P, BARTKOWSKI H et al, MR imaging and spectroscopy in clinical and experimental cerebral ischemia: a review, *AJR* (1987) **148**:579–88.

12 BRADLEY WG, Magnetic resonance imaging of the central nervous system, *Neurol Res* (1984) **6**:91–106.

13 AISEN AM, GABRIELSEN TO, MCCUNE WJ, MR imaging of systemic lupus erythematosus involving the brain, *AJNR* (1985) **6**:197–201.

14 HORNING CR, DORNDORF W, AGNOLI AL, Hemorrhagic cerebral infarction: a progressive study, *Stroke* (1986) **17**:179–84.

15 BRADLEY WG, Pathophysiologic correlates of signal alterations. In: Brant-Zawadzki M, Norman D, eds. *Magnetic resonance imaging of the central nervous system.* (Raven Press: New York 1987) 23–42.

16 FULLERTON GD, CAMERON IL, ORD VA, Frequency dependence of magnetic resonance spin-lattice relaxation of protons in biological materials, *Radiology* (1984) **151**:135–8.

17 SALOMON A, YEATES AE, BURGER PC et al, Subcortical arteriosclerotic encephalopathy: brain stem findings with MR imaging, *Radiology* (1987) **165**:625–9.

18 BILLER J, ADAMS HP, DUNN V et al, Dichotomy between clinical findings and MR abnormalities in pontine infarction, *J Comput Assist Tomogr* (1986) **10**(3):379–85.

19 DIETRICH RB, BRADLEY WG, Iron accumulation in the basal ganglia following severe ischemic-anoxia insults in children, *Radiology* (1988) **168**:203–6.

20 BILLER J, GRAFF-RADFORD NR, SMOKER WRK et al, MR imaging in 'lacunar' hemiballismus, *J Comput Assist Tomogr* (1986) **10**(5):793–7.

21 GOTO K, ISHII N, FUKASAWA H, Diffuse white-matter disease in the geriatric population, *Radiology* (1981) **141**:687–95.

22 ZIMMERMAN RD, FLEMING CA, SAINT-LOUIS LA et al, Periventricular hyperintensity as seen by magnetic resonance: prevalence and significance, *AJR* (1986) **146**:443–50.

23 HEISS WD, HERHOLZ K, BOCHER-SCHWARZ HG et al, PET, CT, and MR imaging in cerebrovascular disease, *J Comput Assist Tomogr* (1986) **19**(6):903–11.

24 DRAYER BP, Imaging of the aging brain. Part I: Normal findings, *Radiology* (1988) **166**:785–96 and Part II: Pathologic findings, *Radiology* (1988) **166**:797–806.

25 AWAD IA, JOHNSON PC, SPETZLER RF et al, Incidental subcortical lesions identified on magnetic resonance imaging in the elderly. II. Postmortem pathological correlations, *Stroke* (1986) **17**(6):1090–97.

26 KIRKPATRICK JB, HAYMAN LA, White-matter lesions in MR imaging of clinically healthy brains of elderly subjects: possible pathologic basis, *Radiology* (1987) **162**:509–11.

27 MARSHALL VG, BRADLEY WG, MARSHALL CE et al, Deep white matter infarction: correlation of MR imaging and histopathologic findings, *Radiology* (1988) **167**:517–22.

28 GEORGE AE, DE LEON MJ, KALNIN A et al, Leukoencephalopathy in normal and pathologic aging. II. MRI of brain lucencies, *AJNR* (1986) **7**:567–70.

29 FAZEKA F, CHAWLUK JB, ALAVI A et al, MR signal abnormalities at 1.5T in Alzheimer's dementia and normal aging, *AJNR* (1986) **8**:421–26

30 BRADLEY WG, WALUCH V, BRANT-ZAWADZKI M et al, Patchy, periventricular white matter lesions in the elderly: a common observation during NMR imaging, *Noninvasive Med Imaging* (1984) **1**(1):35–41.

31 ESCOURELLE R, POIRIER J, *Manual of basic neuropathology,* (Saunders: Philadelphia 1978) 26–7.

32 COLLET A, JACQUE C, Water soluble and insoluble GFA in the brain of patients having had a cerebrovascular accident, *Birth Defects* (1983) **9**:413–23.

33 TSURUDA JS, KORTMAN KE, BRADLEY WG et al, Radiation effects on cerebral white matter: MR evaluation, *AJNR* (1987) **8**:431–7.

34 SOGES LJ, CACAYORIN ED, RAMUCHANDRON TS et al, Migraine: evaluation by MRI, *AJNR* (1988) **9**:425–9.

Cytotoxic Edema

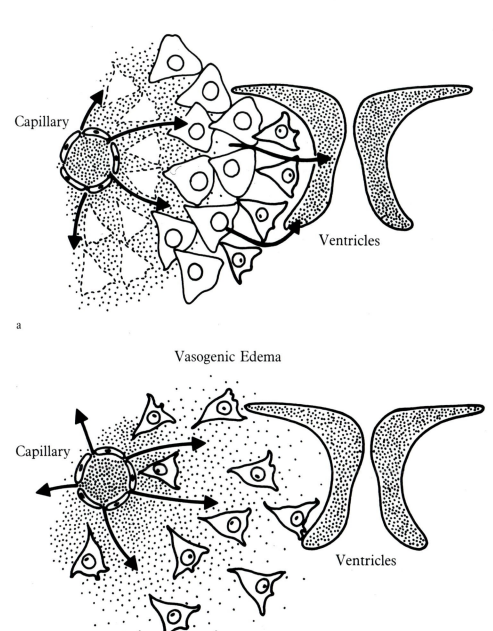

Capillary

Ventricles

a

Vasogenic Edema

Capillary

Ventricles

b

Figure 5.1

Brain edema. (**a**) Cytotoxic edema is produced by ischemia, that is, decrease in the blood supply to a cell. Failure of the sodium/potassium pump results in cellular swelling and local mass effect. If the blood supply to the cell is re-established, function can be restored. (**b**) Vasogenic edema results from cellular death. Blood-brain barrier breakdown results in extravasation of plasma from the disrupted capillaries, that is, increasing proteinaceous fluid in the extracellular space.

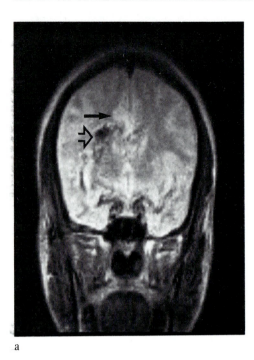

a

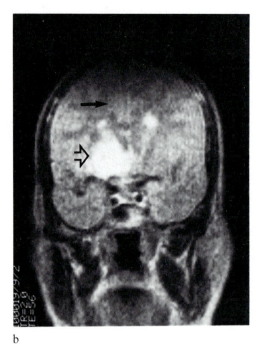

b

Figure 5.2

MR demonstration of cytotoxic edema. (**a**) T$_2$-weighted coronal image through AVM (open arrow) demonstrates high signal and mass effect in the cingulate gyrus (arrow) (SE 2000/56). (**b**) Following embolization of the AVM, the cingulate gyrus (arrow) has returned to normal intensity and a right thalamic infarct has resulted from the embolization (open arrow). Resolution of the high signal in the cingulate gyrus indicates reversible ischemia (with cytotoxic edema) secondary to a vascular steal phenomenon from the AVM (SE 2000/56).

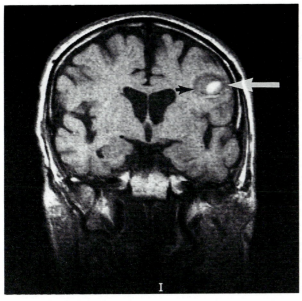

a

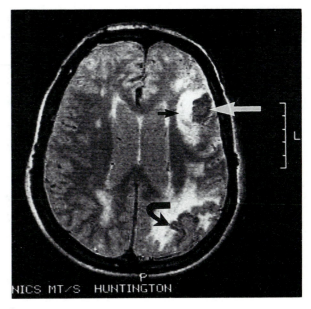

b

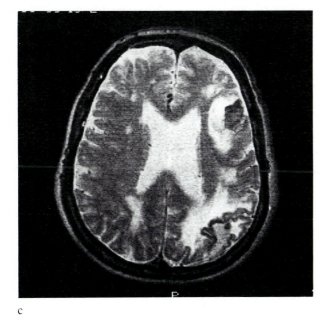

c

Figure 5.3

Hemorrhagic infarction. (**a**) T_1-weighted coronal section demonstrates high-signal intensity (arrow) in left frontal lobe due to methemoglobin in early subacute hemorrhagic infarct. Note medial low-signal intensity (arrowhead) due to associated vasogenic edema (SE 500/30). (**b**) Moderately T_2-weighted axial section through left frontal lesion now demonstrates hypointensity due to short T_2 intracellular methemoglobin (arrow) with hyperintense vasogenic edema (arrowhead) due to its long T_2. Note superficial siderosis posteriorly due to previous hemorrhagic infarct (curved arrow) (SE 3000/40). (**c**) Heavily T_2-weighted axial section through same level as (**b**) demonstrating lower signal in both left frontal hematoma and left parietal superficial siderosis due to magnetic susceptibility effects (SE 3000/80).

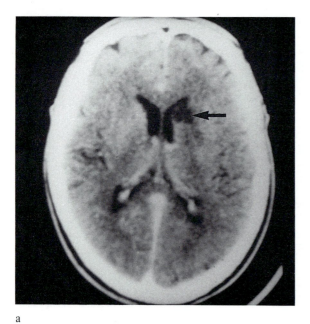

a

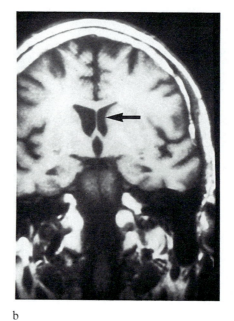

b

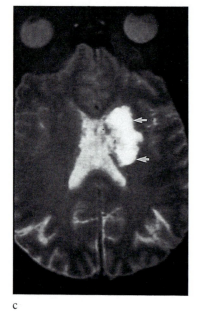

c

Figure 5.4

Petechial hemorrhage in 'bland' infarct. (**a**) Enhanced CT scan demonstrates focal hypodensity in left caudate head (arrow) with mass effect on left frontal horn due to infarction three days earlier. (**b**) T_1-weighted coronal section obtained several hours after CT demonstrates mass effect on left frontal horn (arrow) (SE 600/20).
(**c**) Heavily T_2-weighted axial section through same level as (**b**) demonstrates more diffuse hyperintensity (arrowheads) than suspected on CT scan in (**a**). Note mass effect on left frontal horn. This reflects the presence of vasogenic edema in a bland infarct (SE 2800/80).

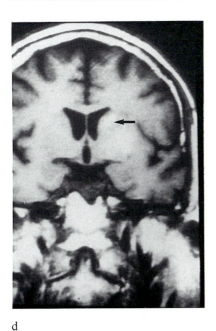

d

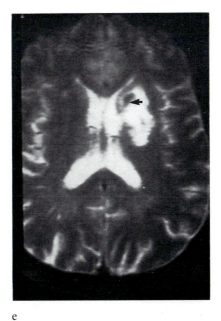

e

(**d**) One week following infarct, T$_1$-weighted coronal section demonstrates less mass effect on left frontal horn than in (**b**), with subtle intensity increase in center of infarct (arrow) (SE 600/20). (**e**) Heavily T$_2$-weighted axial section through infarct demonstrates focal low intensity (arrowhead) within high-intensity edema. The low intensity represents intracellular deoxyhemoglobin or methemoglobin due to petechial hemorrhage in this 'bland' infarct (SE 2800/80). (**f**) Three weeks following infarction, T$_1$-weighted coronal section demonstrates resolution of mass effect on left frontal horn with subtle high signal in left caudate head (arrowhead) due to methemoglobin formation (SE 600/20). (**g**) Heavily T$_2$-weighted image demonstrates increasing low signal in left caudate head (arrowhead) due to continued bleeding with intracellular deoxyhemoglobin and methemoglobin (SE 2800/80). (Courtesy of Jay S Tsuruda, MD, San Francisco, CA.)

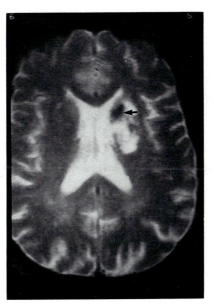

f

g

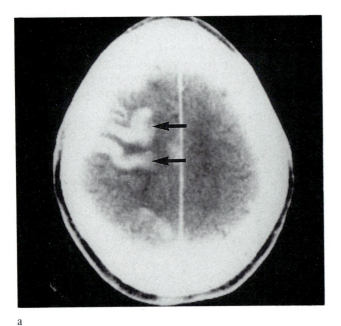

a

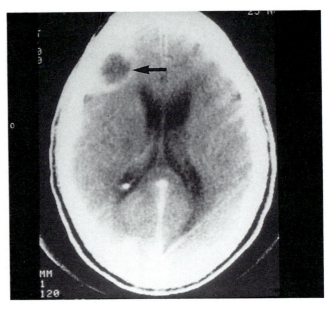

b

c

Figure 5.5

Contrast enhancement of subacute infarction.
(a) Contrast-enhanced CT demonstrates gyral enhancement (arrows) one week following infarction of the right middle cerebral artery.
(b) Enhanced CT through a lower axial section demonstrates enhanced border of subacute hematoma (arrow).

(c) T_1-weighted axial section following intravenous administration of gadolinium-DTPA demonstrates gyral enhancement (arrow) as well as enhanced rim of right frontal hematoma (arrowheads) (SE 800/20). (Courtesy of William Dillon, MD, San Francisco, CA.)

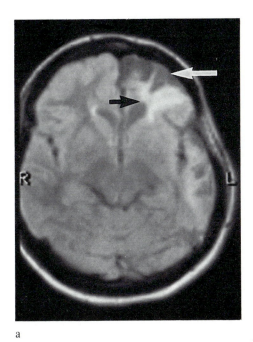

a

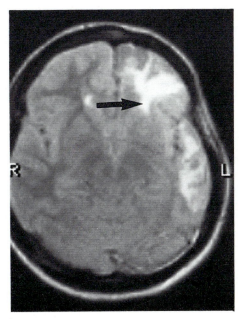

b

Figure 5.6

Post-infarction encephalomalacia. (**a**) Mildly T₂-weighted axial section demonstrates wedge-shaped infarcts in the left frontal and temporal lobes in patient with an occluded left internal carotid artery. The peripheral CSF intensity (arrow) represents macrocystic encephalomalacia which has MR characteristics similar to that of CSF. The more central zone of high-signal intensity (arrowhead) represents microcystic encephalomalacia or 'gliosis' (SE 2000/28). (**b**) On moderately T₂-weighted image, microcystic encephalomalacia (arrow) is more intense than either brain or CSF due to relatively short T₁ and long T₂ (SE 2000/56).

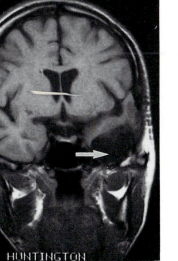

a

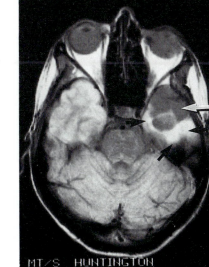

b

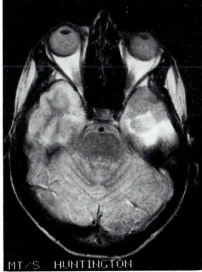

c

Figure 5.7

Postoperative encephalomalacia. (**a**) Coronal T₁-weighted image demonstrates resection of left temporal tip (arrow) for glioma. The subarachnoid space has increased to fill the space previously occupied by the resected brain and tumor (SE 500/30). (**b**) Mildly T₂- weighted axial section through left temporal tip demonstrates peripheral CSF intensity due to enlarged subarachnoid space (arrow) with high-intensity gliosis (arrowheads) between lesion and normal brain (SE 2000/30). (**c**) Moderately T₂-weighted image through same level as (**b**) (SE 2000/60).

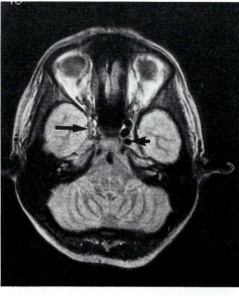

a

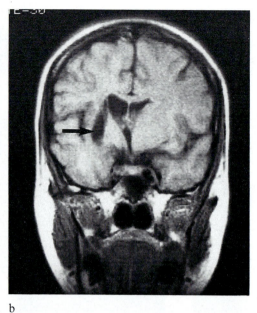

b

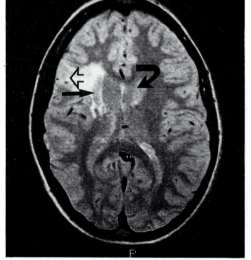

c

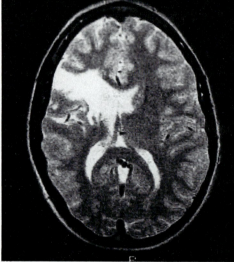

d

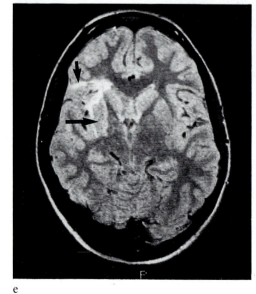

e

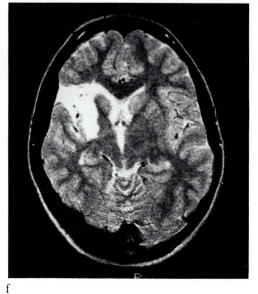

f

Figure 5.8

Middle cerebral artery infarct and porencephaly. (**a**) Axial section through the cavernous sinuses demonstrates absence of flow void in cavernous portion of right carotid artery (arrow) compared to normal flow void on the left (arrowhead) in 19-year-old woman with dissection. (**b**) T_1-weighted coronal section demonstrates porencephalic cyst (arrow) in right basal ganglia. There is also enlargement of the right lateral ventricle and shift of midline structures from left to right due to atrophy (SE 500/30). (**c**) Moderately T_2-weighted axial section through lateral ventricles demonstrates porencephalic cyst (straight arrow) which is isointense with CSF in ventricles (curved arrow). Note also right middle cerebral artery infarct in anterior Sylvian region (open arrow) (SE 3000/40). (**d**) Heavily T_2-weighted image through the lateral ventricles demonstrates uniform high intensity through right frontal horn, porencephalic cyst, and right MCA infarct (SE 3000/80). (**e**) Axial image through the third ventricle demonstrates porencephalic cyst (arrow) and high-intensity gliosis at the border of the infarct (arrowhead). Because CSF and gray matter are isointense on this moderately T_2-weighted sequence, it is difficult to determine exact extent of atrophy of the right Sylvian cistern secondary to the middle cerebral artery infarct (SE 3000/40). (**f**) On heavily T_2-weighted image through the third ventricle, the full extent of the right Sylvian atrophy becomes apparent as does the porencephalic cyst which was isointense with the CSF in the lateral and third ventricles (SE 3000/80).

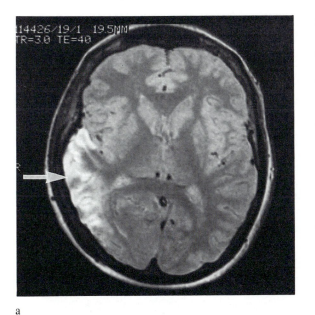

a

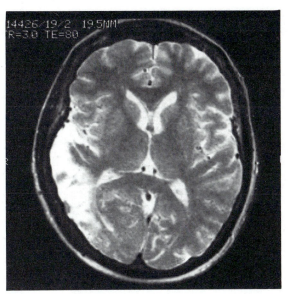

b

Figure 5.9

Chronic right middle cerebral artery infarct. (**a**) Moderately T$_2$-weighted image demonstrates hyperdensity in right temporal lobe following right MCA infarct (arrow). The hyperintensity reflects presence of microcystic encephalomalacia which has a shorter T$_1$ than CSF in the ventricles and therefore appears brighter (SE 3000/40).
(**b**) Heavily T$_2$-weighted axial section also demonstrates hyperintensity in the right temporal lobe which is now indistinguishable from hyperintense CSF within the ventricles (SE 3000/80).

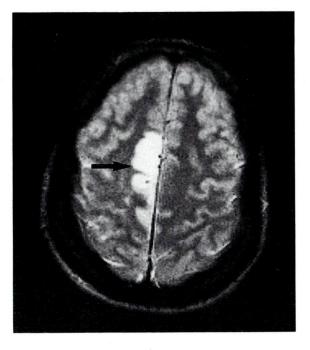

Figure 5.10

Anterior cerebral artery infarct. Parasagittal hyperintensity is noted on moderately T$_2$-weighted image involving the gray matter in the intrahemispheric fissure (arrow). In adults, the gray matter is hypermetabolic relative to white matter and is therefore injured earlier at lower levels of ischemia. The pattern in this case is adjacent to the interhemispheric fissure indicating infarction in the distribution of a branch of the anterior cerebral artery (SE 2000/60).

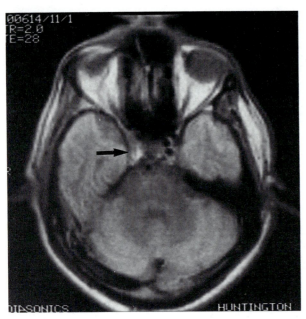

a

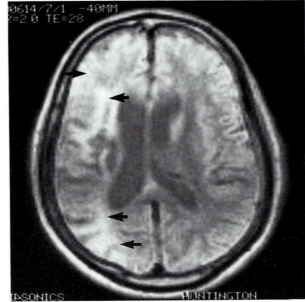

b

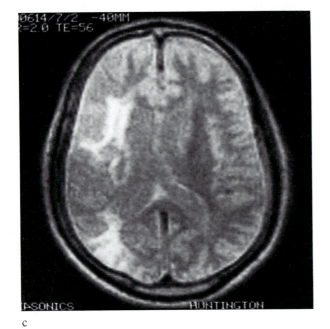

c

Figure 5.11

Middle cerebral infarction. (a) Axial section through the cavernous sinus demonstrates total occlusion of the right internal carotid artery. Note absence of double-barreled 'flow void' on the right (arrow) compared to the normal appearance on the left (SE 2000/28). (b) Mildly T_2-weighted axial section through the level of the lateral ventricles demonstrates high-intensity gliosis in the distribution of the right middle cerebral artery (arrowheads). Note also volume loss with enlargement of the right lateral ventricle and midline shift to the right (SE 2000/28). (c) With additional T_2-weighting, gliosis becomes hyperintense against a relatively featureless background, the CSF and gray matter becoming isointense. This moderate T_2-weighting increases the conspicuity of the infarct (SE 2000/56).

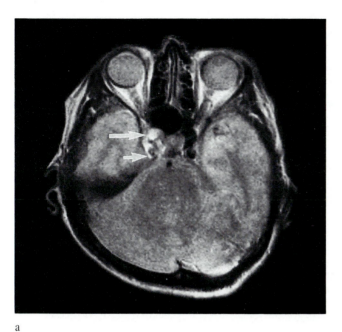

a

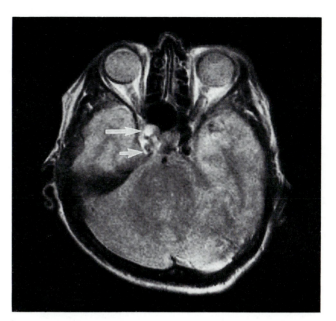

b

Figure 5.12

Slow flow in internal carotid artery. (**a**) First-echo image demonstrates normal double-barreled flow void on the left side of the cavernous sinus due to rapid flow in the internal carotid artery. The flow void on the right side is subtle anteriorly (arrow) and apparently normal posteriorly (arrowhead) (SE 2000/30).

(**b**) On symmetric second-echo image, the subtle flow void anteriorly has now turned bright (arrow) and the flow void posteriorly (arrowhead) has decreased markedly, both due to even-echo rephasing. Note normal appearance of flow void on contralateral left side (SE 2000/60).

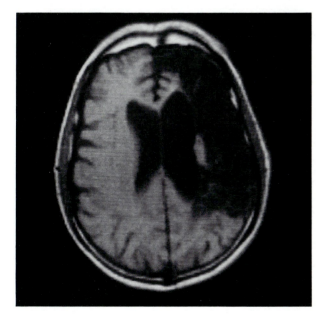

Figure 5.13

Old internal carotid artery infarct. Marked encephalomalacia is noted in the left temporal lobe as well as in the left frontal lobes, reflecting combined infarction in the distributions of the left anterior and middle cerebral arteries without crossover flow through the circle of Willis. Both encephalomalacia and enlarged subarachnoid space have low-signal intensity approaching that of CSF on this T_1-weighted image (SE 500/28).

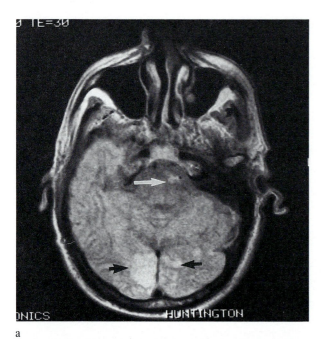

a

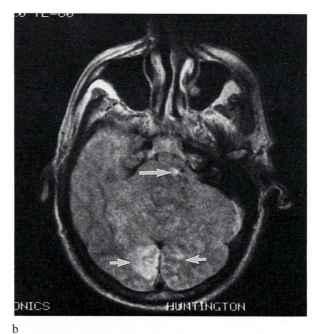

b

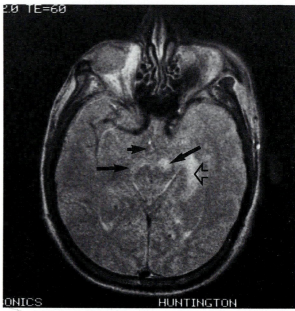

c

d

Figure 5.14

Thrombosis of the basilar artery. (**a**) Mildly T$_2$-weighted axial section through the pons demonstrates high signal (arrow) in the expected position of the flow void of the basilar artery due to recent thrombosis. Note also bilateral infarcts (arrowheads) in the occipital lobes due to markedly decreased flow in the posterior cerebral circulation (SE 2000/30). (**b**) Moderately T$_2$-weighted axial section demonstrates relatively greater intensity in thrombosed basilar artery (arrow) and in infarcted occipital lobes (arrowheads) (SE 2000/60). (**c**) Moderately T$_2$-weighted axial section through the midbrain demonstrates hyperintensity in the anterior aspect of the midbrain representing brainstem infarcts (arrows). Note also high signal in interpeduncular cistern reflecting thrombosed basilar artery (arrowhead)(SE 2000/30). (**d**) Moderately T$_2$- weighted image through the same level as (**c**) demonstrates hyperintensity in the anterior midbrain due to infarction (arrows) and in the basilar artery due to thrombosis (arrowhead). Note also hippocampal infarct (open arrow) due to decreased flow in the anterior choroidal artery (SE 2000/60).

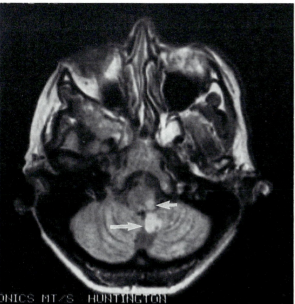

a

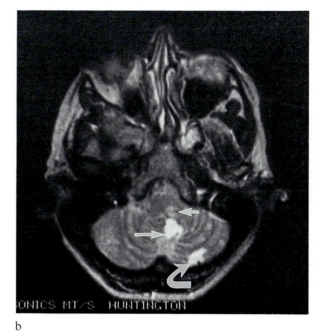

b

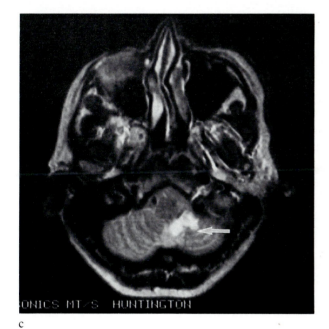

c

Figure 5.15

Infarction in the distribution of the posterior inferior cerebellar artery (PICA). (**a**) Section through the midmedulla demonstrates hyperintensity in the left posterior lateral aspect of the medulla (arrowhead) as well as in the inferior left vermis (arrow) (SE 2000/40). (**b**) With additional T$_2$-weighting, the lateral medullary infarct (arrowhead) becomes somewhat less conspicuous compared to surrounding CSF while the inferior vermian (straight arrow) and inferior cerebellar infarct (curved arrow) become more prominent (SE 2000/80). (**c**) Axial section 5 mm inferior to (**a**) and (**b**) demonstrates hyperintensity in the inferior left cerebellar hemisphere (arrow) due to left PICA branch occlusion (SE 2000/80).

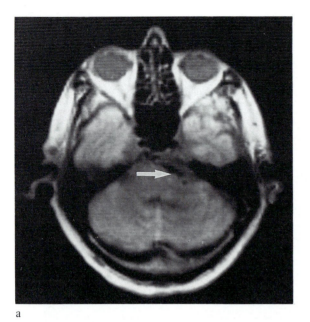

a

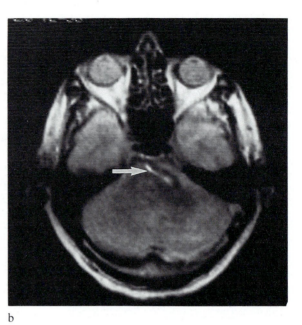

b

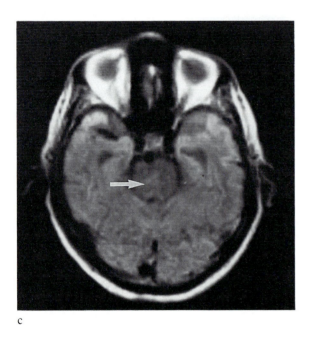

c

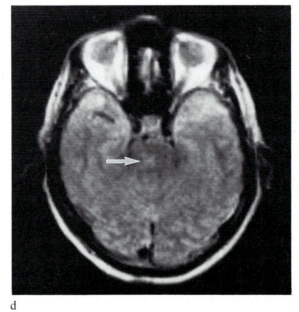

d

Figure 5.16

Vertebrobasilar insufficiency. (a) Mildly T_2-weighted image demonstrates an apparently normal basilar artery (arrow) (SE 2000/28). (b) Symmetric second-echo image demonstrates even-echo rephasing in basilar artery (arrow) indicating unusually slow flow (SE 2000/56). (c) On higher axial section through the upper pons, subtle high-signal intensity is noted, reflecting pontine infarct (arrow) (SE 2000/28). (d) With additional T_2-weighting, pontine infarct (arrow) becomes more conspicuous (SE 2000/56). Subsequent angiography demonstrated high-grade stenoses of the origins of both vertebral arteries.

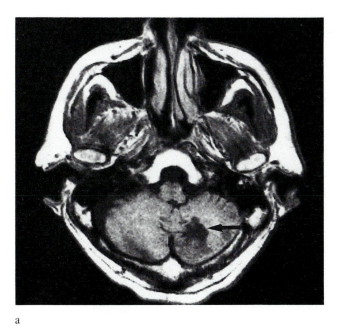

a

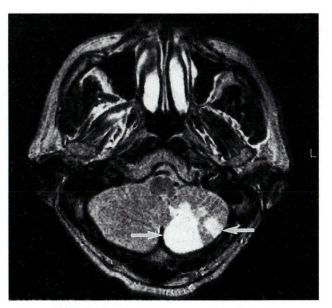

b

Figure 5.17

Cerebellar infarction. (**a**) T_1-weighted axial section through the inferior cerebellum demonstrates focal hypointensity in the inferior left cerebellar hemisphere (arrow) (SE 500/40). (**b**) Heavily T_2-weighted image demonstrates hyperintensity in typical wedge configuration extending to cortex (arrows) due to PICA branch occlusion (SE 2000/80).

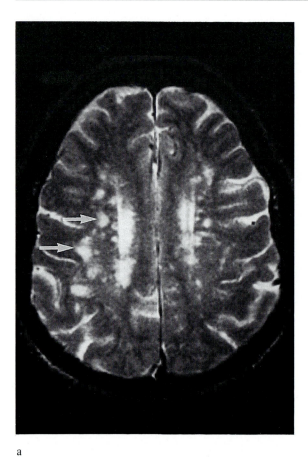

a

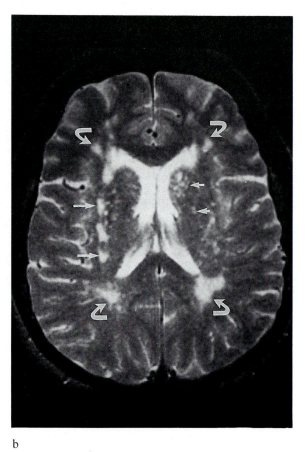

b

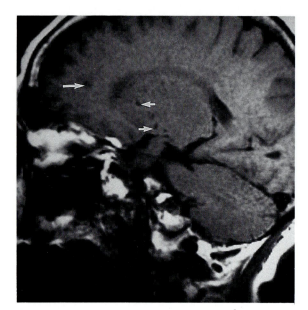

c

d

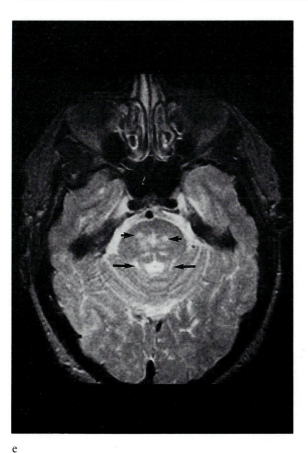

e

Figure 5.18

Subcortical arteriosclerotic encephalopathy in 74-year-old hypertensive woman.
(a) Heavily T_2-weighted axial section through the roofs of the lateral ventricles demonstrates multiple foci of periventricular hyperintensity (arrows). This represents deep white matter infarction due to arteriosclerosis of the long perforating arteries arising at the base of the brain (SE 2500/80). (b) Heavily T_2-weighted axial section through the lateral ventricles demonstrates multiple small lacunar infarcts in the basal ganglia (arrowheads) as well as larger deep white matter infarcts in the right external capsule (straight arrows) and the deep white matter (curved arrows) (SE 2500/80). (c) T_1-weighted parasagittal section through the left basal ganglia demonstrates punctate low-signal intensity secondary to lacunar infarction in the basal ganglia (arrowheads) as well as larger hypointense areas due to deep white matter infarction (arrow). These infarcts tend to appear larger on the T_2-weighted images than on the T_1-weighted images due to the conspicuity of the surrounding isomorphic gliosis on the T_2-weighted images (SE 600/20). (d) Parasagittal section through the right external capsule demonstrates foci of hypointensity corresponding to infarcts (arrowheads) noted in (b) (SE 600/20). (e) Heavily T_2-weighted axial section through the upper pons demonstrates focal hyperintensity in the brainstem secondary to infarction (arrowheads). Obliquely oriented linear structures lateral to the fourth ventricle represent the inferior portions of the wings of the ambient cisterns (arrows) (SE 2500/80).

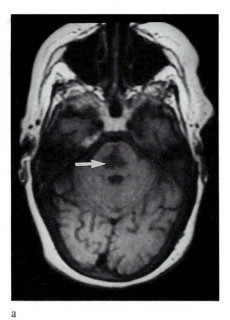

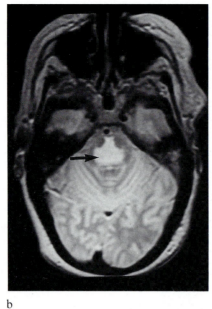

a   b   c

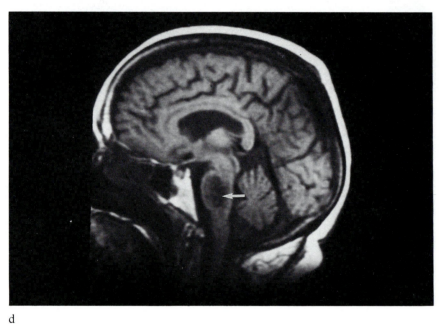

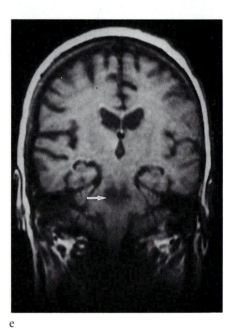

d   e

Figure 5.19

Central pontine myelinolysis.
(a) Axial T_1-weighted section
through the pons demonstrates
marked hypointensity (arrow)
due to central pontine
myelinolysis (SE 600/20).
(b) Heavily T_2-weighted axial
section through the same level
as (a) demonstrates
hyperintensity (arrow) in
central pons due to increased
water content accompanying
loss of hydrophobic myelin (SE
2500/80). (c) Moderately T_2-
weighted axial section through
pontine isthmus demonstrates
hyperintensity in central pons
(arrow) (SE 2500/30). (d) T_1-
weighted sagittal section
demonstrates marked
hypointensity in pons (arrow)
due to T_1 prolongation,
reflecting increased water
content (SE 800/20). (e) T_1-
weighted coronal section
through the pons demonstrates
extensive hypointensity (arrow)
(SE 600/20).

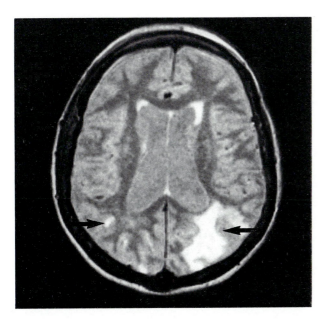

Figure 5.20

Watershed infarction. Bilateral infarcts are noted in the border zone between the posterior cerebral circulation medially and the middle cerebral circulation laterally. The infarcts are hyperintense on this moderately T_2-weighted image (arrows).

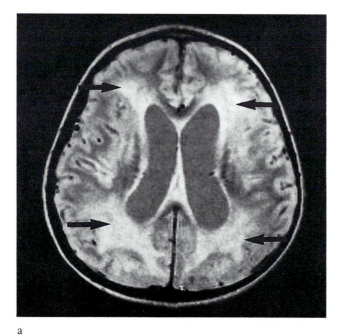

a

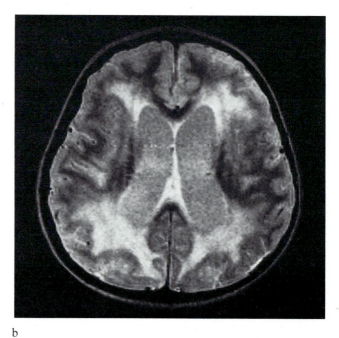

b

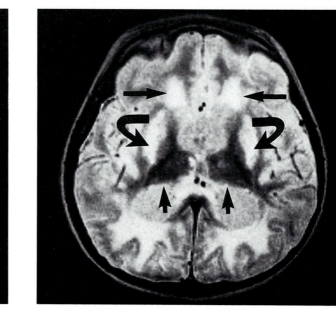

c

d

Figure 5.21

Periventricular leukomalacia. Six weeks following cardiopulmonary arrest, this four-year-old girl was studied by MRI. (**a**) Extensive periventricular hyperintensity is noted (arrows) surrounding enlarged lateral ventricles due to periventricular leukomalacia (SE 3000/40). (**b**) Heavily T$_2$-weighted image through same level as (**a**) (SE 3000/80). (**c**) Axial section through thalami demonstrates periventricular hyperintensity (arrows) with low signal noted in thalami (arrowheads) (SE 3000/40). (**d**) With additional T$_2$-weighting, the thalami become relatively darker due to presumed iron deposition (arrowheads). The greater T$_2$-weighting allows additional infarcts to be seen in the periventricular subfrontal region (arrows) and in the basal ganglia (curved arrows) (SE 3000/80).[19]

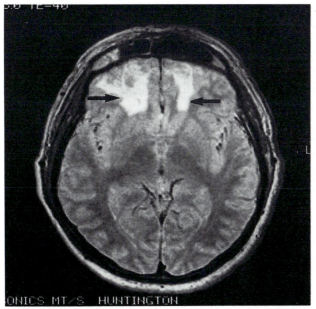

a

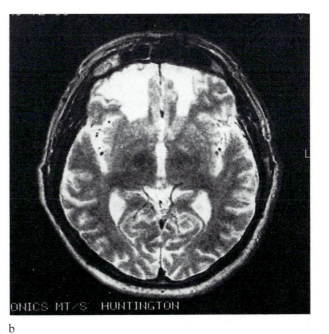

b

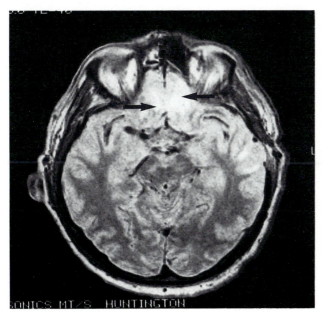

c

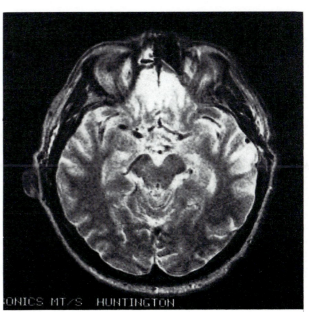

d

Figure 5.22

Subfrontal gliosis secondary to trauma. (**a**) Moderately T₂-weighted image demonstrates gliosis in subfrontal regions bilaterally (arrows) (SE 3000/40). (**b**) Heavily T₂-weighted axial section through the same level as (**a**) (SE 3000/80). (**c**) Axial section through the inferior frontal lobes demonstrates hyperintensity in the gryi recti bilaterally (arrows) due to gliosis from traumatic contusion (SE 3000/40), (**d**) Heavily T₂-weighted axial images through the same level as (**c**) (SE 3000/80).

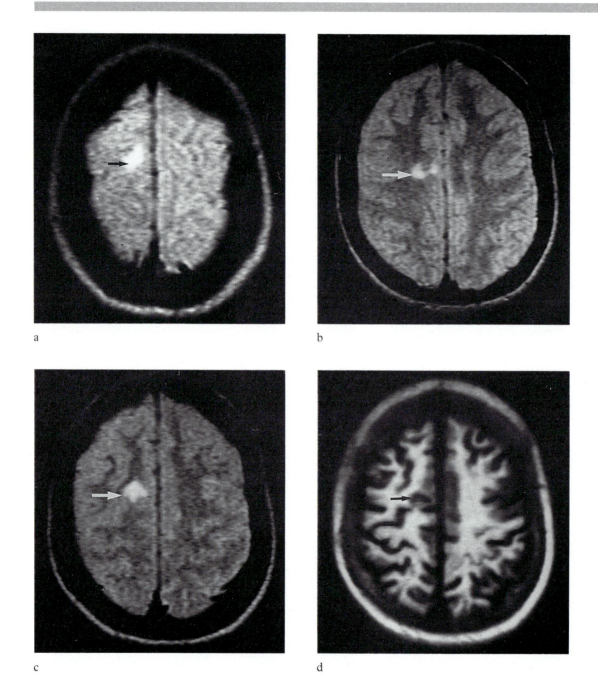

a

b

c

d

Figure 5.23

Mild axonal shearing injury. Following head trauma, 31-year-old woman has longitudinally oriented 'white matter lesion' which simulates single deep white matter infarct. In fact, this lesion extends from vertex through corona radiata to hypothalamus. (a–c) Moderately T_2-weighted axial sections demonstrating 1–2 cm diameter white matter lesions in right periventricular region (arrow) (SE 2550/60).

(d–h) T_1-weighted inversion-recovery images demonstrate abnormal low intensity due to axonal shearing injury extending from vertex (d) through centrum semiovale (e) to corona radiata (f) into thalamus (g) and hypothalamus (h). Low-signal lesion (arrow) reflects T_1 prolongation due to loss of myelin resulting from shearing injury (IR 2400/600/30). (Courtesy of Charles E Seibert, MD, Denver, CO.)

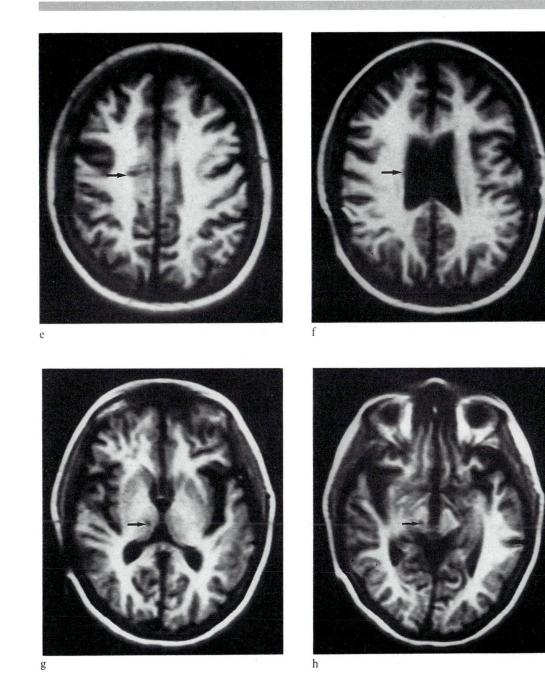

e

f

g

h

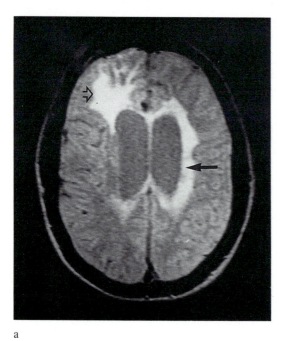

a

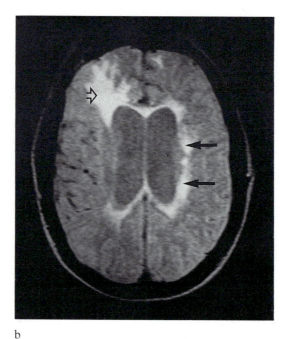

b

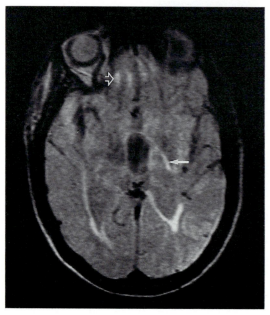

c

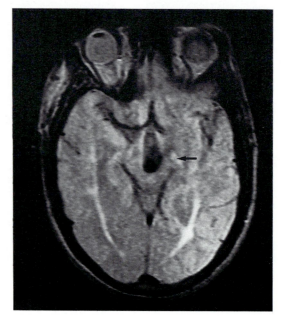

d

Figure 5.24

Moderately severe shearing injury. (**a**) Following head trauma, this 25-year-old male has left-sided periventricular hyperintensity which simulates deep white matter infarction (arrows). In fact, this represents moderately severe axonal shearing injury which occurred at the time of rotatory head trauma. The abnormality (arrow) extends from the left periventricular corona radiata (**a** and **b**) caudally through the left internal capsule (**c**) to the left cerebral peduncle in the midbrain (**d**) (SE 2550/60). Right frontal gliosis also noted from contusion (open arrow in **b**). (Courtesy of Charles E Seibert, MD, Denver, CO.)

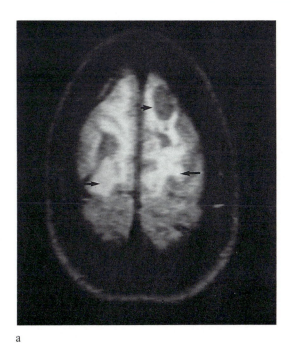

a

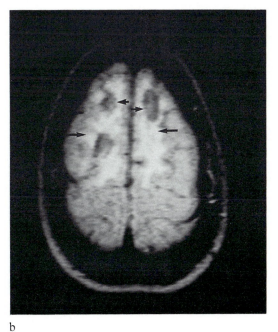

b

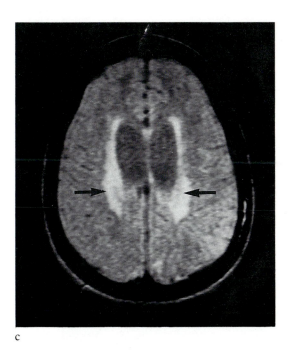

c

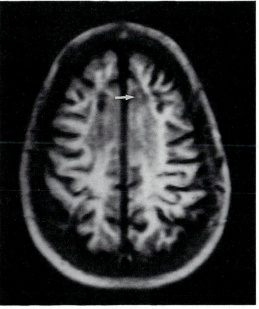

d

Figure 5.25

Severe shearing injury. High-signal intensity (arrow in **b** and **c**) is noted extending from the corticol medullary junction superiorly (**a**) through the centrum semiovale (**b**) to the periventricular corona radiata (**c**) (SE 2550/60). Foci of low-signal intensity (arrowhead in **a** and **b**) noted on the moderately T$_2$-weighted image at the vertex raises the suspicion of hemorrhage. (**d**) Inversion recovery section through same level as **a** confirms presence of methemoglobin (arrow) in left frontal lesion (IR 2400/600/30. (Courtesy of Charles E Seibert, MD, Denver, CO.)

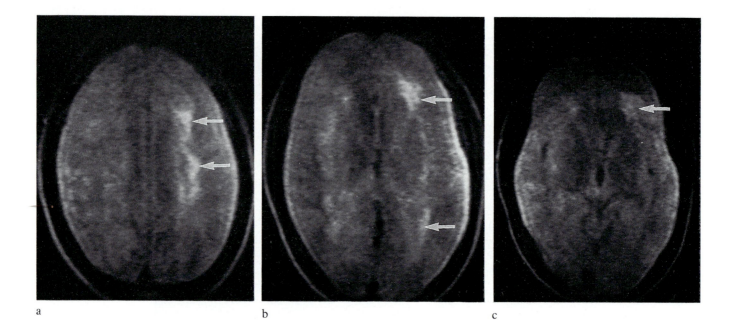

a   b   c

Figure 5.26

Severe axonal shearing injury.
Following severe head trauma
to this 17-year-old male, high
intensity (arrows) is noted at
corticolmedullary junction at
level of roof of lateral ventricles
(**a**) and at level of upper (**b**) and
lower (**c**) third ventricles (SE
2234/80). In an older patient,
this pattern would simulate
infarction. When found in a
trauma victim, it has a very
poor prognosis. (Courtesy of
Charles E Seibert, MD,
Denver, CO.)

Figure 5.27

Lacunar infarction.
(**a**) Hyperintensity is noted in
the right thalamus (arrow) and
posterior limb of the left
internal capsule (arrowhead) in
this hypertensive 55-year-old
male. When these infarcts are
less than one centimeter in
diameter, the adjective
'lacunar' is used. Similar
lacunar infarcts may be found
in the deep white matter in such
hypertensive patients with
subcortical arteriosclerotic
encephalopathy (SE 3000/80).
(**b**) T_1-weighted parasagittal
section through the right
thalamic infarct demonstrates
hypointensity (arrowhead) due
to T_1 prolongation (SE 500/40).

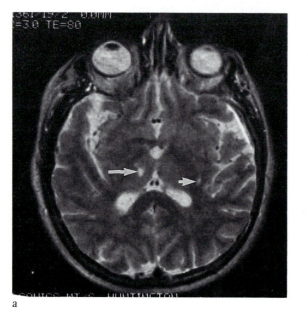

a   b

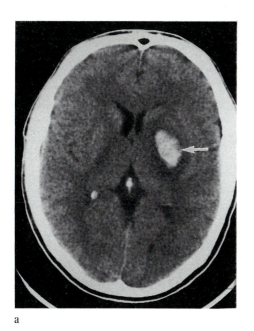

a

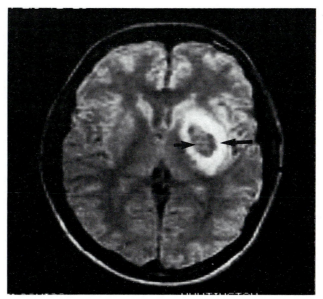

b

Figure 5.28

Hypertensive hemorrhage.
(**a**) Forty-eight hours following hypertensive bleed, high density is noted on CT (arrow). (**b**) High-signal rim (arrow) is noted surrounding lower-intensity center (arrowhead) in this mildly T_2-weighted image (SE 2000/28). (**c**) Even with moderate T_2-weighting at intermediate field (0.35 Tesla), hematoma is seen to become less intense (arrowhead) due to presence of intracellular deoxyhemoglobin. Vasogenic edema surrounding hematoma becomes more intense (arrow) with greater T_2-weighting (SE 2000/56).

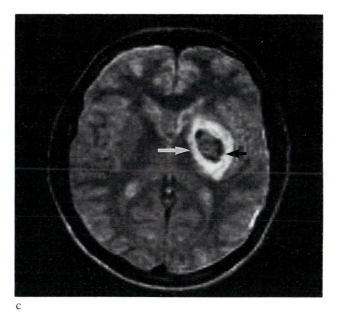

c

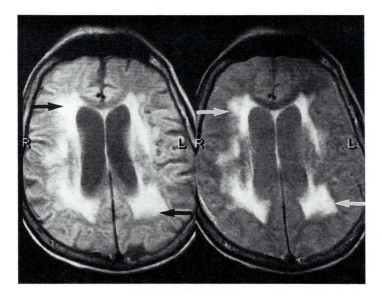

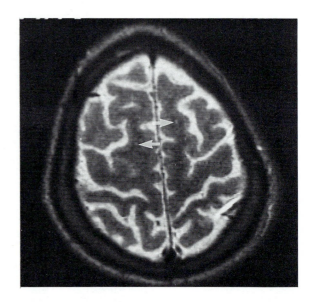

Figure 5.29

Deep white matter infarction. Mildly T_2-weighted image (left side) demonstrates periventricular hyperintensity (arrows) secondary to deep white matter infarction. In the more advanced stages, this becomes confluent as shown here. While this pattern tends to be more pronounced in hypertensive patients, it may be seen in elderly patients without a history of significant hypertension (SE 2000/30). On moderately T_2-weighted image on right through same level as (**a**), periventricular hyperintensity is displayed to greater advantage. This represents isomorphic gliosis surrounding smaller central infarct cavities (SE 2000/60).

Figure 5.30

Enlarged perivascular space at the vertex. Well-defined punctate high-signal intensity at the vertex (arrowheads) represents enlarged perivascular spaces. These tend to increase with age and should not be confused with deep white matter infarcts (SE 3000/80).

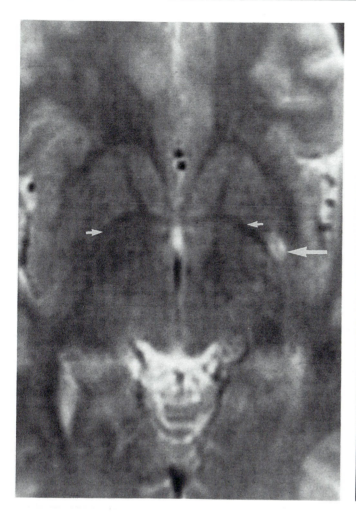

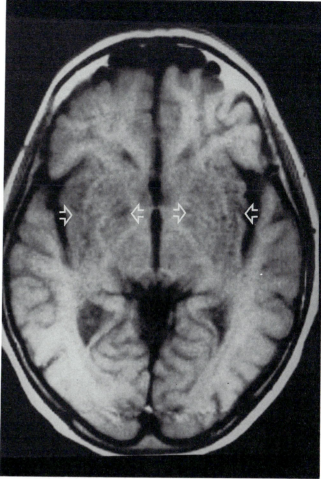

Figure 5.31

Enlarged perivascular space near the base of the brain. Well-defined focal high-signal intensity (arrow) is noted immediately anterior to the anterior commissure (arrowheads). This is a typical location for an enlarged perivascular space and should not be confused with lacunar infarct (SE 2500/80).

Figure 5.32

Etat criblé. On this T_1-weighted axial section, multiple, small, well-defined foci of low intensity are noted throughout the basal ganglia and insular cortex (open arrows). This represents multiple enlarged perivascular spaces. It is known as the cribriform state or 'état criblé' (SE 800/25).

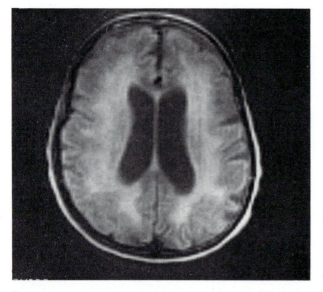

a

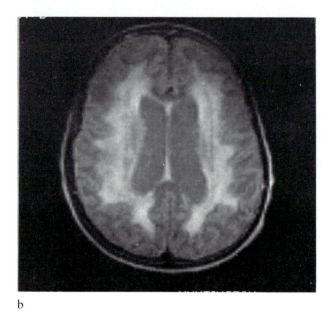

b

Figure 5.33

Radiation changes in the deep white matter. (**a**) Mildly T$_2$-weighted axial image demonstrates extensive periventricular hyperintensity in this 70-year-old woman treated with 3000 rads to the brain for metastatic lung carcinoma two years and eight months previously. This represents a combination of deep white matter infarction due to radiation-induced swelling of the long penetrating vessels as well as the direct effect of periventricular demyelination (SE 2000/28). (**b**) Moderately T$_2$-weighted axial image through the same level as (**a**) demonstrates periventricular radiation changes to better advantage (SE 2000/56).

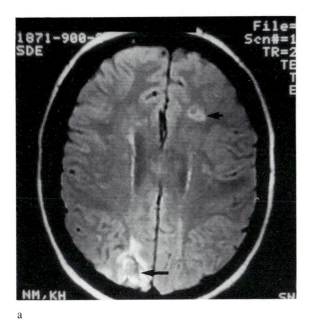

a

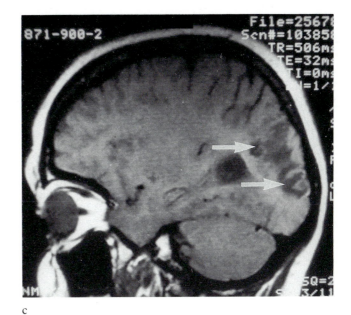

c

b

Figure 5.34

Lupus cerebritis. Combination of periventricular (arrowhead) and cortical (arrow) infarcts in this 43-year-old woman suggest vasculitis. (**a**) Mildly T_2-weighted axial image through the top of the lateral ventricles demonstrates deep white matter infarct in left frontal white matter (arrowhead) as well as cortical infarct in right parieto-occipital lobe (arrow) (SE 2110/32). (**b**) Heavily T_2-weighted image through the same level as (**a**) demonstrates white matter infarct (arrowhead) and cortical infarct (arrow) to better advantage (SE 2010/120). (**c**) T_1-weighted right parasagittal section demonstrates low signal in region of right parieto-occipital infarct (arrows) secondary to T_1 prolongation (SE 506/32). (Courtesy of Meredith A Weinstein, MD, Cleveland, OH.)

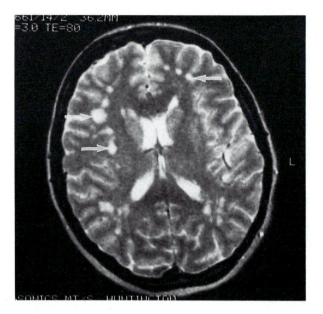

Figure 5.35

Lupus sclerosis. Multiple focal white matter lesions (arrows) are noted in this 36-year-old woman with known lupus cerebritis. These white matter infarcts result from an autoimmune vasculitis and produce a pattern similar to the demyelination seen in multiple sclerosis (SE 3000/80).

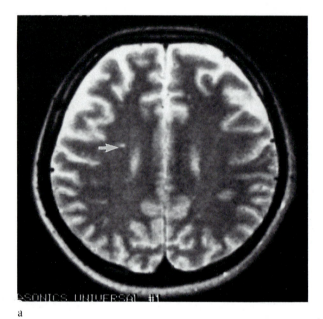

a

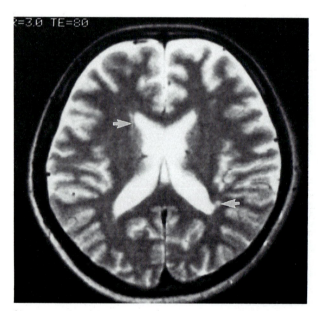

b

Figure 5.36

Deep white matter abnormalities associated with migraine headaches. Multiple foci of high-signal intensity are noted (arrowheads) in the periventricular region in this 40-year-old woman with a long history of classic migraine. There was no history of hemiplegia or hemisensory deficit at the time of the attack or subsequently at the time of the MR evaluation. (a) Section through the centrum semiovale. (b) Section through the lateral ventricles (SE 3000/80).

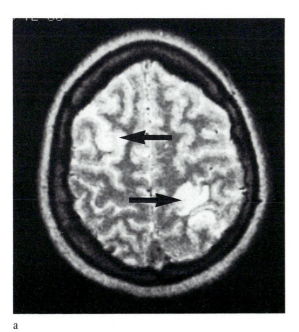

a

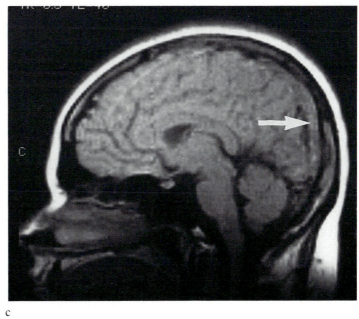

c

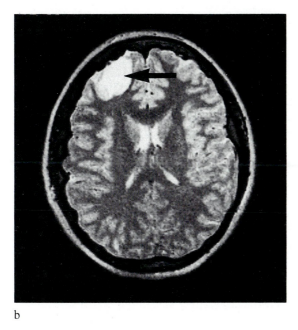

b

Figure 5.37

Venous infarction. Multiple
cortical infarcts (arrows) are
noted at vertex (**a**) and in right
frontal lobe (**b**) (SE 3000/80).
(**c**) Absent flow void in superior
sagittal sinus (arrow) (SE 500/
40).

6

Demyelinating disease and infection

Graeme Bydder

Introduction

Differences in the relaxation times of gray and white matter of the brain were first described in 1974,[1] when proton spectroscopy of human autopsy samples performed at a frequency of 60 MHz showed that the T_1 and T_2 of white matter were less than that of gray matter.

In 1978, Clow and Young used a highly T_1-dependent inversion-recovery sequence to produce an image of the brain displaying a high level of contrast between gray and white matter.[2] Figure 6.1 shows an early inversion recovery scan in a normal volunteer. The level of contrast between these two tissues was greater than that of contemporary X-ray CT images, and this stimulated considerable interest in the potential of MRI to detect changes in demyelinating disease. It was known at this time from post-mortem studies that in multiple sclerosis (MS), many more lesions were usually present in the brain than were suspected during life.[3] It was also known that X-ray CT studies were a relatively insensitive technique for the detection of these lesions.[4] Within two years it was shown that MRI displayed more lesions than contrast-enhanced CT in MS, although considerable care was necessary to avoid misdiagnosis of partial-volume effects as lesions.[5] Multiple sclerosis lesions not seen with contrast-enhanced CT were also detected by Buonanno et al in 1981, with the use of an inversion-recovery sequence.[6]

The clinical use of spin-echo sequences in early 1982 provided a new approach to the diagnosis of MS plaques with MRI. These sequences produced images with lower contrast between gray and white matter, but with high sensitivity to a wide variety of pathological change. Because of the lower level of contrast

between the gray and white matter with these sequences, partial-volume effects between these two tissues did not make diagnosis difficult. In addition, TR and TE could be selected to keep the signal from CSF less than that from adjacent brain, while providing higher T_2-dependent contrast. Partial-volume effects were thus easily differentiated from MS lesions, which produced higher signal than brain. The greater sensitivity of MRI compared with X-ray CT was again demonstrated.[7,8] Further confirmation of this sensitivity was provided by a number of other groups.[9–12] Preliminary studies also showed that the activity of MS lesions could be followed by serial measurement of T_1.[13] The range of demyelinating disease recognized by MRI was also extended to include acute disseminated encephalomyelitis.[14]

Over the next year (1983), the range of demyelinating disease studied widened further and some comparison of different sequences in MS was performed.[15] The normal development of myelination was also studied in vivo, and delays or deficits in this process were recognized.[16]

During 1984 there was a general improvement in MR image quality, with many groups using a 256 × 256 matrix for image reconstruction to provide images of similar resolution to X-ray CT but with generally greater soft tissue contrast. More detailed comparisons of pulse sequences were performed.[17] Multiple sclerosis lesions were also recognized in the spinal cord,[18] and follow-up studies were published.[19]

More recent developments have included the use of intravenous gadolinium-DTPA (Gd-DTPA) in MS in order to determine the activity of the lesions.[20] Two groups of authors have now observed that the T_1 of the apparently normal white matter in the brain may be elevated in patients with MS in the absence of any overt lesions.[21,22] The use of short TI inversion-recovery sequences has enabled plaques to be seen in the optic nerves in MS. Studies at high field have also indicated an apparent increase in iron content in MS.[23] Pediatric studies have been extended to include periventricular leukomalacia, where characteristic changes have been observed with MRI.[24]

The widespread dissemination of MRI systems has led to a greater appreciation of the differential diagnosis of periventricular lesions,[25] and an increase in reports of patients with unusual forms of demyelinating disease.[26]

Classification of white matter disease

It is useful to divide disease of white matter into a myelinoclastic (or demyelinating) group, in which myelin is formed normally but is later destroyed, and a dysmyelinating group in which normal myelin is not formed or at best, if formed is not maintained. This classification is listed in more detail in Table 6.1. The demyelinating disease may be primary or of unknown etiology (such as MS), or secondary when associated with a variety of infections, toxic, anoxic-ischemic, or other factors. The dysmyelinating disease is often due to a specific enzyme deficiency.

Table 6.1 Classification of white matter disease.

Myelinoclastic disease
Multiple sclerosis
Progressive multifocal leukoencephalitis (PML)
Subacute sclerosing panencephalitis (SSPE)
Acute disseminated encephalomyelitis (ADE)
Radiation damage
Central pontine myelinolysis (CPM)
Marchiafava-Bignami disease
Subcortical arteriosclerotic encephalopathy (SAE)
Anoxic damage
Methotrexate damage

Dysmyelinating disease
Many Leucodystrophies
Adrenoleucodystrophy
Anderson-Faby disease
Alexander's disease
Metachromatic leucodystrophy

Multiple sclerosis

Features of multiple sclerosis on MRI

Focal areas of increased T_1 and T_2 are observed at the anterolateral angles of the lateral ventricle in normal volunteers. Other features which may be mistaken for focal lesions include the tail of the caudate nucleus, the superior aspect of the thalamus in mid-ventricular section, and the red nucleus. A band of increased T_2 within the centrum semiovale, just lateral to the lateral ventricles and extending into the frontal lobes, representing the body of the caudate nucleus, is another normal finding which is particularly prominent in younger patients. Very fine areas of tissue with slightly increased T_2 may also be seen around the margins of the posterior aspect of the lateral ventricles as normal features.

Abnormal findings include periventricular lesions (single, multiple, or confluent), illustrated in Figures 6.2 and 6.3, isolated lesions within the hemispheres, and brainstem or cerebellar lesions. Cerebral atrophy may also be seen. Care must be taken to exclude the normal features described above as well as partial-volume effects and artifacts.

Table 6.2 Differential diagnosis of periventricular lesions (short list)

Multiple sclerosis
Other demyelinating disease
Vascular disease
Systemic lupus erythematosis
Sarcoidosis
Infective disease
Periventricular edema associated with hydrocephalus
Multiple metastases
Radiation damage

Periventricular lesions similar or identical to those seen in MS have been seen in a variety of other diseases, examples given in Table 6.2, and in older patients MS and vascular disease are often bracketed as diagnostic possibilities.

Patterns of remission, fluctuating exacerbation, and remission and progression can be identified, as in Figure 6.4, although it is difficult to obtain exact correspondence with the position of previous scans. Advances in technique may also cause problems in the assessment of lesions.

The most important aspect of MRI in MS is that it provides access to clinically silent lesions. Many lesions in MS characteristically occur in the periventricular regions around the lateral ventricles. The clinical features resulting from these lesions may be subtle or absent, and provide little or no indication of the number or extent of the lesions. The discrepancy between clinical manifestations and the extent of the underlying disease is important in early diagnosis, when subtle signs may be present although the disease is in fact well established. It is also important in research applications in monitoring therapeutic response where the clinical signs may poorly reflect changes within the brain or spinal cord.

Choice of pulse sequences in MS

Early studies were performed which indicated that spin-echo sequences are more sensitive than inversion-recovery sequences. Other studies subsequently confirmed this result, with the exception of the brainstem, where inversion recovery may have an advantage. The choice of a spin-echo sequence is dictated by the behaviour of CSF. Sequences in which the CSF signal is lower than brain are of value in the resolution of partial-volume effects between brain and CSF. Although sequences with CSF signal higher than that of brain may display high sensitivity, there may also be considerable difficulty in differentiating periventricular lesions from partial-volume effects between CSF and brain. This problem is more common at higher fields, as the T_1 of brain increases more than that of CSF with increasing field strength, so that it becomes more difficult to allow a high level of recovery of brain magnetization between 90° pulses whilst keeping CSF in a state of incomplete recovery.

There are several additional classes of image which may be of value in the detection of lesions in MS. One is the short TI inversion-recovery sequence, which has the advantage that T_1 and T_2 contrast are additive around the 90° pulse. These sequences show a high level of gray/white matter contrast and if TR and TE are reduced, the CSF signal may be made less than that of brain.[27]

Another approach is the double inversion-recovery sequence, which can be designed so that the CSF signal is very low and partial-volume effects between brain and CSF do not cause confusion with lesions.[27] This may be of value at higher fields.

An additional approach is the use of chemical-shift imaging. It has been suggested that the lipid seen in demyelinating lesions may be of different quality to that in other pathological processes (such as infarction) and that this may be detectable with chemical-shift imaging and so may be of value in differential diagnosis.

Rapid versions of the partial-saturation sequence, including FLASH, GRASS, CE-FAST, etc, which are modified to display high T_2-dependent contrast, are useful for detecting MS lesions, but it may be difficult to keep the CSF signal lower than that of brain.

Spinal cord lesions

Spinal cord lesions have been described for MS and have a fairly typical appearance, although they may also be associated with a mass effect. Figure 6.5 illustrates these lesions. Silent lesions are not as frequent within the spinal cord as in the brain. The role of MRI may be more useful in the identification of associated lesions in the brain, than in the identification of MS lesions in the cord, although exclusion of tumor or other lesions within the cord may also be of value.

Differential diagnosis

The differential diagnosis of periventricular lesions is quite extensive, some of the possibilities are listed in Table 6.2. So far no pathognemonic features have been identified, but certain features can change the priorities within the differential diagnosis.

Binswangers and leucodystrophies may produce confluent lesions. Sometimes vascular lesions are confined largely to gray matter. In some cases, such as post-infectious demyelinating disease, the disease may be very largely restricted to specific white matter tracts.

Contrast agents

Intravenous Gd-DTPA has been used in tumors, and in general terms its action tends to parallel that seen with iodinated contrast agents used with CT.

The increased diagnostic accuracy of contrast-enhanced CT with double dosage and delayed examination has been well documented. In general, the yield of the lesion is not increased by the use of Gd-DTPA-enhanced MRI. Gd-DTPA may still be useful in the assessment of lesion activity. Unfortunately, the spin-echo sequence which is usually of most value in the diagnosis of MS lesions (the long TE long TR spin echo) is relatively insensitive to contrast enhancement; inversion-recovery and highly T_1-dependent spin-echo sequences are the patterns of choice for enhancement demonstration.

Lacunar infarction

Focal lesions are often seen in lacunar infarctions in the central deep white matter of the brain, as shown in Figure 6.6. The distribution may not be as specifically periventricular as in MS, but there is considerable overlap in the appearance of the two entities.

Subcortical arteriosclerotic encephalopathy (SAE)

Cases of SAE typically display bilateral, confluent, long T_1 regions with loss of gray/white matter contrast and increased T_2 regions within the centrum semiovale (Figure 6.7), as well as multiple periventricular lesions elsewhere. This diagnosis is difficult in the presence of less severe disease, and isolated periventricular lesions may be seen in a number of diseases.

Anoxic disease

Diffuse and symmetrical changes may be seen in the subcortical regions as well as the basal ganglia following anoxic damage. More focal changes due to infarction in vulnerable areas within the brain can also be found.

Age-related periventricular changes

Quite extensive periventricular changes may be seen in apparently normal adults in older age groups.[28] These changes are akin to those of periventricular leukomalacia, which are frequently seen in similar circumstances with X-ray CT.

The pathological basis includes infarction and demyelination, with emphasis on the former. As with lesions in MS, there may be no close correlation with clinical features.

Central pontine myelinolysis

This condition is usually associated with excessive alcohol consumption. Characteristic lesions are seen in the pons and brainstem, as shown in Figure 6.8.

Leucodystrophy

Leucodystrophy is the term used to describe disseminated disease in the white matter. Extensive bilateral changes are often seen in the white matter of the hemispheres, although the cerebellum and brainstem may be spared. Less severe involvement is also seen. Figure 6.9 illustrates white matter changes in Alexander's disease.

Adrenoleucodystrophy is characterized by dilated posterior horns with periventricular lesions in this region.

Radiation damage

Changes are seen within white matter in radiation damage. In the case illustrated in Figure 6.10, the cerebellum beneath the carcinoma of the mastoid shows increased T_2 in the region of the radiation field. Diagnosis depends on a review of the patient's radiation plan and the geometrical shape of the lesion. Changes may be delayed some months or a few years after the therapy.

Methotrexate-treated patients

Patients treated with prophylactic intrathecal methotrexate for acute lymphatic leukaemia may display areas of increased T_2 at the ventricular margins.

Post-infectious demyelinating disease

A variety of different viral infections result in extensive white matter demyelination due to the effects of the virus itself and viral-induced immune changes. Typical examples of the first group are progressive multifocal leukoencephalopathy (PML) and subacute sclerosing panencephalitis (SSPE). Acute disseminated encephalomyelitis (ADE) is an example of the second category.

Progressive multifocal leukoencephalopathy affects immunocompromised patients such as those receiving immunosuppressive therapy and those with carcinoma, leukaemia, and other malignancies. A papova virus is responsible for the production of variable regions of demyelination. The lesions may be subcortical, symmetrical, or ring-shaped. Typical lesions are illustrated in Figures 6.11 and 6.12.

Subacute sclerosing panencephalitis may follow many years after exposure to the measles virus. The clinical cause progressively worsens over months or years. Extensive changes may be seen in white matter accompanied by cerebral atrophy.

Acute disseminated encephalomyelitis is a devastating illness which may follow a few days or weeks after exposure to vanceller influenza or other viruses. Widespread and frequently symmetrical changes are seen in the brain.

Post-infectious demyelinating disease displays extensive abnormalities, which may be seen on a lobar basis (Figure 6.13), confined very largely to the white matter tracts (Figure 6.14).

Encephalitis

Herpes simplex virus is the commonest carrier of encephalitis in the child and adult, and appears to be a reactivation of a latent infection. It may be preceded by skin lesions or a flu-like illness.

The temporal lobes show hemorrhagic or necrotic changes. Magnetic resonance imaging demonstrates high-signal intensity regions with T_2-weighted sequences; it appears to be an early and sensitive monitor of disease, as shown in Figure 6.15.

Focal brainstem encephalitis may be seen in children and young adults as illustrated in Figure 6.16. Changes in T_1 and T_2 are in Figure 6.17. The differential diagnosis includes brainstem tumor. With time, the changes of encephalitis resolve and there is usually less mass effect than with tumors.

Acquired immunodeficiency syndrome (AIDS)

The features of AIDS are variable, reflecting the pattern of underlying disease and the effect of opportunistic infections and associated malignancies.

Toxoplasma gondii may produce abscesses, as may cytomegalovirus (CMV), but even prior to these changes diffuse involvement of the frontal white matter may be seen, as in Figure 6.18.

Subacute encephalitis may also occur, with extensive white matter changes and some sparing of gray matter (Figure 6.19).

There is a relatively high incidence of primary lymphoma and metastatic Kaposi's sarcoma. The pattern of lymphoma may principally involve white matter. Biopsy studies may be necessary to establish a definitive diagnosis.

Abscess

Bacterial infection usually begins as a cerebitis. Pathologically, there is often an ill-defined edematous area with some associated hemorrhage. With MRI, areas of increased T_2 are usually seen. If the condition evolves, liquefaction may follow and reactive changes may lead to localization of infection, as illustrated in Figures 6.20 and 6.21.

Magnetic resonance imaging is very sensitive in the demonstration of edema and the central cavity with any associated hemorrhage. The central cavity generally has a long T_1 and T_2, but this may vary depending on the nature of the fluid contents.

Intracranial tuberculosis usually results from hematogenous spread. The lesion is typically fairly well defined and displays contrast enhancement with Gd-DTPA. Characteristic lesions are shown in Figures 6.22 and 6.23. Fungal abscess may also occur, illustrated in Figure 6.24. However, non-specific changes are also seen as in Figure 6.23.

Meningitis

Leptomeningitis may be acute, subacute, or chronic. The changes in the meninges may be demonstrated with intravenous Gd-DTPA, but they can also be seen less frequently on T_2-weighted images without enhancement, as in Figure 6.25. No consistent changes have been seen with viral meningitis.

Ear, nose and throat

Acute and chronic infection involving the nasal sinuses is very common. Infection of the mastoid is shown in Figure 6.26.

Conclusion

The investigation of demyelinating disease has proved an important application of MRI, and the technique has also been successful in the diagnosis of a wide variety of infectious disease. Although the sensitivity of MRI is not in question, its lack of specificity may mean that additional information from clinical and other sources is necessary to make a definitive diagnosis.

References

1 PARRISH RG, KURLAND RJ, JANESE WW et al, Proton relaxation rate of water in brain and brain tumour, *Science* (1974) **483**:349.

2 Britain's brains produce first NMR scans *New Scientist* (1978) **80**:588.

3 LUMSDEN CE, The neuro-pathology of multiple sclerosis. In: Vinken PJ, Bruyn GW, eds. *Handbook of clinical neurology*, 217–309.

4 HAUGHTON VM, HO KC, WILLIAMS AL et al, CT detection of demyelinated plaques in multiple sclerosis, *AJR* (1979) **132**:213–15.

5 YOUNG IR, HALL AS, PALLIS CA et al, Nuclear magnetic resonance imaging of the brain in multiple sclerosis, *Lancet* (1981) **ii**:1063–6.

6 BUONANNO FS, PYKETT IL, VIELMA J et al, Proton NMR imaging of normal and abnormal brain. Experimental and clinical observation in NMR imaging. In: Witcofski RL, Karstaedt N, Partain CL, eds. *NMR imaging.* (Bowman-Gray School of Medicine: Winston Salem 1982) 147–57.

7 BAILES DR, YOUNG IR, THOMAS DJ et al, NMR imaging of the brain using spin-echo sequences, *Clin Radiol* (1982) **23**:395–414.

8 BYDDER GM, STEINER RE, YOUNG IR et al, Clinical NMR imaging of the brain: 140 cases, *AJR* (1982) **139**:215–36.

9 LUKES SA, AMINOFF MJ, MILLS C et al, Nuclear magnetic resonance imaging of multiple sclerosis, *J Comput Assist Tomogr* (1983) **7**:180.

10 BRANT-ZAWADSKI M, DAVIS PL, CROOKS LE et al, NMR demonstration of cerebral abnormalities: comparison with CT, *AJR* (1983) **140**:847–54.

11 BRYAN RN, KELLEY GR, WILLCOTT RW et al, CT–NMR imaging of multiple sclerosis – A comparative study, *Magn Reson Imaging* (1982) **1**:231.

12 ZEITLER E, SCHUIERER G, NMR clinical results: Nuremburg. In: Partain CL, James AE, Rollo FD et al, eds. *Nuclear magnetic resonance (NMR) imaging.* (Saunders: Philadelphia 1983) 267–75.

13 NEW PFJ, BUONANNO FS, BRADY TJ et al, Proton (^{1}H) NMR imaging in multiple sclerosis: potential characterisation of activity using in vivo T_1 mapping, *J Comput Assist Tomogr* (1983) **7**:180.

14 LUKES SA, NORMAN D, MILLS C, Acute disseminated encephalomyelitis: CT and NMR findings, *J Comput Assist Tomogr* (1983) **7**:182.

15 YOUNG IR, RANDELL CP, KAPLAN PW et al, NMR imaging in white matter disease of the brain using spin echo sequences, *J Comput Assist Tomogr* (1983) **7**:182–7.

16 JOHNSON MA, PENNOCK JM, BYDDER GM et al, Clinical NMR imaging of the brain in children: normal and neurological disease, *AJNR* (1984) **4**(5):1013–26.

17 RUNGE VM, PRICE AC, KISHNER HS et al, Magnetic resonance imaging of multiple sclerosis: A study of pulse-technique-efficiency, *AJNR* (1984) **5**:691–702.

18 MARAVILLA KR, WEINREB JC, SUSS R et al, Magnetic resonance demonstration of multiple sclerosis plaques in the cervical cord, *AJNR* (1984) **5**:685–9.

19 JOHNSON MA, LI DKB, BRYANT DJ et al, NMR imaging: serial follow-up in multiple sclerosis, *AJNR* (1984) **5**(5):495–9.

20 GROSSMAN RI, GONZALEZ-SCARANO F, ATLAS SW et al, Multiple sclerosis: gadolinium enhancement in MR imaging, *Radiology* (1986) **161**:721.

21 LACOMIS D, OSBAKKEN MD, BROSS G, Spin-lattice relaxation (T_1) times of cerebral white matter in multiple sclerosis, *Magn Reson Med* (1986) **3**:194–201.

22 OMEROD IEC, MILLER DH, MCDONALD WI et al, The role of NMR imaging in the assessment of multiple sclerosis and isolated neurological lesions, *Brain* (1987) **110**:1579–1616.

23 DRAYER BP, BURGER P, HURWITZ B et al, Reduced signal intensity on MR images of thalamus and putamen in multiple sclerosis: increased iron content? *AJNR* (1987) **8**:413–17.

24 DEVRIES LS, DUBOWITZ LMS, PENNOCK JM et al, Extensive cystic leukomalacia: correlation of cranial ultrasound, magnetic resonance imaging and clinical findings in sequential studies, *Clin Radiol* (1989) **40**(2):158–66.

25 GEORGE AE, DE LEON MJ, KALNIN A et al, Leukoencephalopathy in normal and pathological aging 2:MRI of brain lucencies, *AJNR* (1986) **7**:567–72.

26 HOWELL MA, GROSSMAN RI, HACKNEY DB et al, Imaging of white matter disease in children, *AJNR* (1988) **9**:503–9.

27 BYDDER GM, YOUNG IR, MRI: clinical use of the inversion recovery sequence, *J Comput Assist Tomogr* (1985) **9**:659–75.

28 BRADLEY WG, WALUCH V, BRANT-ZAWADSKI M et al, Patchy periventricular white matter lesions in the elderly: a common observation during NMR imaging, *Non-invasive imaging* (1984) **1**:35–42.

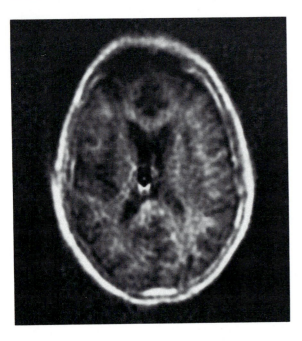

Figure 6.1

Normal volunteer. IR 1400/5/
400 image, showing a high level
of contrast between gray and
white matter (image taken in
1979).

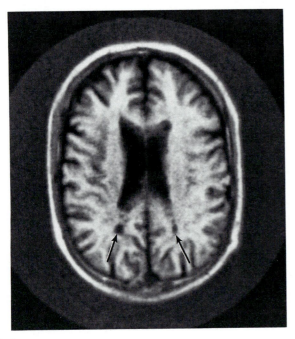

a

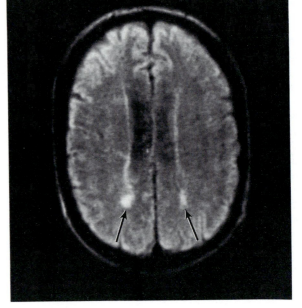

b

Figure 6.2

Multiple sclerosis. IR 1500/44/
500 (**a**) and SE 1500/80 (**b**)
images. Lesions are seen
posteriorly in a periventricular
location (arrows).

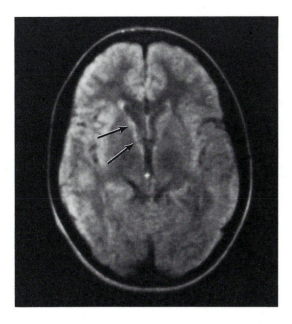

Figure 6.3

Multiple sclerosis (SE 1500/80). Subtle periventricular changes are seen (arrows).

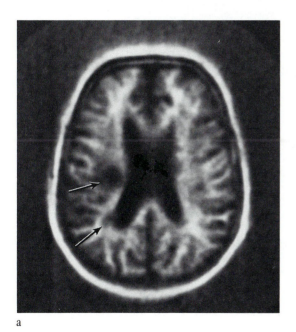

a

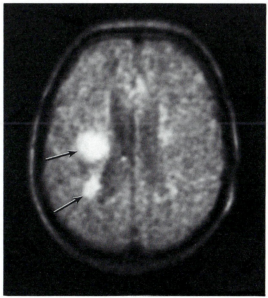

b

Figure 6.4

Multiple sclerosis. Serial follow-up IR 1400/5/400 (**a**) and SE 1080/80 (**b**) series followed eight months later by IR 1400/5/400 (**c**) and SE 1080/80 (**d**) series. Seventeen months after the initial scans IR 1400/13/400 (**e**) and SE 1580/80 (**f**) images were obtained. Note the improvement in signal-to-noise between the first and second pair of images and the increase in spatial resolution from the second to the third pair. The right-sided periventricular lesions (arrows) in (**a**) and (**b**) have resolved in (**c**) and (**d**) but the left-sided posterior ventricular lesions appear to have increased in size. The last pair of images indicate remission.

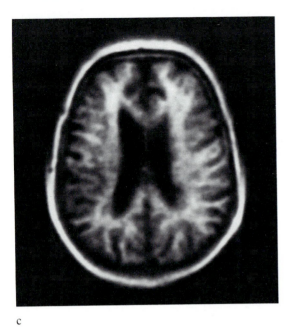

c

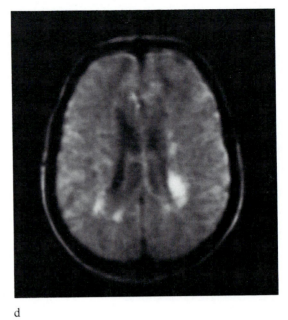

d

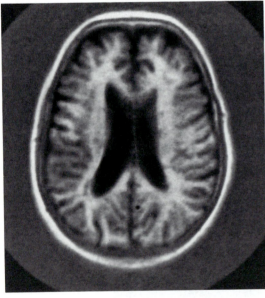

e

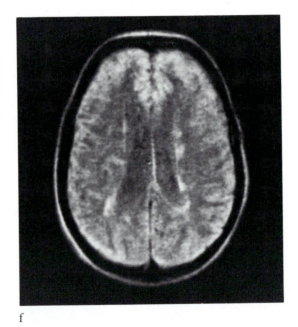

f

Figure 6.4 *continued*

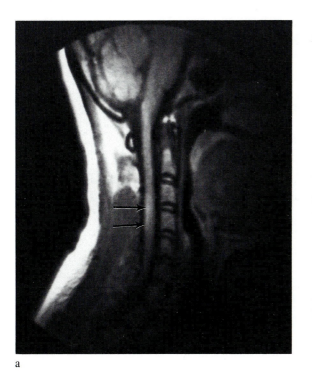

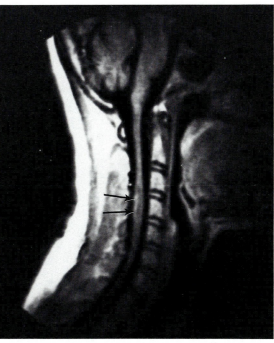

a

b

Figure 6.5

Multiple sclerosis. Images of
the spinal cord, after
intravenous Gd-DTPA, SE
544/44 (**a**) and IR 1500/44/500
(**b**). Enhancement of the lesion
is seen posteriorly (arrows).

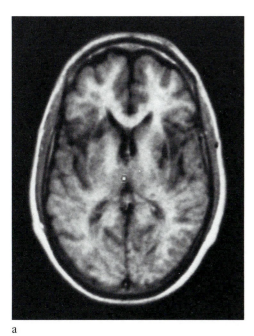

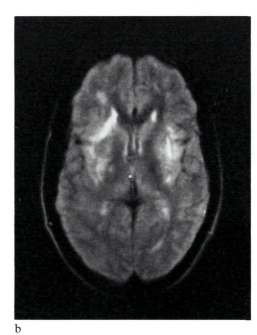

Figure 6.6

Cerebrovascular disease. IR
1500/44/500 (**a**) and SE 1500/80
(**b**) images. Multiple focal
lesions are seen in the deep gray
and white matter of the brain as
well as in the periventricular
regions.

a

b

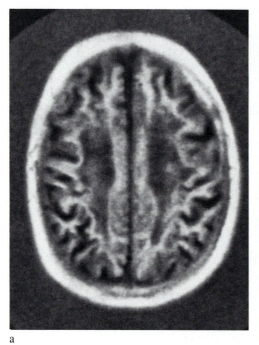

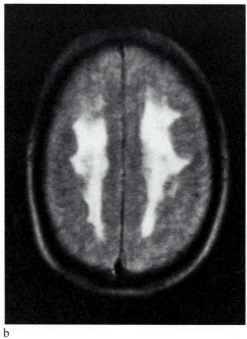

a

b

Figure 6.7

Subacute arteriosclerosis encephalopathy. IR 1500/44/500 (**a**) and SE 1500/80 (**b**) images. Extensive confluent changes are seen in the white matter.

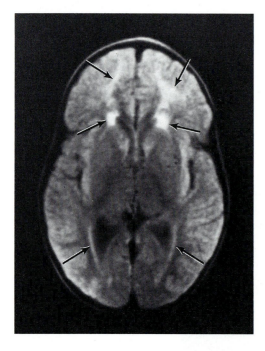

Figure 6.8

Alexander's disease (SE 1500/80). Changes are seen in the white matter of both frontal lobes (arrows).

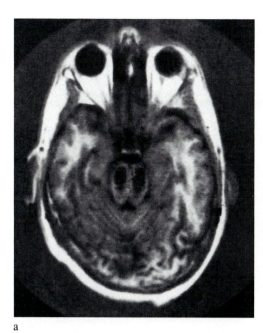

a

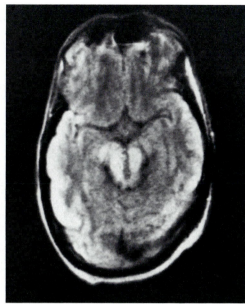

b

Figure 6.9

Central pontine myelinolysis. IR 1500/44/500 (**a**) and SE 1500/80 (**b**).

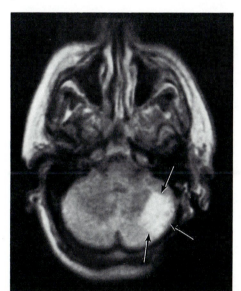

Figure 6.10

Radiation damage (SE 1500/80). Changes are seen in the cerebellum (arrows) medial to a carcinoma of the mastoid which was irradiated.

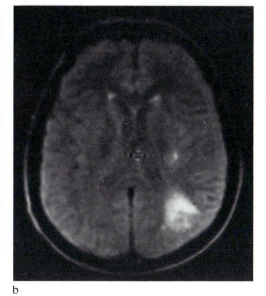

a   b

Figure 6.11

Progressive multifocal leukoencephalopathy. (**a–b**) SE 1580/80. Multiple confluent and ring-shaped lesions are seen.

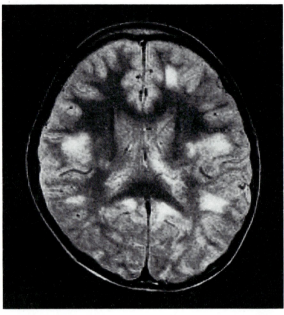

a

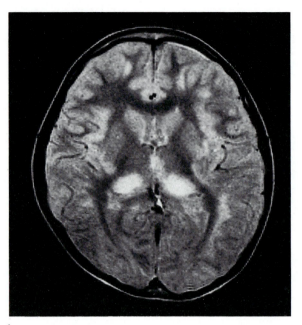

b

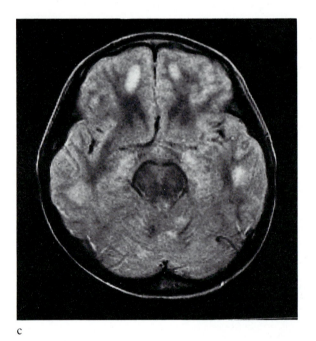

c

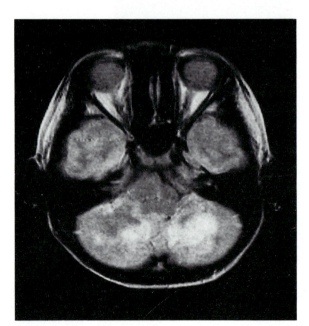

d

Figure 6.12

Progressive multifocal
leukoencephalitis. (**a–b**) SE
2000/60. Multifocal lesions are
present.

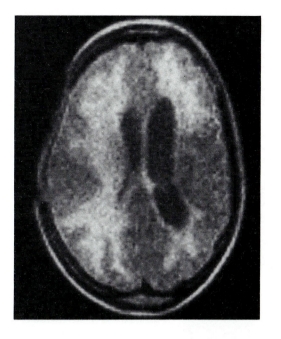

Figure 6.13

Post-infectious demyelinating disease (SE 1000/56). Extensive changes are seen in both hemispheres.

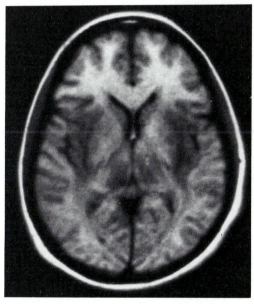

a

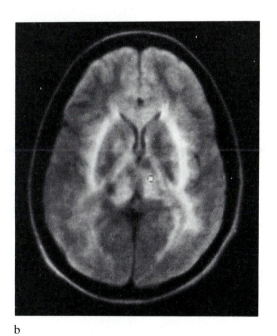

b

Figure 6.14

Post-infectious demyelinating disease. IR 1500/44/500 (**a**) and SE 1500/80 (**b**) images. The disease is largely confined to white matter tracts.

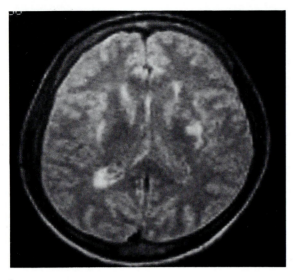

a

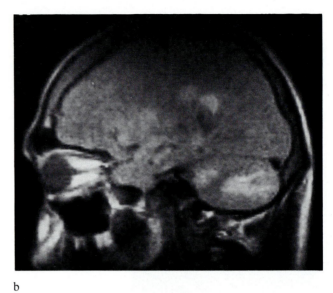

b

Figure 6.15

Encephalitis. SE 2000/56 (**a**) and SE 1000/56 (**b**) sagittal images. Early changes are seen.

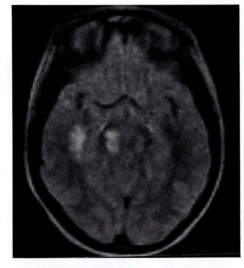

Figure 6.16

Brainstem encephalitis (SE 2000/56). Focal changes are seen.

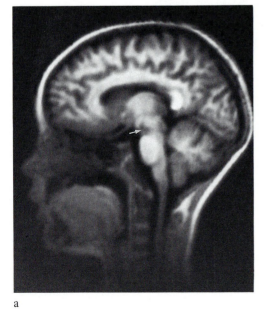

a

b

Figure 6.17

Brainstem encephalitis. IR 1400/13/400 (**a**) and SE 1080/80 (**b**) sagittal images. Changes are seen in the mesencephalon.

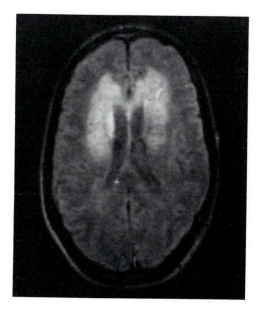

Figure 6.18

Acquired immunodeficiency
syndrome (SE 1500/80).
Extensive changes are seen in
the white matter of both frontal
lobes.

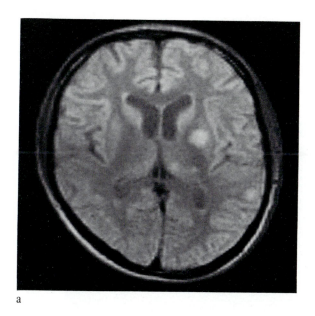

a

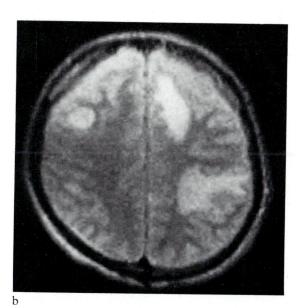

b

Figure 6.19

Acquired immunodeficiency
syndrome. SE 2000/28 (**a**) and
SE 2000/56 (**b**). Extensive focal
changes are present.

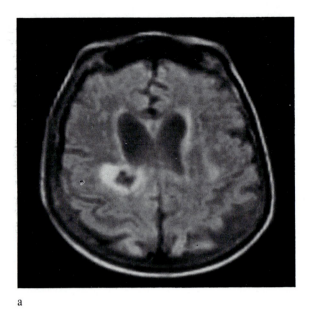
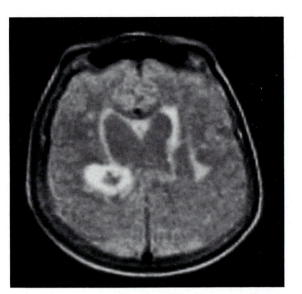

a   b

Figure 6.20

Bacterial abscess. SE 2000/28
(**a**) and SE 2000/56 (**b**) images.
Focal ring-shaped lesions are
seen.

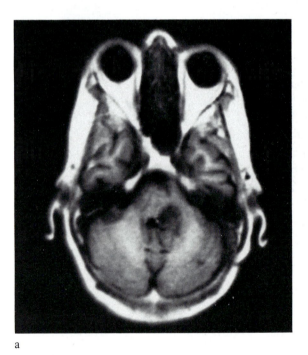
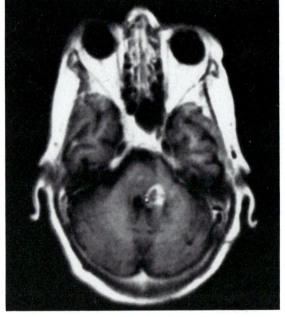

a   b

Figure 6.21

Bacterial abscess. IR 1500/44/
500 images before (**a**) and after
(**b**) iv Gd-DTPA. Ring
enhancement is seen at the
margins of the lesions.

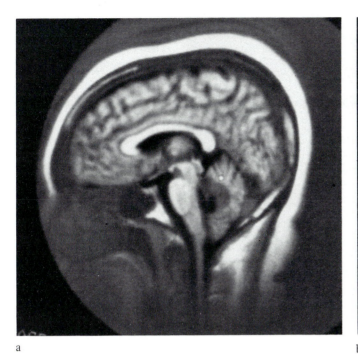

a

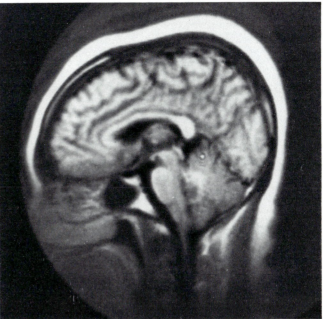

b

Figure 6.22

Tuberculous abscess. IR 1500/
44/500 before (**a**) sagittal images
and after (**b**) iv Gd-DTPA.
Ring enhancement is seen
around the lesion.

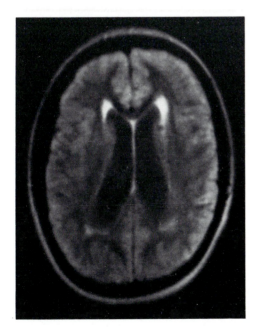

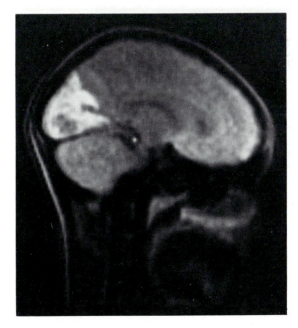

Figure 6.23

Tuberculous infection. (SE
1580/80). Changes are seen at
the periventricular margins.

Figure 6.24

Fungal abscess (SE 1080/80).
Sagittal image. The disease is
anterior to the occipital lobe.

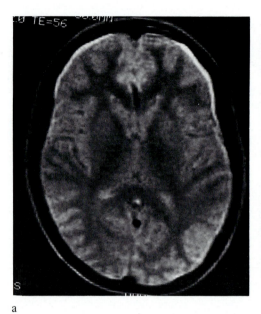

a

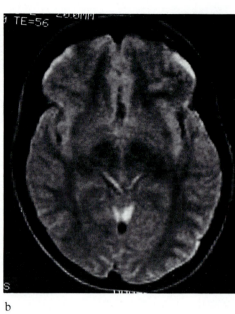

b

Figure 6.25

Meningitis. SE 2000/56 (**a**) and SE 2000/56 (**b**) images. Changes are seen in the cisterns and at the brain margin.

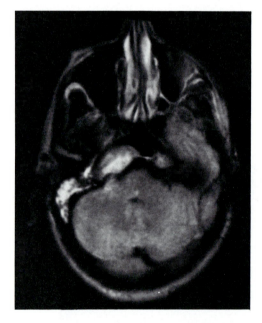

Figure 6.26

Infection of the left mastoid (SE 1500/80). Fluid is seen at the left mastoid.

7

Hemorrhage and vascular abnormalities

William G Bradley

While many brain lesions have a similar appearance on MRI and CT, this is certainly not true of hemorrhage.[1] On CT, acute hemorrhage becomes hyperdense within an hour as the clot forms. This lasts for several days and then fades to isodensity and eventually hypodensity. On MRI, hemorrhage less than 12 to 24 hours old may not be distinguishable from vasogenic edema. Its appearance subsequently is an evolving pattern of variable signal intensity which depends on the specific form of hemoglobin which is present (Figure 7.1), or whether the red cells are intact or lysed, on the operating field strength, on the type of signal (that is, spin echo or gradient echo), and on contrast (that is, T_1- or T_2-weighting). The appearance of hemorrhage also depends on the compartment of the brain involved—subarachnoid, subdural, or intraparenchymal. Finally, for parenchymal hematomas, different zones may be defined from the inner core to the outer rim which all vary in appearance depending on field strength and imaging technique.

The MR appearance of most lesions in the brain has a direct correlate in CT. Edematous or encephalomalacic lesions, which appear relatively dark on non-enhanced CT, generally appear dark on T_1-weighted images (due to relative T_1 prolongation), and bright on T_2-weighted images (due to T_2 prolongation). The degree of T_1 and T_2 prolongation depends primarily on water content and secondarily on molecular environment, that is, specifically, on the percentage of hydration-layer water (see Chapter 1). The appearance of hemorrhage, on the other hand, requires an understanding of not only the evolving pathophysiology of a hematoma, but also the complex NMR chemistry of hemoglobin oxidation.[1] Because the heme iron may have unpaired electrons, the concept of 'paramagnetism' must be understood to appreciate

fully the MR appearance of evolving hemorrhage. Paramagnetic concepts such as the 'electron–proton dipole–dipole interaction' and 'magnetic susceptibility effects' all enter into an MR discussion of hemorrhage. Such concepts have necessitated the increasing collaboration of chemists and radiologists in the understanding of these phenomena. Because the mechanisms responsible for the variable appearance of hemorrhage include those which affect the appearance of physiologic and pathologic iron deposition, the two topics are combined in this chapter.

The earliest reports of intracranial hemorrhage suggested a relatively intense MR appearance of all hemorrhage relative to surrounding brain, as in Figure 7.2.[2,3] This was attributed to the short T_1 of the presumably paramagnetic, iron-containing hemoglobin. The short T_1 character of hemorrhage could be particularly enhanced relative to surrounding brain on a T_1-weighted spin-echo image, also shown in Figure 7.2.

As experience was gained, subsequent reports indicated that acute intracranial hemorrhage could be much more difficult to detect by MRI.[4,5] This was attributed to a lack of T_1-shortening during the acute phase; however, no explanation of this phenomenon was given.[4] Acute subarachnoid hemorrhage in particular was said to be difficult to detect, particularly in comparison with CT.[5] Although these two reports agreed that acute intracranial hemorrhage was difficult to detect on MR images, they disagreed as to the mechanism by which hemorrhage subsequently became intense. While the data of a number of workers suggested a T_1-shortening process,[2,3,4,6] other results suggested no change in T_1 but rather a prolongation of T_2,[5] both explanations which increase the signal intensity on spin-echo images. Subsequently, the short

T_2, long T_1 appearance of an acute intracranial hematoma was described at 1.5 Tesla.[7] It was noted that the subsequent intensity increase in the hematoma reflected both a shortening of T_1 and a prolongation of T_2. While there is now general agreement on the MR *appearance* of intracranial hemorrhage, the biochemical mechanisms involved continue to be a matter of debate. Appreciation of the subtleties of this complex topic requires a working understanding of the mechanisms of enhancement of proton relaxation.[8,9]

Mechanisms of proton relaxation enhancement

At present, most high-quality MR images are still produced by a traditional 90°/180° spin-echo technique in which the spins are rephased both by gradient reversal and by the 180° RF pulse. The gradient reversal causes spatial rephasing, for example, from left to right, and the 180° pulse causes temporal rephasing. To generate a spin-echo signal, spatial and temporal rephasing must occur simultaneously. The dependence of signal intensity I on T_1 and T_2 in a spin-echo image can be approximated:[10]

$$I = N(H) \, f(v) \, (1 - e^{-TR/T_1}) \, (e^{-TE/T_2})$$

Where N(H) is the proton density, f(v) is a function of flow, TR and TE are the programmable repetition and echo-delay times, respectively, and e is the base of the natural logarithm.

The newer fast scanning or 'gradient-echo' techniques utilize flip angles θ less than 90° and gradient reversal alone without 180° pulses to temporally rephase the spins. Signal intensity for such techniques can be approximated:[11]

$$I = \frac{N(H) \, f(v) \sin \theta \, [1 - e^{-TR/T_1}] \, e^{-TE/T_2^\star}}{1 - \cos \theta \, e^{-TR/T_1}}$$

Notice that signal intensity for these fast scanning techniques depends not on T_2 but on $T_2^\star$.

The relationship between T_2 and $T_2^\star$ is shown in Figure 1.6, page 14. $T_2^\star$ is the exponential time constant of the envelope of the free induction delay (FID) which incorporates all causes of dephasing due to non-uniform magnetic fields.[10] These fields can be constant over the time course of an echo or they can fluctuate randomly. Fixed non-uniformities can result from a poorly wound magnet or from focal areas of iron deposition which become relatively more magnetized than the non-iron-containing areas around them.

Fluctuating non-uniformities are due either to the random thermal motions of flipping hydrogen nuclei, or to the random diffusion of protons through regions of different magnetic field strengths. Only randomly fluctuating fields produce T_2 decay. Both fixed and fluctuating non-uniformities contribute to loss of signal in the FID, that is, to $T_2^\star$ decay.[10]

Both fixed and fluctuating non-uniformities cause signal loss on a gradient-echo image.[11] The fixed non-uniformities, on the other hand, can be rephased by the 180° pulse in a traditional spin echo. Spin-echo images, therefore, are only sensitive to the fluctuating non-uniformities which produce T_2 decay. In a perfectly uniform external magnetic field, T_2 is equal to $T_2^\star$, since all dephasing is due to fluctuations of the internal magnetic fields of the sample.[10] In a real magnet, however, $T_2^\star$ is shorter than T_2 because of the inevitable non-uniformities in the main magnetic field.

The molecules which contain hydrogen nuclei are constantly in motion—translating, vibrating, and rotating.[12] The time constants for these motions depend on the size of the parent molecules and on the strength of the local chemical bonds and intra- and intermolecular forces. The reciprocal of a time constant of motion is frequency. One can describe certain aspects of molecular behaviour in terms of these intrinsic motional frequencies. The T_1 relaxation time usually reflects the component of these natural motional frequencies at the operating (Larmor) frequency of the MR imager. Most MR imagers in clinical practice today operate in the frequency range of 2 to 65 MHz. To the extent that there is a large component of motion at the Larmor frequency, T_1 relaxation is efficient and T_1 is short. If the predominant motional frequencies of the protons are too high or too low, T_1 is long. Water (being a very small molecule) has very high natural motional frequencies (small component at the Larmor frequency) and, therefore, water has a long T_1. Large protein molecules tumble very slowly with frequency components far below the usual Larmor frequency. They are equally inefficient at T_1 relaxation and also have large T_1 values. The water in proteinaceous solutions has a shorter T_1 time than pure (bulk-phase) water because of the hydration-layer environment.[13] This is due to the slowing of the naturally rapid motions as a result of attraction of the water molecules to the charged side groups of the protein. Therefore, they have a frequency closer to that of the Larmor frequency. While the above discussion has centered on the motion of the proton or of the molecule to which the proton is attached, relaxation really results from the natural motional frequencies of the magnetic moments.[12]

Any motion of the magnetic moments that contributes to T_1 relaxation also contributes to T_2 relaxation; however, the converse is not true. There are motions which contribute to T_2 relaxation which do not affect T_1 relaxation at all. For example, T_2 relaxation can result from slowly fluctuating internal fields which cause local magnetic field inhomogeneity at the molecular level. Liquids tend not to have significant components of motion at the usual Larmor frequencies, nor do they have significant, fixed internal fields. They thus have long T_2 times. Solids and viscous materials have stationary internal fields which force spin–spin exchange (leading to dephasing), and thus they have much shorter T_2 times.[14,15]

Processes which shorten either T_1 or T_2 are said to 'enhance' proton relaxation.[8,9] Paramagnetic substances dissolved in water expose the water protons to fluctuating magnetic fields from unpaired electrons flipping up and down. When these electronic magnetic moments fluctuate at or near the Larmor frequency, both T_1 and T_2 are shortened. Such substances are said to cause 'proton relaxation enhancement' (PRE). Since T_1 times in biological substances are almost always longer than T_2 times, however, T_1-shortening is observed at a lower concentration of the paramagnetic agent than is needed to produce T_2-shortening (as discussed below).

When discussing the effects of paramagnetic substances, it is useful to consider the reciprocals of the T_1 or T_2 relaxation times which are called the R_1 and R_2 'relaxation rates', respectively.[9] The addition of a paramagnetic substance to an aqueous solution affects the R_1 and R_2 relaxation rates to the same degree, thus

$$R_{net} = R_{substance} + R_{paramagnetic\ agent}$$

where $R = R_1$ or R_2. The effect on the T_1 or T_2 relaxation times differs markedly, however. For example, if a substance (like brain) has a T_1 of 600 msec and a T_2 of 50 msec, then $R_1 = 1/T_1 = 1.66\ sec^{-1}$ and $R_2 = 1/T_2 = 20\ sec^{-1}$. If the paramagnetic agent increases both relaxation rates by $1\ sec^{-1}$, then $R_{1_{net}} = 2.66\ sec^{-1}$ and $R_{2_{net}} = 21\ sec^{-1}$. As a result, $T_{1_{net}} = 1/2.66 = 376\ msec$ and $T_2 = 1/21\ sec^{-1} = 48\ msec$. Thus T_1 has decreased by 37.4 per cent while T_2 has decreased by only 4 per cent, despite the 'equal' additive effect on the relaxation rates.

In biological substances which do not contain iron or other paramagnetic species, the proton–proton–dipole–dipole interaction between nuclear magnetic moments is the principal mechanism for T_1 and T_2 relaxation. When paramagnetic substances with unpaired electrons are present, these can have a profound effect on T_1 and T_2 because the electron magnetic moment is some 700 times greater than that of the proton. Unpaired electrons are necessary to produce electronic paramagnetism. The greater the number of unpaired electrons, the greater will be the magnetic effect. Unpaired electrons in the outer shell of an atom undergo relaxation processes just like the nuclei. These processes are characterized by T_1 and T_2

values for electrons, called the 'electron spin relaxation times'. How rapidly electronic relaxation occurs can be a major determinant of the magnetic influence of the dissolved paramagnetic substance on the water protons.[6]

Just as proton magnetic moments fluctuating at the Larmor frequency are most efficient at T_1 relaxation,[12] flipping electrons at or near the Larmor frequency enhance T_1 relaxation of the nearby water protons. When the T_1 time of the electron corresponds to a natural frequency much higher than the Larmor frequency (short electronic T_1), the efficiency of PRE is reduced.[6] Because the interaction between the dipole of the electron and that of a local hydrogen nucleus falls off as the sixth power of the distance between them, hydrogen nuclei must be able to approach the paramagnetic center within a distance of several angstroms,[8] or there will be a negligible enhancement of relaxation.

Proton–electron–dipole–dipole interactions occur when the water protons in an aqueous solution have access (within 3 angstroms) to the paramagnetic center. Since the T_1 of most biologic tissues is significantly longer than the T_2, the effect of addition of a paramagnetic agent is initially one of visible T_1-shortening and, as the concentration increases, T_2-shortening.[12] T_1-shortening increases the signal intensity, particularly on T_1-weighted spin-echo images. At higher concentrations of the paramagnetic substances, however, the effect of T_2-shortening is to decrease the intensity due to increased dephasing and loss of coherence, as shown in Figure 1.13, page 19.

With paramagnetic substances in aqueous solution, T_1-shortening is expected to dominate over T_2-shortening at the concentrations usually encountered. There are other types of paramagnetic PRE mechanisms, however, where T_2 can be selectively shortened without affecting T_1.[7] The T_2 relaxation time of a substance reflects internal magnetic field inhomogeneities which lead to irreversible loss of phase coherence.[10] Such local non-uniformity can be produced by unpaired electrons which become aligned in a magnetic field. The greater this magnetic non-uniformity, the more rapid the dephasing, and the shorter the T_2 time, as illustrated in Figure 1.15, page 20.

One property of *paramagnetic* substances is that, when placed in a magnetic field, they become more strongly magnetized than *diamagnetic* substances. (Diamagnetic substances have no unpaired electrons and are repelled from the strong part of a magnetic field.) This magnetization is quantified by the 'magnetic susceptibility' which is the ratio of the induced over the applied magnetic field. Iron-containing molecules such as ferritin have high magnetic susceptibilities and create local regions of magnetic non-uniformity. These lead to more rapid $T_2^\star$ decay (producing signal loss on gradient-echo images,[16] and also shorten the T_2 times of the nuclear moments diffusing through these regions, decreasing the signal of a traditional spin-echo image.[7,17] Because the induced field (and thus the induced non-uniformity) is proportional to the strength of the applied magnetic field (through the magnetic susceptibility coefficient), both T_2^*- and T_2-shortening are greater at higher fields.[7] To the extent that dephasing results from diffusion through the field gradients,[17] T_2 decreases as the square of the field strength.[7] This quadratic dependence of dephasing on field strength has also been noted in the phenomenon of slow flow into a gradient which produces first-echo dephasing and even-echo rephasing,[18] as discussed in Chapter 3. Dephasing can also result from the diffusion of water molecules across cell membranes when the intracellular magnetic susceptibility differs from that outside the cell.[19] For example, when paramagnetic deoxyhemoglobin or methemoglobin molecules (see below) are contained within intact red blood cells in an acute or subacute hematoma, the induced magnetic field inside the red cell is much greater than that outside the red cell. Water molecules diffusing across the red cell membrane thus experience a magnetic field gradient which may result in dephasing, as shown in Figure 1.16, page 21, and thus T_2-shortening.[1] The influence of fibrin clot retraction on T_2-shortening has also been noted recently.[20,21] Specifically, when the clot does not retract, there is less T_2 shortening.[21] Patients with hemorrhagic diatheses or those on anticoagulants, therefore, may not demonstrate the expected T_2-shortening following acute hemorrhage. Obviously, much remains to be learned about this complicated process.

Oxidation of hemoglobin

In order to understand the variable MR appearance of intracranial hemorrhage, the structure of hemoglobin and its various oxidation products[22] must be considered, as shown in Figure 7.1. Circulating in blood, hemoglobin alternates between the oxy and deoxy forms as oxygen is exchanged during transit through the high oxygen environment of the lungs and lower oxygen environment of the capillaries. To bind oxygen irreversibly, the iron in the hemoglobin (the 'heme iron') must be in the reduced, ferrous (Fe^{2+}) state.[22] The red cell has several metabolic pathways to inhibit various oxidizing agents from converting its heme iron to the non-functional ferric (Fe^{3+}) state. These include the Embden-Mayerhof pathway (anaerobic glycolysis which produces NADH) and the hexose monophosphate shunt (aerobic glycolysis which produces NADPH), both of which power methemoglobin

reductase systems.[23] When the red cell is removed from the circulation, these metabolic pathways fail and the hemoglobin undergoes oxidative conversion to methemoglobin.

The heme iron is normally held in a non-polar crevice in the hemoglobin molecule by a covalent bond to histidine attached at the F8 position of the globin chain and by four hydrophobic van der Waals forces to non-polar groups on the globin molecule. The sixth coordination site of the heme iron is occupied by molecular oxygen in oxyhemoglobin and is vacant in deoxyhemoglobin, as illustrated in Figure 7.1. If the ferrous heme iron is oxidized to the ferric state, methemoglobin is formed.[6] Although the five bonds to the globin molecule are unchanged, the sixth coordination site of the heme iron is now occupied by either a water molecule or a hydroxyl ion, depending on whether the methemoglobin is in the acid or base form, respectively. At physiologic pH, the acid form predominates. With continued oxidative denaturation, methemoglobin is subsequently converted to derivatives known as hemichromes.[22] The iron in these compounds remains in the ferric state. However, an alteration of the tertiary structure of the globin molecule occurs such that the sixth coordination site of the heme iron becomes occupied by a ligand from within the globin molecule (most likely the distal histidine at E7). Unlike methemoglobin, there are no unpaired electrons in hemichromes, that is, they are not paramagnetic.

As noted in Figure 7.1, the oxidation of deoxyhemoglobin to methemoglobin is a reversible reaction. While the factors affecting the conversion of deoxyhemoglobin to methemoglobin (or vice versa) are incompletely described at this time, several statements can be made empirically. *Some* oxygen is needed to oxidize the heme iron to the ferric form, yet normal levels of oxygen allow the methemoglobin reductase systems to reduce it back to the ferrous form. Methemoglobin formation thus appears to occur most rapidly when there is a small amount of oxygen available. Methemoglobin formation is retarded when the oxygen tension is both normal and very low.

The magnetic properties of dried blood were first evaluated by Faraday 140 years ago.[24] However, it was not until 90 years later that Pauling and Coryell considered the magnetic properties of blood in the fluid state and showed that deoxyhemoglobin was paramagnetic, while oxyhemoglobin was diamagnetic.[25] These observations enabled them to describe the various electron spin states of oxy- and deoxyhemoglobin. In deoxyhemoglobin, the heme iron is in the high-spin ferrous state, characterized by four unpaired electrons. When oxygen is added to form oxyhemoglobin, one of the electrons is partially transferred to the oxygen molecule resulting in a low-spin ferrous form without any unpaired electrons.[22]

Although Pauling and Coryell demonstrated that deoxyhemoglobin is paramagnetic, the paramagnetism by itself does not ensure proton paramagnetic enhancement in aqueous solution. As discussed above, the paramagnetic center must also be accessible to surrounding water protons. Quantitation of PRE requires consideration of the magnitude of the magnetic moment of the paramagnetic dipole (that is, the number of unpaired electrons), the electron-spin relaxation time, the concentration of paramagnetic dipoles, the average distance from surrounding water protons, and the rates of the relative motions of the proton and paramagnetic centers.[6,8,9] Theories of proton relaxation by paramagnetic solutes are based on translational diffusion and the distance of closest approach of the proton and paramagnetic ions, which determines an 'outer sphere' of influence.[26] It has also been shown that there can be a contribution to the relaxation from exchange between solvent and water ligands in the first coordination sphere of the paramagnetic ion, that is, 'inner-sphere effects'.[26]

Although deoxyhemoglobin is paramagnetic, this only means that there are unpaired electrons. Because the T_1 of the electrons in deoxyhemoglobin is very short and because water molecules are unable to approach the heme iron within a distance of three angstroms, the T_1 of an aqueous solution of deoxyhemoglobin is not particularly short, thus it does not manifest enhanced proton paramagnetic relaxation.[27] Methemoglobin, on the other hand, has a much longer electronic T_1 (this means there is a frequency component of motion closer to the Larmor frequencies used in MRI) and water molecules are better able to approach the paramagnetic center.[26] Thus, methemoglobin causes significant T_1-shortening in aqueous solutions because of a combination of both inner-sphere and outer-sphere effects.[26] Water proton T_1 relaxation by methemoglobin results from a combination of ligand exchange effects (from the water molecule at the sixth coordination site) and from outer-sphere diffusional effects, perhaps by virtue of increased access of solvent protons to the heme iron through the non-polar crevice.[26]

With this physiologic and chemical background, we can now examine the variable appearance of hemorrhage and brain iron on MR images.

Intraparenchymal hematoma

When describing intraparenchymal hematomas (IPHs), it is useful to consider four separate factors: the form of hemoglobin present, the state of the red cells, ie intact or lysed, the MR technique (spin echo or gradient echo and T_1- or T_2-weighting), and the strength of the magnetic field. Table 7.1 lists the T_1 and T_2 characteristics of IPHS.

Four stages in the aging of the hematoma can be described:[1] hyperacute (first 24 hours), acute (beginning at 24 hours), subacute (more than 3 days), and chronic (older than 1 week). Four zones can be

Table 7.1 MR appearance of intraparenchymal hematomas.

Stage	Time	Compartment	Hemoglobin	T1	T2
Hyperacute	<24 Hours	Intracellular	Oxyhemoglobin	Med	Med
Acute	1–3 Days	Intracellular	Deoxyhemoglobin	Long	Short
Subacute:					
Early	3+ Days	Intracellular	Methemoglobin	Short	Short
Late	7+ Days	Extracellular	Methemoglobin	Short	Long
Chronic:					
Center	14+ Days	Extracellular	Hemichromes	Med	Med
Rim		Intracellular	Hemosiderin	Med	Short

described: inner core, outer core, rim, and reactive brain.[28] During the first 24 hours (hyperacute phase), the hematoma consists of a mixture of oxy- and deoxyhemoglobin, initially as a liquid suspension of intact red cells and, as thrombosis progresses and plasma is resorbed, an increasingly solid conglomerate of intact red cells.[1,21] Over the next several days (acute phase), the hematoma consists primarily of deoxy-hemoglobin within intact red cells, as illustrated in Figure 1.16. Over the subacute period, which begins after several days, deoxyhemoglobin undergoes oxidative denaturation, forming methemoglobin, first at the periphery (outer core) and then in the center (inner core).[7] Early in this phase, the red cells are intact. Later in this phase (at approximately one week), red cell lysis occurs. At the end of the first week, modified macrophages (glitter cells) begin to remove the iron from the hemoglobin within the hematoma.[1] This marks the beginning of the chronic phase. The heme iron is deposited at the periphery as a rim of hemosiderin and ferritin within the macrophages surrounding the hematoma.[7] The center of the hematoma[1] is eventually left with a non-iron-containing, non-paramagnetic heme pigment, such as hematoidin.[28] During the hyperacute and acute phases, the hematoma is surrounded by vasogenic edema which gradually resorbs during the subacute phase and is essentially absent during the chronic phase.

A note of caution: although it is useful to describe the evolution of a hematoma in these well-defined stages, in fact they may coexist. For example, at the time hemosiderin is first deposited at the periphery of a hematoma (indicating the beginning of the chronic stage), free methemoglobin may be present in the outer core (late subacute stage) and intracellular methemoglobin or even deoxyhemoglobin may still be present in the inner core from the early subacute and acute stages, respectively. By convention, the hematoma is described in terms of the most mature form present.

On T_1-weighted images, the hematoma and reactive vasogenic edema are iso- to hypointense with brain during the first three days (approximately) due to their longer T_1 times, as shown in Figure 7.3a. As the deoxyhemoglobin is oxidized to methemoglobin peripherally during the subacute stage, T_1 is markedly shortened, resulting in increased intensity on T_1-weighted images, as in Figure 7.4a.[6] During the early chronic stage,[1] hemosiderin is first seen in the rim and the vasogenic edema starts to be resorbed, as in Figure 7.5. Subsequently, the deoxyhemoglobin in the inner core is also oxidized to methemoglobin, illustrated in Figure 7.6, which can persist for years following the initial hemorrhage. Eventually the methemoglobin is either oxidized to hemichromes (which have no paramagnetic properties),[22] or the iron is removed by macrophages leaving non-iron-containing heme pig-

ments such as hematoidin. Moderate T_1-shortening remains, however, because of the protein content which increases the percentage of water in the hydration-layer environment.[15] The T_1 changes in evolving hemorrhage do not depend on field strength over the range of field strengths currently used for routine MR imaging, although this statement may not be true for the ultralow field scanners now being increasingly used.

On T_2-weighted images, the changing temporal appearance of a hematoma depends on the field strength of the particular MR imaging system being used.[7] During the initial 24 hours (hyperacute phase), the T_2 relaxation time reflects both the fluid–solid character of the fresh hematoma,[21] and the state of oxygenation of the hemoglobin. As the clot contracts over the first few hours, it initially becomes visible on CT due to the protein content of the hemoglobin. Until a significant amount of deoxyhemoglobin is formed on MR, however, T_2-shortening is not seen.[29] Over 95 per cent of arterial blood is oxyhemoglobin,[23] which is diamagnetic and, therefore, does not cause T_2-shortening. Over 70 per cent of venous blood is normally in the oxy form, depending upon the pH.[23] Because most non-traumatic hematomas arise from arterial blood (such as microaneurysms in hypertension, true aneurysms, and AVMs), the fraction of deoxyhemoglobin in the hematoma may initially be well below 5 per cent and there may be no significant PRE.[30] The minimum concentration of deoxyhemo-globin which produces visible T_2-shortening depends on the field strength,[7] and on the imaging technique, the gradient echo being more sensitive than the traditional spin echo.[16,31]

In a recent presentation, it was reported that hyperacute arterial hemorrhage blood appears black on $T_2^\star$-weighted gradient echo images.[30] This would suggest that these sequences are sensitive to the magnetic susceptibility effects in the small amount of deoxyhemoglobin (5 per cent) present in arterial blood. If these results are verified clinically, then such sequences will render MR as sensitive as CT in the detection of hyperacute parenchymal hemorrhage.

The rate at which deoxyhemoglobin is formed from oxyhemoglobin depends on the local oxygen tension.[31] This tends to be lower in non-perfused hemorrhagic tumors,[32] as well as in extra-axial and extracranial hematomas (see below). The oxygen tension tends to be higher in hemorrhagic cortical infarction.[31] Petechial hemorrhages in hemorrhagic cortical infarcts in normally oxygenated brain may remain in the oxy-hemoglobin state for a much longer period of time.[31] Interstitial hemorrhage, for example, that arising from venous infarcts (Figure 7.7) and hemorrhagic contusions (Figures 7.8–7.10), will have a somewhat lower partial pressure of oxygen. Large hematomas and tumors have a lower oxygen tension still.[33–35]

Even after deoxyhemoglobin has been formed, T_2-shortening is not ensured.[20] Deoxyhemoglobin in unclotted blood does not have a short T_2 relaxation time.[21] The red cells must be further concentrated by thrombosis to cause T_2-shortening.[21,36] Stated differently, T_2 shortens progressively as hematocrit approaches 100%.[20] Prior to clot retraction during the hyperacute phase, therefore, T_2-shortening may be minimal or absent.[21]

While certain causes of T_2-shortening in an acute hematoma are field strength-dependent, several others are not. The T_2-shortening produced by the conversion of oxy- to deoxyhemoglobin and that due to increasing hematocrit both depend on field strength.[20] However, the formation and retraction of the fibrin clot alone account for 18% of the T_2-shortening observed at 90 MHz (2.1 Tesla).[20] These causes of T_2-shortening are not field-dependent and thus are expected to have a proportionally greater influence at lower fields.[20]

After the initial 24 hours, magnetically-susceptible deoxyhemoglobin should be present within clotted, intact red cells (acute phase). The dephasing (T_2 decay) resulting from diffusion of water molecules in and out of the red cell increases as the square of the applied magnetic field.[7] Thus the low-intensity appearance in the center of an acute hematoma is more obvious at 1.5 Tesla (Figure 7.10) than at 0.35 Tesla. However, the decreased signal is also easily seen at midfield using a routine T_2-weighted spin-echo technique (Figure 7.9). Even at fields as low as 0.15 Tesla,[37] however, acute hemorrhages which are subtle by CT are obvious when a T_2-weighted gradient echo technique is used (Figure 7.8). Since high-field and gradient-echo techniques increase the sensitivity to magnetic susceptibility effects through different mechanisms, they are additive,[1] and produce marked signal loss when used together, as shown in Figure 7.11.

The subacute phase is defined by the oxidation of deoxyhemoglobin to methemoglobin.[6] Early in the subacute phase the red cells are still intact.[33] When methemoglobin is present within intact red cells, there is both T_1- and T_2-shortening.[33] The T_1-shortening can be enhanced on T_1-weighted inversion recovery (Figure 7.12) or short TR/short TE spin-echo (Figure 7.13) images. The T_2-shortening becomes apparent on long TR/long TE T_2-weighted images (Figure 7.4). Since the dipole–dipole interaction (resulting in T_1-shortening) occurs over a typical distance of 3 angstroms and the T_2-shortening (resulting from magnetic non-uniformity) occurs over 25 angstroms, the T_2-shortening effect predominates on long TE images (Figure 7.4). The T_2-shortening observed during the acute phase may actually increase during the subacute phase,[33] if deoxyhemoglobin is oxidized to methemoglobin while the red blood cells remain intact. This reflects the five unpaired electrons on methemoglobin as compared to the four unpaired electrons on deoxyhemoglobin. (Other factors being equal, T_2-shortening should be proportional to the square of the number of unpaired electrons.) Early in the subacute phase deoxyhemoglobin may still be present within intact red cells in the inner core and a low-intensity, short T_2 appearance will persist (Figure 7.4). Thus, the transition from acute to subacute hemorrhage may be difficult to document by MRI on T_2-weighted images alone.

Later in the subacute phase, red cell lysis occurs, first peripherally (Figure 7.5),[33] and then centrally (Figure 7.6). As lysis occurs, the T_2-shortening resulting from compartmentalization of methemoglobin is lost and the short T_1 characteristics predominate, leading to high signal on short TR/short TE image (Figure 7.14). The high water content leads to prolongation of both T_2 and proton density,[38] thus late subacute (and chronic) IPH also has high intensity on long TR/long TE images (Figures 7.6 and 7.14). As much now seen obvious, both T_1- and T_2-weighted images are necessary to accurately stage hemorrhage.

In the chronic stage, hemosiderin and ferritin are found within macrophages in the rim surrounding the hematoma.[28] In order for hemosiderin to be formed, red cells containing methemoglobin must first lyse. Thus, there is always a bright ring of free methemoglobin just inside the darker hemosiderin ring. Like deoxyhemoglobin, intracellular, paramagnetic hemosiderin causes preferential T_2-shortening,[7] as in Figures 7.5 and 7.6. Since this is also a magnetic susceptibility effect, the low-intensity rim is more apparent on spin-echo images at high field (Figures 7.5 and 7.6) and on gradient-echo images at any field (Figure 7.15). Such magnetic susceptibility effects offer additional sensitivity in the detection of hemosiderin staining the cortex following subarachnoid hemorrhage (Figures 7.16 and 7.17), that is 'superficial siderosis'.[39] High-field and gradient-echo techniques are also more sensitive for the detection of parenchymal hemosiderin deposition associated with venous angiomas, shown in Figure 7.18, and angiographically occult AVMs which have bled previously.[39–42] It should be emphasized that the staging of parenchymal hematomas is based on the most 'mature' hemoglobin product present. Thus, a 'chronic' hematoma (which is defined by the presence of a hemosiderin rim) may well have less 'mature' forms centrally, for example the oxyhemoglobin in Figure 7.5 or the methemoglobin in Figure 7.6.

Subdural and epidural hematomas

Like parenchymal hemorrhage, subdural hematomas (SDH) have four stages of evolution and thus four different appearances on MRI.[1] Hyperacute SDHs are comprised of a mixture of oxy- and deoxyhemoglobin in semi-clotted blood. They appear slightly more intense than brain on T_1- and T_2-weighted images. Acute SDHs contain deoxyhemoglobin within intact red cells. As noted above, this results in T_2-shortening. Thus, acute SDHs will have low intensity on T_2-weighted images, particularly at higher fields,[7] and when gradient echoes are used at any field strength.[37] They will be isointense with brain on T_1-weighted images.

During the subacute stage (CT isodense), the red cells lyse and deoxyhemoglobin becomes oxidized to methemoglobin. If they occur synchronously, these effects tend to shorten the T_1 and lengthen the T_2, both of which will increase the intensity on either T_1- or T_2-weighted images, as shown in Figures 7.19 and 7.20.

The definition of a chronic SDH depends on whether the determination is being made clinically or by CT hypointensity (both of which suggest onset at three weeks). Continued oxidative denaturation of methemoglobin forms hemichromes, which are low-spin, non-paramagnetic ferric compounds.[22] The T_1 of such compounds is greater than that of paramagnetic methemoglobin, thus the intensity of chronic subdural hematomas (Figure 7.20) is less than that of subacute subdural hematomas, particularly on T_1-weighted images. Chronic SDHs are still more intense than CSF, however, due to their higher protein concentration.[13]

Most elderly patients present in the subacute phase several weeks after the veins bridging the subdural space have been torn by relatively minor trauma. Subdural hematomas are often bilateral, as illustrated in Figure 7.20, and may be of different ages. In this setting, the more intense collection is generally due to the more recent subacute event, while the less intense collection is due to a more chronic bleed. When recurrent bleeding occurs in the same subdural hematoma, the different events may be distinguishable by the variable signal intensities on MRI, as shown in Figure 7.21.

Variable signal intensity in a subdural hematoma need not imply multiple events. An in vivo hematocrit can often be observed in the trauma setting (Figure 7.22) or following shunting for hydrocephalus (Figure 7.23). In such cases, the intact red cells containing either deoxyhemoglobin or methemoglobin fall to the dependent position and have a short T_2 due to magnetic susceptibility effects. The supernatant contains free methemoglobin and thus has a short T_1. The short TR/short TE images have high signal in the non-dependent collection and are isointense to slightly hypointense (depending on the TE) in the dependent collection. As T_2-weighting is increased on long TR/long TE images, the non-dependent portion of the

subdural hematoma retains its high signal but the dependent collection of intact red cells becomes markedly hypointense, shown in Figures 7.22 and 7.23.

Epidural hematomas (EDHs) evolve in a manner similar to SDHs. They are distinguished from the latter by the low intensity of the fibrous dura mater[1] between the hematoma and the brain, as in Figure 7.24. Like an acute SDH, an acute EDH has deoxyhemoglobin within intact red blood cells resulting in T_2-shortening and low intensity on T_2-weighted images, particularly at high fields. On the basis of intensity characteristics alone, it may be difficult to separate the low-intensity dura from the low-intensity hematoma during this phase and to distinguish accurately a subdural from an epidural collection. In the subacute phase of an epidural hematoma, methemoglobin is formed and the diagnosis is obvious on both T_1- and T_2-weighted sequences, regardless of field strength.

In the setting of trauma, subdural and epidural hematomas may be found in combination with hemorrhagic contusions and frank intraparenchymal hematomas, as illustrated in Figure 7.25, either of which may be coup or contrecoup to the point of impact. Hematomas in different intracranial compartments tend to mature at different rates; that is, they have different rates of oxidation and red cell lysis. Figure 7.25 demonstrates variable maturation of several intraparenchymal hematomas, two subdural hematomas, and a cephalohematoma. In vivo hematocrits can be seen not only in subdural hematomas (Figures 7.22 and 7.23), but also in traumatic parenchymal hematomas (Figure 7.24), in hematomas due to amyloid angiopathy (Figure 7.16) or to arteriovenous malformations, and in hemorrhagic metastases (Figure 7.11). The lower intensity, dependent collection always represents intact red cells containing either paramagnetic deoxyhemoglobin or methemoglobin. The low signal arising from such magnetic susceptibility effects can be elicited on T_2-weighted spin-echo and gradient-echo images.

Subarachnoid hemorrhage

Subarachnoid hemorrhage differs significantly from intraparenchymal, subdural, or epidural hemorrhage in that it may be admixed with CSF.[43] Immediately after subarachnoid hemorrhage, there is a small decrease in T_1,[6,43,44] which most likely reflects the increase in hydration-layer water due to the elevated protein content of the bloody CSF. As has been shown in vitro,[6] significant quantities of methemoglobin are not formed until several days after the hemorrhage. Several days to a week post ictus, signal intensity increases in the subarachnoid space due to methemo-globin formation, shown in Figures 7.26–7.28. In cases of milder subarachnoid hemorrhage, red cells may have been resorbed by the time significant methemoglobin formation has occurred and, there-fore, the anticipated short T_1 appearance will not be seen. For these reasons, CT is advocated for the early diagnosis of subarachnoid hemorrhage in the clinical setting.[1,6] As noted above, the short T_2 properties of a hematoma require both formation of deoxyhemoglo-bin and clot retraction,[20] that is, resorption of plasma.[21] For both reasons, the short T_2 appearance is rarely observed in subarachnoid hemorrhage unless massive bleeding has occurred in which case a subarachnoid thrombus is present.[6,44] In addition, the oxygen tension in the subarachnoid space is higher than that in the center of a hematoma or a tumor, thus, deoxyhemoglobin (and eventually methemoglobin) forms more slowly than in the lower oxygen environments.[35]

In the subacute phase following subarachnoid hemorrhage, CT with contrast may show meningeal enhancement due to the chemical meningitis. Gadolinium-enhanced MRI is equally efficacious in this setting.[45] Should communicating hydrocephalus result from subarachnoid hemorrhage at a later stage, both CT and MRI are capable of demonstrating ventricular enlargement. However, MRI may be superior to CT in suggesting the degree of elevation of intraventricular pressure through the thickness of the rim of interstitial edema (see Chapter 8). In addition, recent MR studies have noted the presence of a hyperdynamic CSF flow state in patients with chronic communicating hydrocephalus.[46]

Hemorrhagic neoplasms

The hemorrhage associated with primary or metastatic tumors may appear quite similar to nonneoplastic parenchymal hemorrhage. The two may be disting-uished by the greater signal heterogeneity[32] due to the presence of additional soft tissue in the case of neoplasms, as shown in Figures 7.29 to 7.30, particu-larly if it enhances with gadolinium immediately post ictus. When followed over time, the vasogenic edema tends to persist longer with neoplastic hemorrhage than with non-neoplastic bleeds. While the progres-sion of hemoglobin oxidation is similar in tumors and benign hematomas, the oxygen tension in the center of a tumor is less than in the center of a non-neoplastic hematoma of comparable size when the neoplastic hematoma is surrounded by necrotic, devascularized tissue.[34,35] This low-oxygen environment results in a delay in the normal progression of hemoglobin oxygenation.[32] Indeed, deoxyhemoglobin has been

noted[32] two months following the acute bleed and methemoglobin has been found years after initial detection. The delayed oxygenation of deoxyhemoglo-bin to methemoglobin and of methemoglobin to hemichromes is presumably due to the low-oxygen environment.

The rim of hemosiderin-laden macrophages noted in chronic hematomas may also be seen in neoplastic hemorrhage where it abuts normal brain, shown in Figure 7.31. With the use of T_2-weighted images at high field, it has been suggested that an intact hemosiderin rim is suggestive of a non-neoplastic hematoma, while the presence of a discontinuous rim (secondary to episodic tumor growth) suggests a neoplastic origin.[32]

Hemorrhagic metastases (Figure 7.11) are generally easier to distinguish from the non-malignant causes of hemorrhage on the basis of their multiplicity. Metasta-tic melanoma, in particular, has a tendency to bleed and will be associated with methemoglobin formation (Figure 7.29). While the high-signal intensity of melanomas has been previously attributed to the free radical (one unpaired electron) on the melanin,[47] the short T_1 observed in melanomas is more likely due to the five unpaired electrons of the methemoglobin which has resulted from previous hemorrhage.[48]

Vascular abnormalities

Once hemorrhage has been detected in a particular compartment, it is then necessary to determine its source. Nontraumatic hemorrhage can result from rupture of aneurysms or bleeding from vascular malformations. Rapidly flowing blood produces a 'flow void', which allows both aneurysms (Figures 7.32–7.34) and AVMs (Figure 7.35) to be detected without the necessity of intravenous contrast injection (see Chapter 3). Even echo rephasing may be seen (Figure 7.36) in the lumen of aneurysms due to slow laminar flow if a symmetric double-echo technique is used.[49,50] Although it currently lacks the spatial resolution of cut film magnification angiography, MRI may be useful as a non-invasive screening procedure for such abnormalities. On the other hand, mural thrombi are not visualized on angiography and are easily seen on MRI, as illustrated in Figures 7.32 and 7.36. While routine MRI demonstrates such abnorma-lities on the basis of the flow void on multiple images (Figure 7.37), it is also possible to display the abnormalities as projectional images, as in Figure 7.38, with the use of MR angiography.[51] At the present, however, the complete preoperative evalua-tion of an aneurysm requires angiography.

Hemorrhage of unknown etiology in certain loca-tions, such as near the circle of Willis or in the Sylvian cistern (Figure 7.39) should suggest aneurysmal rupture as a cause. Hematomas associated with multiple flow voids, illustrated in Figures 7.40 and 7.41 suggest bleeding from an AVM. Subacute hematomas contain predominately methemoglobin (Figure 7.40), while chronic hematomas can have significant hemosiderin staining (Figure 7.41). AVMs may bleed into more than one intracranial compartment, as in Figure 7.42, for example, parenchymal, subdural, and subarachnoid. Hemorrhage can be particularly prominent following surgery for such vascular malformations, as illustrated in Figure 7.43. New cine MR techniques have also been found useful in the evaluation of larger intracranial aneurysms, particularly when interventional balloons are used for management.[52] Signal void areas on routine spin-echo images which could be due to rapid flow, dystrophic calcification, or hemosiderin may be distinguished by the use of single-slice, gradient-echo techniques, as in Figure 7.44. On such images, flowing blood appears bright due to flow-related enhancement (covered in Chapter 3) while calcium and hemosiderin remain dark.

In certain cases, giant intracranial aneurysms may simulate parenchymal hematomas or even hemorrhagic neoplasms, as in Figure 7.45.[50] In such cases, the oxygen gradient may provide a clue to the correct diagnosis.[53] In giant intracranial aneurysms, the highest oxygen tension is in the center near the patent lumen. In intraparenchymal hematomas or hemorrhagic neoplasms, however, the center of the lesion has the lowest oxygen tension while the periphery is better oxygenated due to contiguity with normally perfused tissue. Since the oxidative denaturation of deoxyhemoglobin and methemoglobin requires some oxygen, methemoglobin formation is first found centrally in giant intracranial aneurysms with a patent lumen and peripherally in hematomas and tumors.[53]

MRI may be useful when subarachnoid hemorrhage is associated with *multiple* intracranial aneurysms. The finding of a small subarachnoid thrombus may be helpful in determining the exact site of bleeding.[54] In one case report,[54] this finding resulted in a more accurate diagnosis by MRI than by either CT or angiography. MRI is complementary to angiography in the evaluation of arteriovenous malformations.[52] The feeding arteries and draining veins are visualized by virtue of the flow void produced, as illustrated in Figure 7.35. MRI is superior to angiography in the demonstration of the nidus as well as the degree of mass effect and encephalomalacia resulting from the AVM (Figure 7.44). MRI is certainly more sensitive for the detection of associated hemorrhage.[52]

There are three categories of angioma: capillary, cavernous, and venous.[55] While venous angiomas may be distinguished angiographically, in certain cases the other two forms may only be distinguished histologically. The central draining vein associated with venous angiomas may be visualized by virtue of its flow void (Figure 7.46a) or by the presence of even-echo rephasing on MRI (Figure 7.46b).[39] Capillary and cavernous angiomas are indistinguishable on MRI and may be angiographically occult, as demonstrated in Figures 7.47 to 7.49. Their presence is inferred from the finding of parenchymal hemorrhage,[39,40] or merely hemosiderin staining, although similar findings are seen with hemorrhagic neoplasms.[56] Such lesions may be prone to recurrent bleeding, thus there may be evidence of both acute and chronic hemorrhage, as in Figure 7.47.

Brain iron

Soon after the introduction of 1.5 Tesla imaging systems, low intensity was reported in the basal ganglia on T_2-weighted images which was attributed to iron deposition.[57] Such iron deposition was confirmed using Perls stains on autopsy specimens and the iron presumed to be in the form of ferritin. Ferritin deposits can be visualized after age six months and generally increase until 20 years of age, with a further increased noted after the age of 60. In order of appearance, the normal sites for ferritin deposition (by both MRI and pathologic studies) are the globus pallidus, red nucleus, reticular portion of the substantia nigra, dentate nucleus in the cerebellum, and the putamen (Figure 7.50). Thus in elderly patients, low intensity is generally found in these structures on T_2-weighted images acquired at high field. Iron is present in many enzyme systems in the brain. The increasing iron deposition in the brain normally seen by MRI may reflect alteration of these enzyme systems with advancing age.

Iron has also been noted in specific locations with certain disease states using high-field systems and midfield systems with gradient echoes.[58] In neuroaxonal dystrophy or Hallervorden-Spatz disease,[59] there is marked ferritin deposition in the globus pallidus and the reticular portion of the substantia nigra.[57] In Huntington disease, increased ferritin deposits have been found pathologically in the caudate nucleus and in the putamen. The putamen and globus pallidus are involved in Parkinson's disease and its variants (for example, Shy Drager syndrome, multisystem atrophy, progressive supranuclear palsy, and Parkinson-plus).[60,61]

Abnormal iron deposition has been demonstrated in other movement disorders (such as hemiballismus and dystonia), as well at high field.[62] When only hemosiderin staining is seen, this may be evidence of old hemorrhage from an angioma.[39–41] It has also been noted, however, that such lesions may not be of such a relatively benign vascular etiology, but rather may represent hemorrhagic tumors.[56]

T_2-shortening has been found in association with multiple sclerosis plaques[57] at high field.[63] This presumably reflects iron deposition secondary to prior hemorrhage during the acute inflammatory stage.

Focal T_2-shortening has also been noted in the thalami in children, as illustrated in Figure 7.51, after severe ischemic-anoxic events.[64] Pathologic studies have shown ferruginated or mineralized neurons containing iron in the thalami in this clinical setting. The mechanism for this focal iron deposition in this setting is speculative, although three possibilities have been suggested.[64] Concomitant ganglionic hemorrhage (too mild to be seen by CT) could easily produce T_2-shortening on MR images acquired in the chronic stage. Concomitant bland ganglionic ischemia-infarction has been shown to cause delocalization of tissue iron stores, leading to additional lipid perioxidation and infarction. Redeposition of iron in this setting could produce the T_2-shortening noted above. A third intriguing possibility for focal iron deposition is the disruption of normal axonal transport. In a rat model, it has been shown that iron is transported along GABAergic axons from sites of uptake in the caudate nuclei to sites of utilization elsewhere in the basal ganglia. Should similar axonal transport be demonstrated between sites of uptake in the basal ganglia and sites of utilization in the cortex, then any process leading to axonal disruption, such as periventricular leukomalacia, could lead to iron accumulation at the point of uptake in the basal ganglia.

References

1 BRADLEY WG, MRI of hemorrhage and iron in the brain. In: Stark DD, Bradley WG, eds. *Magnetic resonance imaging.* (CV Mosby and Co: St Louis 1988) Chapter 20.

2 BAILES DR, YOUNG, IR, THOMAS DJ et al, NMR imaging of the brain using spin-echo sequences, *Clin Radiol* (1982) 33:395–414.

3 BYDDER GM, STEINER RE, YOUNG IR et al, Clinical NMR imaging of the brain: 140 cases, *AJR* (1982) 139:215–36.

4 SIPPONEN JT, SEPPONEN RE, SIVULA A, Nuclear magnetic resonance (NMR) imaging of intracerebral hemorrhage in the acute and resolving phases, *J Comput Assist Tomogr* (1983) 7(6):954–9.

5 DELAPAZ RL, NEW PFJ, BUONANNO FS et al, NMR imaging of intracranial hemorrhage, *J Comput Assist Tomogr* (1983) 8(4):599–607.

6 BRADLEY WG, SCHMIDT PC, Effect of methemoglobin formation on the MR appearance of subarachnoid hemorrhage, *Radiology* (1985) 156:99–103.

7 GOMORI JM, GROSSMAN RI, GOLDBERG HI et al, Intracranial hematomas: imaging by high field MR, *Radiology* (1985) 157:87–92.

8 BLOEMBERGEN N, PURCELL E, POUND RV, Relaxation effects in nuclear magnetic resonance absorption, *Phys Rev* (1948) 73:679–712.

9 WOLF GL, BURNETT KR, GOLDSTEIN EJ et al, Contrast agents for magnetic resonance imaging. In: Kressel HY, ed. *Magnetic resonance annual 1985* (Raven: New York 1985) 231–66.

10 BRADLEY WG, CROOKS LE, NEWTON TH, Physical principles of NMR. In: Newton TH, Potts PG, eds. *Modern neuroradiology: advanced imaging techniques*, Vol II. (Clavadel Press: San Francisco 1983) Chapter 3.

11 MILLS TC, ORTENDAHL DA, HYLTON NM et al, Partial flip angle MR imaging, *Radiology* (1987) 162:531–9.

12 BRADLEY WG, Fundamentals of MR image interpretation. In: Bradley WG, Adey WR, Hasso AN, eds. *Magnetic resonance imaging of the brain, head and neck: a text atlas.* (Aspen: Rockville 1985) Chapter 1.

13 FULLERTON GD, CAMERON IL, ORD VA, Frequency dependence of magnetic resonance spin-lattice relaxation of protons in biological materials, *Radiology* (1984) 151:135–8.

14 FULLERTON GD, Physiologic basis of magnetic relaxation. In: Stark DD, Bradley WG, eds. *Magnetic resonance imaging.* (CV Mosby and Co: St Louis 1988) Chapter 3.

15 FULLERTON GD, FINNIE MF, HUNTER KE et al, The influence of macromolecular polymerization on spin-lattice relaxation of aqueous solutions, *Magn Reson Imaging* (1987) 5(5):353–70.

16 EDELMAN RR, JOHNSON K, BUXTON R et al, MR of hemorrhage: a new approach, *AJNR* (1986) 7:751–6.

17 WESBEY GE, MOSELEY ME, EHMAN RL, Translational molecular self-diffusion in magnetic resonance imaging: effects and applications. In: James TL, Margulis AR, eds. *Biomedical magnetic resonance.* (University of California Press: San Francisco 1984) 63–78.

18 WALUCH V, BRADLEY WG, NMR even echo rephasing in slow laminar flow, *J Comput Assist Tomogr* (1984) 8:594–8.

19 PACKER KJ, The effects of diffusion through locally inhomogeneous magnetic fields on transverse nuclear spin relaxation in heterogeneous systems: proton transverse relaxation in striated muscle tissue, *J Magn Reson* (1973) 9:438–43.

20 CLARK RA, ROBERTS JD, BRADLEY WG et al, The influence of fibrin clot retraction on the short T_2 appearance of an acute hematoma, *Magn Reson Imaging,* (abstract), (1989) 7:74.

21 HAYMAN LA, MCARDLE C, TABA K et al, Role of clot formation in MR imaging of blood, (abstract) *Radiology* (1987) 165(P):402.

22 WINTROBE MM, LEE GR, BOGGS DR et al, *Clinical hematology* (Lea Febiger: Philadelphia) 88–102.

23 RAPOPORT SI, *Introduction to hematology,* (Harper and Row: New York 1971).

24 PAULING L, CORYELL C, The magnetic properties and structure of hemoglobin, oxyhemoglobin and carbonmonoxyhemoglobin, *Proc Natl Acad Sci* (1936) 22:210–16.

25 PAULING L, CORYELL C, The magnetic properties and structure of the hemochromogens and related substances, *Proc Natl Acad Sci* (1936) 22:159–63.

26 KOENIG SH, BROWN RD, LINDSTROM TR, Interactions of solvent with the heme region of methemoglobin and fluoromethemoglobin, *Biophys J* (1981) 34:397–408.

27 SINGER JR, CROOKS LE, Some magnetic studies of normal and leukemic blood, *J Clin Eng* (1978) 3:357–63.

28 THULBORN KR, MCKEE A, KOWALL NW et al, Magnetic susceptibility of ferritin as the primary determinant of the appearance of late phase cerebral hematoma on T_2-weighted

magnetic resonance images. Presented at SMRM, 7th Annual Meeting, 22–26 August 1988, San Francisco, CA. Book of abstracts, 583.

29 WHISNANT JP, SAYER GP, MILLIKAN CH, Experimental intracerebral hematoma, *Arch Neurol* (1963) **9**:586–92.

30 WEINGARTEN K, ZIMMERMAN RD, MARKISZ J et al, The effect of hemoglobin oxygenation on the MR intensity of experimentally produced intracerebral hematomas at 0.6 T and 1.5 T. Presented at SMRM, 7th Annual Meeting, 22–26 August 1988, San Francisco, CA. Book of abstracts, 58.

31 HECHT-LEAVITT C, GOMORI JM, GROSSMAN RI et al, High-field MR imaging of hemorrhagic cortical infarction, *AJNR* (1986) **7**:587–94.

32 ATLAS SW, GROSSMAN RI, GOMORI JM et al, Hemorrhagic intracranial malignant neoplasms: spin-echo MR imaging, *Radiology* (1987) **164**:71–7.

33 GOMORI JM, GROSSMAN RI, Head and neck hemorrhage. In: Kressel HY, ed. *Magnetic resonance annual.* (Raven Press: New York 1987) 71–112.

34 GATENBY RA, COIA LR, RICHTER MP et al, Oxygen tension in human tumors: in vivo mapping using CT-guided probes, *Radiology* (1985) **156**:211–14.

35 GROSSMAN RI, KEMP SS, YU IP C et al, The importance of oxygenation in the appearance of acute subarachnoid hemorrhage on high field magnetic resonance imaging, *Acta Radiol* (in press).

36 RAPOPORT S, SOSTMAN HD, POPE C et al, Venous clots: evaluation with MR imaging, *Radiology* (1987) **162**(2):527–30.

37 BYDDER GM, PAYNE JA, COLLINS AG et al, Clinical use of rapid T_2-weighted partial saturation sequences in MR imaging, *J Comput Assist Tomogr* (1987) **11**:17.

38 HACKNEY DB, ATLAS SW, GROSSMAN RI et al, Subacute intracranial hemorrhage: contribution of spin density to appearance of spin-echo images, *Radiology* (1987) **165**:99–202.

39 GOMORI J, GROSSMAN RI, BILANIUK LT et al, High-field MR imaging of superficial siderosis of the central nervous system, *J Comput Assist Tomogr* (1985) **9**:972–5.

40 GOMORI J, GROSSMAN R, GOLDBERT H et al, Occult cerebral vascular malformations: high-field MR imaging, *Radiology* (1986) **158**:707–13

41 LEMME-PLAGHOS L, KUCHARCZYK, BRANT-ZAWADZKI M et al, MR imaging of angiographically occult vascular malformations, *AJNR* (1986) **7**:217–22.

42 KUCHARCZYK W, LEMME-PLEHOS L, USKE A et al, Intracranial vascular malformations: MR and CT imaging, *Radiology* (1985) **156**:383–9.

43 CHAKERES DW, BRYAN RN, Acute subarachnoid hemorrhage: in vitro comparison of magnetic resonance and computed tomography, *AJNR* (1986) **7**:223–8.

44 YOON HC, LUFKIN RB, VINUELA F et al, MR of acute subarachnoid hemorrhage, *AJNR* (1988) **9**:405–8

45 BURKE JW, PODRASKY AE, BRADLEY WG, Meningeal enhancement by Gd-DTPA in postoperative brain MR imaging (abstract), *Magn Reson Imaging*, (1989) **7**:4.

46 BRADLEY WG, WHITTEMORE AR, JINKINS JR, CSF flow pattern in hydrocephalus: correlation of clinical and phantom studies using MRI, (abstract), *Radiology*, (1987) **78**:165(P).

47 GOMORI JM, GROSSMAN RI, SHIELDS JA et al, Choroidal melanomas: correlation of NMR spectroscopy and MR imaging, *Radiology* (1986) **158**:443–5.

48 WOODRUFF WW, DJANG WT, MCLENDON RE et al, Intracerebral malignant melanoma: high-field-strength MR imaging, *Radiology* (1987) **165**:209–13.

49 ALVAREZ O, HYMAN RA, Even echo MR rephasing in the diagnosis of giant intracranial aneurysm, *J Comput Assist Tomogr* (1986) **10**(4):699–701.

50 OLSEN WL, BRANT-ZAWADZKI M, HODES J et al, Giant intracranial aneurysms: MR imaging, *Radiology* (1987) **163**:431–5.

51 MASARYK TJ, MODIC MT, ROSS JS et al, MR Angiography of the intracranial circulation: clinical utility. Presented at SMRM, 7th Annual Meeting, 22–26 August 1988, San Francisco, CA. Book of abstracts, 117.

52 SMITH HJ, STROTHER CM, KIKUCHI Y et al, MR imaging in the management of supratentorial intracranial AVMs, *AJNR* (1988) **9**(2):225–36.

53 ATLAS SW, GROSSMAN RI, GOLDBERG HI et al, Partially thrombosed giant intracranial aneurysms: correlation of MR and pathologic findings, *Radiology* (1987) **162**:111–14.

54 HACKNEY DB, LESNICK JE, ZIMMERMAN RA et al, MR identification of bleeding site in subarachnoid hemorrhage with multiple intracranial aneurysms, *J Comput Assist Tomogr* (1986) **10**(5):878–80.

55 RAO KCV, LEE SH, Cerebrovascular anomalies. In Stark DD, Bradley WG, eds. *Magnetic resonance imaging.* (CV Mosby and Co: St Louis 1988) 473–505.

56 SZE G, KROL G, OLSEN WL et al, Hemorrhagic neoplasms: MR mimics of occult vascular malformations, *AJNR* (1987) **8**:795–802.

57 DRAYER B, BURGER P, DARWIN R et al, Magnetic resonance imaging of brain iron, *AJNR* (1986) **7**:373–80.

58 NORFRAY JF, CHIARADONNA NL, HEISER WJ et al, Brain iron in patients with Parkinson disease: MR visualization using gradient modification, *AJNR* (1988) **9**(2):237–40.

59 LITTRUP PJ, GEBARSKI SS, MR imaging of Hallervorden-Spatz disease, *J Comput Assist Tomogr* (1985) **9**(3):491–3.

60 DRAYER BP, OLANOW W, BURGER P et al, Parkinson plus syndrome: diagnosis using high field MR imaging of brain iron, *Radiology* (1986) **159**:493–8.

61 PASTAKIA B, POLINSKY R, DICHIRO G et al, Multiple system atrophy (Shy-Drager syndrome): MR imaging, *Radiology* (1986) **159**:499–502.

62 RUTLEDGE JN, HILAL SK, SILVER AJ et al, Study of movement disorders and brain iron by MR, *AJR* (1987) **149**:365–79.

63 DRAYER B, BURGER P, HURWITZ B et al, Reduced signal intensity on MR images of thalamus and putamen in multiple sclerosis: increased iron content? *AJR* (1987) **149**:357–63.

64 DIETRICH RB, BRADLEY WG, Iron accumulation in the basal ganglia following severe ischemic-anoxia insults in children, *Radiology* (1988) **168**:203–6.

Oxyhemoglobin

Deoxyhemoglobin

Methemoglobin

Reversible
Hemichromes

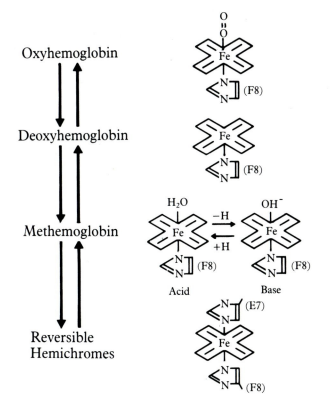

Figure 7.1

Hemoglobin oxidation. Molecular oxygen (O_2) is attached to the heme iron (Fe) at the sixth coordination site in oxyhemoglobin. This site is vacant in deoxyhemoglobin. The heme iron is in the low-and high-spin ferrous (Fe^{2+}) forms in oxyhemoglobin and deoxyhemoglobin, respectively. The heme iron becomes oxidized to the ferric (Fe^{3+}) state in methemoglobin. The iron in methemoglobin is in the high-spin form and contains water (H_2O) at the sixth coordination site in the acid form, which predominates at physiologic pH. Continued oxidative denaturation forms low-spin ferric compounds called 'hemichromes', in which the sixth coordination site is occupied by a histadine from the denatured globin molecule.

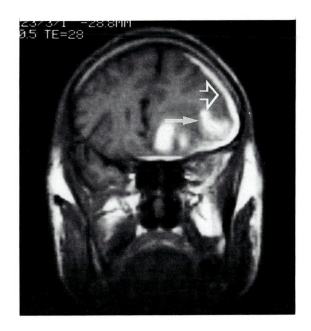

Figure 7.2

Subacute hemorrhage. T_1-shortening is noted in the parenchymal (arrow) and subdural (open arrow) compartments due to methemoglobin formation in this subacute trauma case. The short T_1 character of the hemorrhage is enhanced on this short TR/short TE image (SE 500/28).

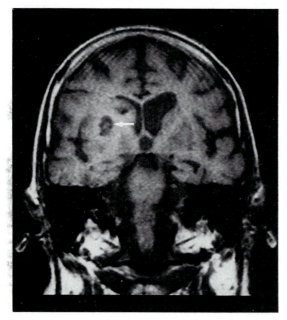

a

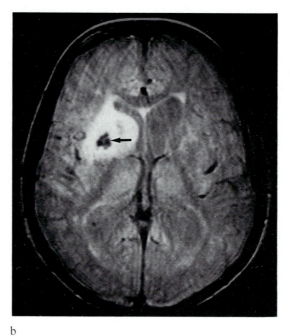

b

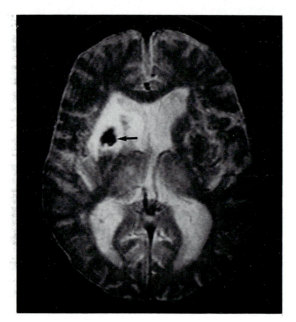

c

Figure 7.3

Acute intraparenchymal hematoma. Two days post ictus, hypertensive hematoma in right putamen contains deoxyhemoglobin within intact red cells. (**a**) Coronal T_1-weighted image demonstrates low signal in region of hematoma (arrow) (SE 600/30). (**b**) Axial moderately T_2-weighted image demonstrates hypointensity in hematoma (arrow) relative to hyperintense edema (SE 2500/30). (**c**) With increasing T_2-weighting (SE 2500/60), hematoma (arrow) becomes even darker due to its short T_2 relaxation time.

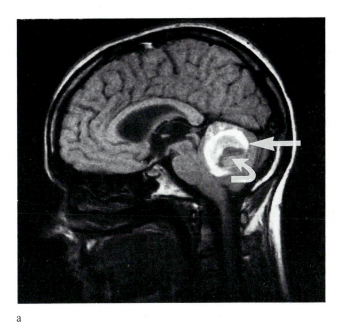

a

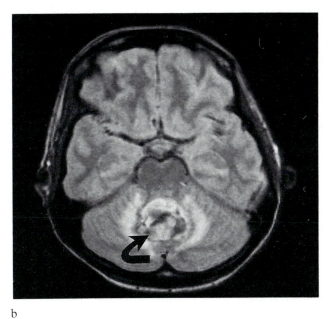

b

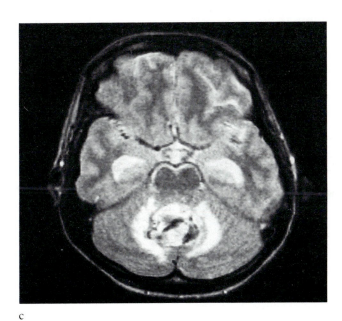

c

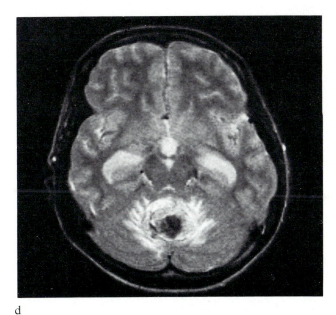

d

Figure 7.4

Early subacute hematoma. Four days following cerebellar hemorrhage, hematoma contains free methemoglobin peripherally and deoxyhemoglobin within intact red cells centrally. This combination results in T_1-shortening (due to a dipole–dipole interaction) peripherally, and in T_2-shortening (due to magnetic susceptibility effects) centrally. (a) T_1-weighted sagittal image demonstrates high-signal intensity in peripheral portion of hematoma (arrow) due to methemoglobin, while central portion remains dark due to persistent deoxyhemoglobin (curved arrow) (SE 500/40). (b) Mildly T_2-weighted axial image demonstrates hypointensity in center of hematoma (curved arrow) (SE 3000/40). (c–d) More heavily T_2-weighted images (SE 3000/80) result in additional signal loss in the center of the hematoma where the deoxyhemoglobin-containing red cells remain intact.

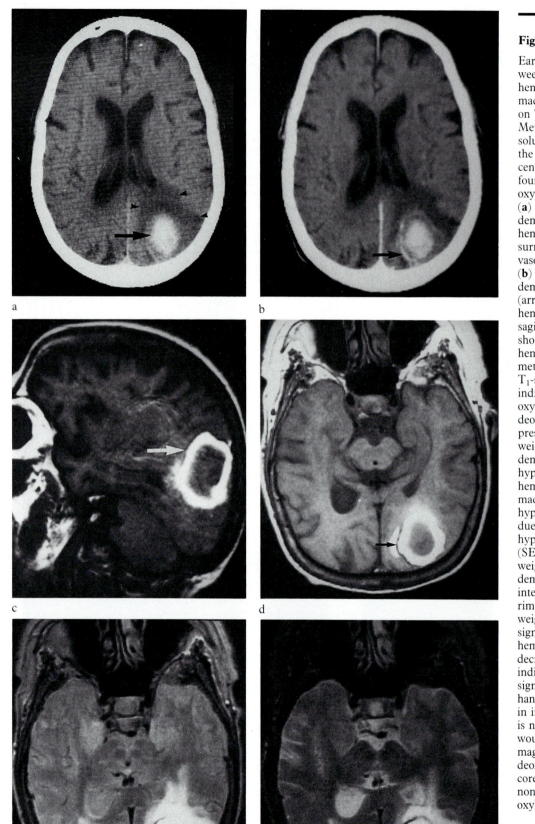

a

b

c

d

e

f

Figure 7.5

Early chronic hematoma. One week post ictus, a rim of hemosiderin-laden macrophages becomes apparent on T_2-weighted images. Methemoglobin is found free in solution in the outer portion of the hematoma, while in the central core, intact red cells are found still containing oxyhemoglobin. (**a**) Unenhanced CT demonstrating hyperdensity in hematoma (arrow) with surrounding hypodense vasogenic edema (arrowheads). (**b**) Contrast-enhanced CT demonstrates rim enhancement (arrow) surrounding week-old hematoma. (**c**) T_1-weighted sagittal image demonstrates T_1-shortening in the outer core of hematoma (arrow) due to methemoglobin. The lack of T_1-shortening in the inner core indicates that either oxyhemoglobin or deoxyhemoglobin are still present (SE 600/25). (**d**) T_1-weighted axial image demonstrates peripheral rim of hypointensity (arrow) due to hemosiderin-laden macrophages. Again noted is hyperintensity in the outer core due to free methemoglobin and hypointensity in the inner core (SE 600/25). (**e**) Moderately T_2-weighted image (SE 2500/40) demonstrates decreasing signal intensity in the hemosiderin rim (arrow). (**f**) On heavily T_2-weighted image (SE 2500/80), signal intensity in the hemosiderin rim (arrow) has decreased relative to **c** and **d** indicating a short T_2. The low signal in the core, on the other hand, has not decreased further in intensity, indicating that T_2 is not particularly shortened as would be expected from magnetically susceptible deoxyhemoglobin. The inner core must therefore contain nonparamagnetic oxyhemoglobin.

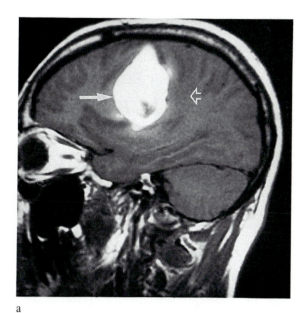

a

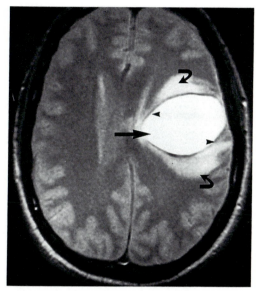

b

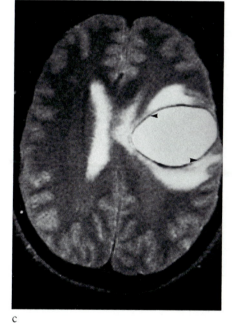

c

Figure 7.6

Late chronic hematoma. (a) Two weeks following hemorrhage, left parasagittal T_1-weighted section demonstrates hyperintensity (arrow) due to methemoglobin formation. Vasogenic edema is subtly hypointense relative to normal white matter (open arrow) (SE 600/20). (b) On moderately T_2-weighted axial section, central free methemoglobin (arrow) is more intense than surrounding vasogenic edema (curved arrows). At this later stage, the red cells have all lysed so the center is homogeneously hyperintense due to free methemoglobin. Low-intensity rim of hemosiderin-laden macrophages is noted (arrowheads) with additional T_2-weighting (SE 2700/30). (c) On heavily T_2-weighted axial sections through same level as (b) center of hematoma and surrounding vasogenic edema are isointense with CSF. Hemorrhage cannot therefore be specifically diagnosed. Note increasing hypointensity in hemosiderin rim (arrowheads) (SE 2700/80).

Figure 7.7

Superior sagittal sinus
thrombosis with venous
infarcts. (**a–d**) Several axial
sections from the vertex
through the lateral ventricles
demonstrate multiple
hemorrhagic infarcts (arrows)
which manifest very high signal
intensity due to presence of
extracellular methemoglobin.
The normal flow void in the
superior sagittal sinus is
replaced by intermediate signal
from the thrombosis (open
arrow) (SE 3000/80)

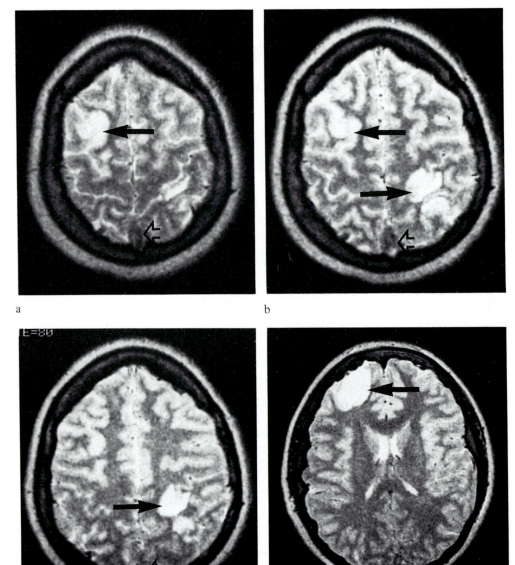

a

b

c

d

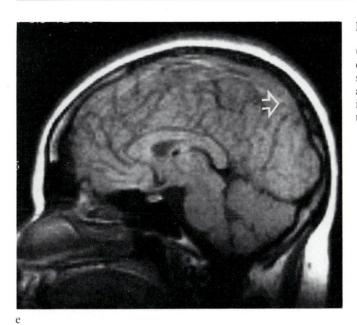

e

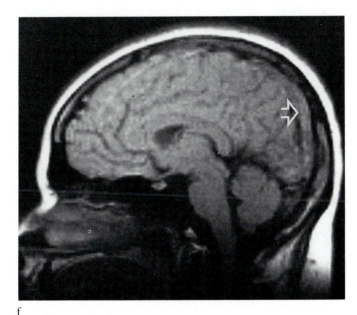

f

Figure 7.7 *continued*

(**e–f**) Adjacent sagittal sections demonstrate lack of flow void in superior sagittal sinus (open arrows) which is replaced by intermediate signal due to thrombosis (SE 500/40).

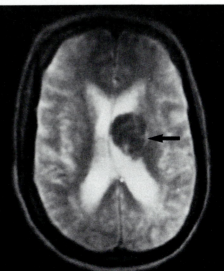

a   b

Figure 7.8

Acute hematoma on gradient-echo image at low field (0.15 Tesla). (**a**) On T_1-weighted gradient-echo image (PS 250/22, $\theta = 90°$), hematoma (arrow) has signal intensity between that of brighter brain and darker CSF. (**b**) On T_2^*-weighted gradient-echo image (PS 250/113, $\theta = 90°$), hematoma (arrow) has lower signal than either brain or CSF. The short T_2^* of acute hematomas is obvious even at low field using a long TE, gradient-echo technique.

Figure 7.9

Acute hemorrhagic contusion at midfield (0.35 Tesla). Three days following trauma, hemorrhagic contusions are noted in the subfrontal regions bilaterally and in the high left parietal lobe. (a) Mildly T_1-weighted coronal section demonstrates slight peripheral hyperintensity due to long T_2 vasogenic edema (arrow) with central mild hypointensity. The marked high-signal intensity which would indicate methemoglobin formation is not observed (SE 1000/30). (b) Mildly T_2-weighted high-axial image demonstrates central hypointensity (arrow) due to intact red cells containing deoxyhemoglobin with peripheral hyperintensity due to surrounding vasogenic edema (SE 3000/40). (c) On more heavily T_2-weighted image (SE 3000/80), the short T_2 center of the hematoma becomes even darker due to the magnetic susceptibility effects of the intracellular deoxyhemoglobin. (d) Subfrontal axial section demonstrates multiple acute hematomas with surrounding vasogenic edema (SE 3000/80). (e) One month following trauma at the same level as (b) and (c), the peripheral vasogenic edema has resolved, the deoxyhemoglobin has been oxidized to methemoglobin, and the red cells within the hematoma have lysed, producing a short T_1, long T_2 appearance (arrow) (SE 3000/40).

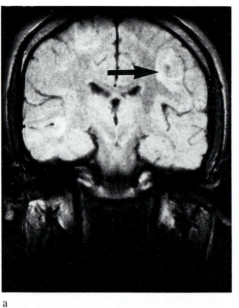

a

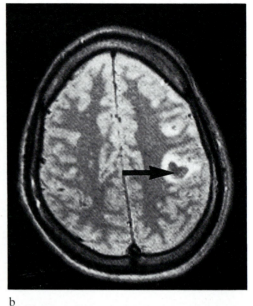

b

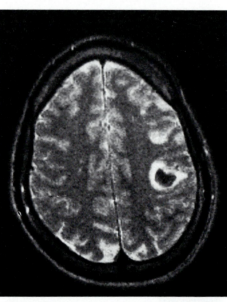

c

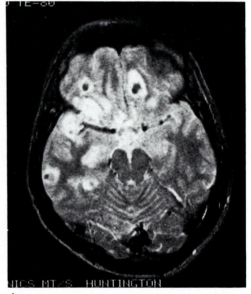

d

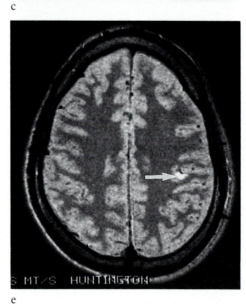

e

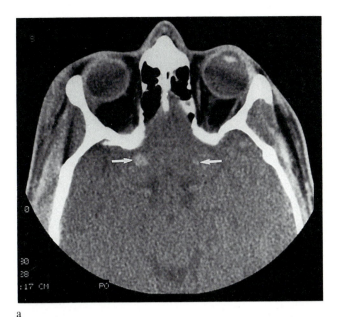

a

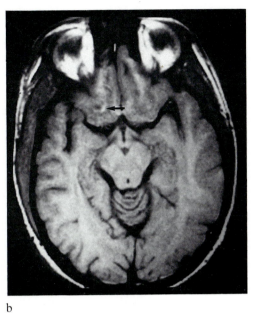

b

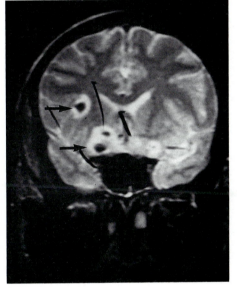

c

d

Figure 7.10

Acute hemorrhagic contusion at high field (1.5 Tesla). (**a**) Several hours after motor-vehicle accident, small foci of high density are noted on unenhanced CT secondary to hemorrhagic contusion (arrows). (**b**) T_1-weighted MR image three days after trauma demonstrates subtle foci of low signal with surrounding rims of high signal in right subfrontal region (arrow) (SE 800/20). (**c**) Higher axial T_1-weighted image demonstrates scattered foci of high signal due to presence of methemoglobin (arrow) (SE 800/20). (**d**) Heavily T_2-weighted coronal section demonstrates multiple foci of low signal (arrows) secondary to intracellular deoxy- or methemoglobin, with surrounding rims of hyperintensity due to edema. (Case and tick marks courtesy of Michael Brant-Zawadzki, MD, Newport Beach, CA.)

Figure 7.11

Acute hemorrhage on high-field, gradient-echo images. This 55-year-old woman presented with headaches without focal neurologic findings. Subsequent workup revealed hemorrhagic metastases to the brain from small-cell carcinoma of the lung. (**a**) CT demonstrates left frontal, high-density lesions (arrows) on unenhanced scan suggesting acute hemorrhage. (**b**) T_1-weighted coronal section demonstrates scattered foci of high-signal intensity (arrows) due to methemoglobin formation (SE 1000/20). (**c**) Mildly T_2-weighted axial MR image (SE 2500/25) demonstrates additional abnormalities, some of them having a low-intensity rim (arrow). (**d**) On heavily T_2-weighted image (SE 2500/80) at higher axial level, low-intensity rim becomes darker due to short T_2 (arrowhead). Note also 'in vivo hematocrit' effect due to settling of intact red cells in larger left frontal hematoma (arrow). (**e**) GRASS image (PS 200/80, $\theta = 10°$) demonstrates multiple additional foci of low intensity due to additional sensitivity of this technique to magnetic susceptibility effects. This leads to 'blueberry muffin' appearance of multiple hemorrhagic metastases. (Courtesy of Edward Behnke, MD, Whittier, CA.)

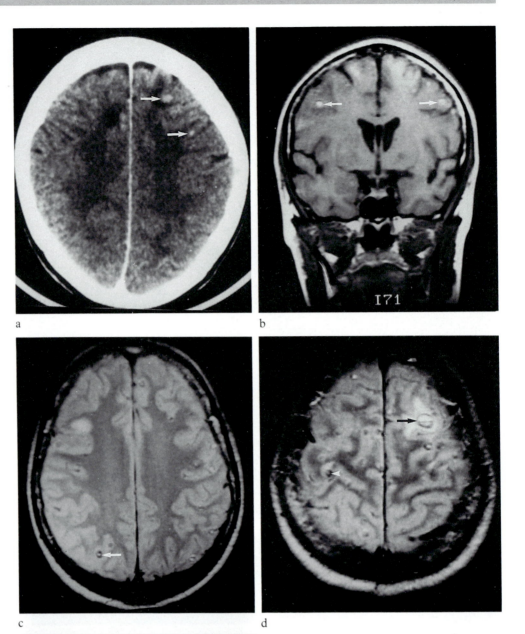

a

b

c

d

e

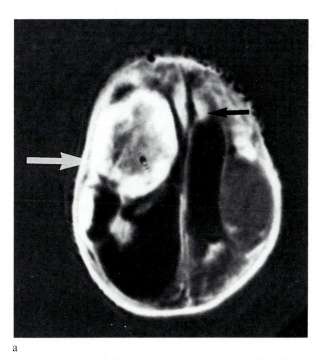

a

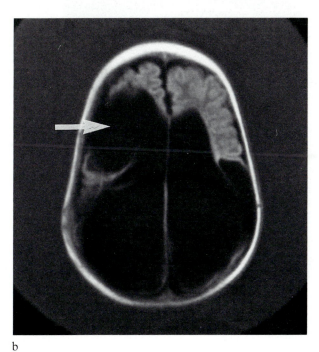

b

Figure 7.12

Evolution of hematoma on inversion-recovery images. (**a**) T_1-weighted inversion-recovery image (IR 2400/800/ 44) demonstrates multiple high-signal hematomas in seven-day-old infant (arrows). High signal in right frontal hematoma is due to the short T_1 of methemoglobin, which is particularly prominent on this T_1-weighted inversion-recovery image. (**b**) At five months of age, porencephalic cyst (arrow) is noted at site of previous right frontal hematoma. This has CSF intensity on T_1-weighted inversion-recovery image (IR 1800/600/44). Note also dilated ventricles due to communicating hydrocephalus.

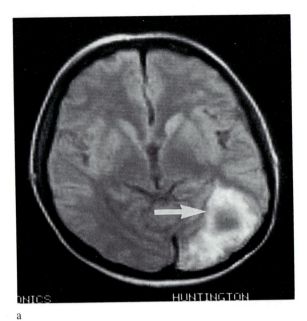

a

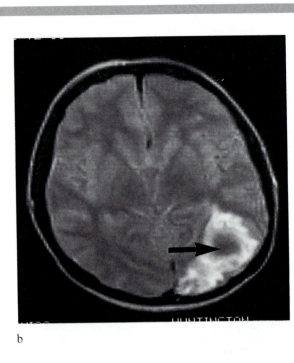

b

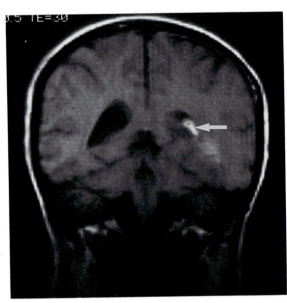

c

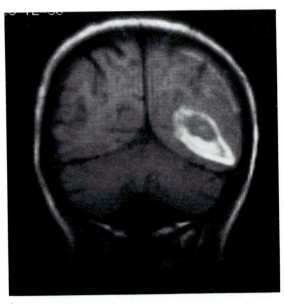

d

Figure 7.13

Parenchymal-intraventricular hemorrhage. Images acquired in 44-year-old woman with vasculitis one week following onset of right homonymous hemianopsia. (**a**) Left occipital hematoma has peripheral high-signal intensity (arrow) due to methemoglobin and edema (SE 2000/30). (**b**) Inner core darkens with additional T_2-weighting (SE 2000/60) due to presence of intracellular deoxyhemoglobin (arrow). (**c**) High-intensity hematoma extends into occipital horn of left lateral ventricle (arrow) on T_1-weighted coronal section (SE 500/30). (**d**) More posterior coronal section demonstrates peripheral high intensity due to methemoglobin in parenchymal hematoma (SE 500/30).

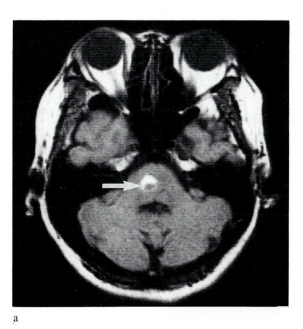

a

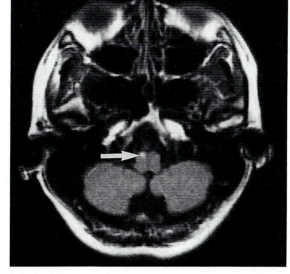

b

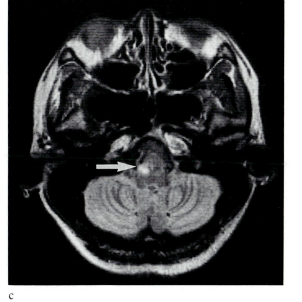

c

Figure 7.14

Brainstem hemorrhage in late subacute phase. Subject was 45-year-old hypertensive male who had developed acute brainstem symptoms two weeks earlier. (**a**) Transaxial section through the pons demonstrates high-signal intensity (arrow) with subtle mass effect on fourth ventricle in the basilar portion of the pons (SE 500/40). (**b**) T_1-weighted section through the caudal medulla demonstrates high-signal intensity (arrow) in the right corticospinal tract due to T_1-shortening (SE 500/40). (**c**) T_2-weighted image through the caudal medulla demonstrates persistent high signal (arrow). There is no T_2-shortening because the red cells have already lysed (SE 3000/40).

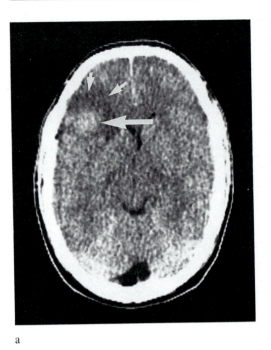
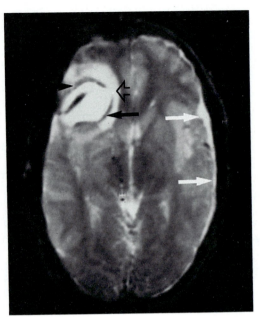

a

b

Figure 7.15

Chronic hemorrhage on
gradient-echo image at 0.15
Tesla. Twenty-one-year-old
male suffered right frontal
hematoma during trauma two
weeks earlier. (**a**) CT
demonstrates persistent high
density (arrow) and edema
(arrowheads) in right frontal
hematoma. (**b**) T_2-weighted
gradient-echo image (PS 250/
113, $\theta = 90°$) demonstrates
hemosiderin rim (black arrows)
between central
methemoglobin (in lysed red
cells) and peripheral vasogenic
edema (open arrow). Note also
small left-sided subdural
hematoma (white arrows)
which cannot be seen on CT.

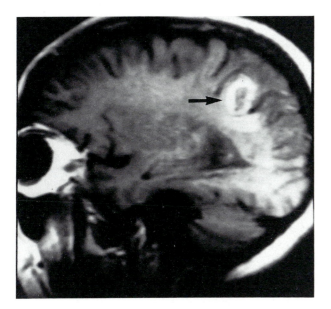

a

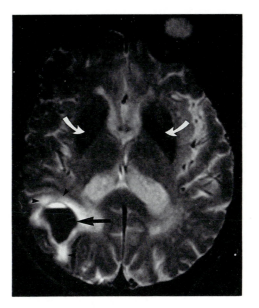

b

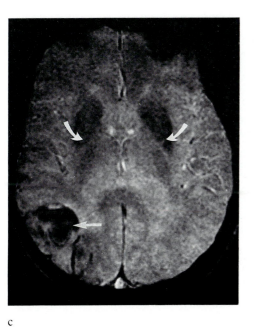

c

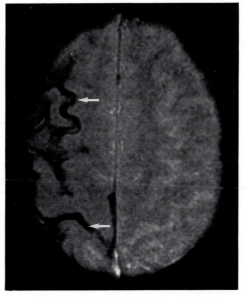

d

Figure 7.16

Parenchymal hematoma and superficial siderosis from presumed amyloid angiopathy. (a) Parasagittal T_1-weighted section demonstrates parenchymal hematoma in high right parietal lobe one week following hemorrhage (arrow). Peripheral high intensity reflects presence of methemoglobin while central lower intensity is due to deoxyhemoglobin (SE 800/20). (b) Heavily T_2-weighted axial section through right parietal hematoma (straight arrow) demonstrates in vivo hematocrit effect. The larger hypointense posterior collection reflects intracellular deoxyhemoglobin and methemoglobin, while the non-dependent high-intensity collection represents free methemoglobin. Note also surrounding edema (arrowheads) and normally hypointense basal ganglia due to physiologic ferritin deposition (curved arrows) (SE 2800/70). (c) T_2^*-weighted GRASS image through the same level as (b) demonstrates similar hypointensity in parenchymal hematoma (straight arrow) and in basal ganglia (curved arrows). GRASS image is less sensitive to the vasogenic edema noted in (b) (PS 75/20, $\theta = 10°$). (d) Higher axial GRASS image demonstrates superficial siderosis (arrows) following previous bleed (PS 75/20, $\theta = 10°$). (Courtesy of Michael Brant-Zawadzki, MD, Newport Beach, CA.)

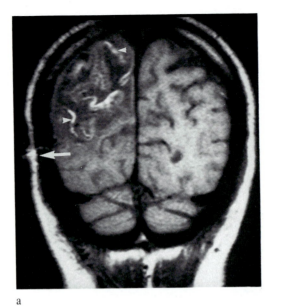

a

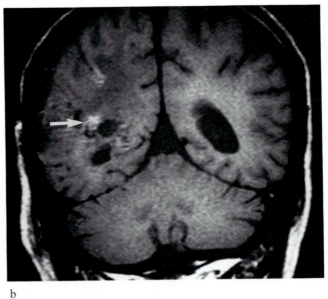

b

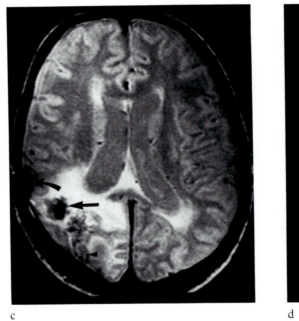

c

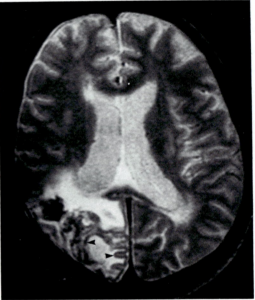

d

Figure 7.17

Chronic hemorrhage and superficial siderosis. (**a**) T₁-weighted coronal section demonstrates high intensity conforming to gyri (arrowheads). This is due to methemoglobin formation. Note metallic artifact at craniectomy site (arrow) following evacuation of hematoma one year previously (SE 600/30). (**b**) More anterior coronal section demonstrates globular high-signal intensity (arrow) due to methemoglobin (SE 600/30). (**c**) Moderately T₂-weighted axial section demonstrates hypointensity in globular lesion (arrow) noted in (**b**). This indicates that methemoglobin is within intact red cells. Note also superficial siderosis (arrowheads) posterior to residual hematoma. Metallic artifact at craniectomy site (curved arrow) is increased with additional T₂-weighting (SE 2500/30). (**d**) On more heavily T₂-weighted image through same level as (**c**), gyral low-signal intensity (arrowheads) becomes more hypointense due to presence of intracellular methemoglobin (as noted in **a**) and hemosiderin (SE 2500/60).

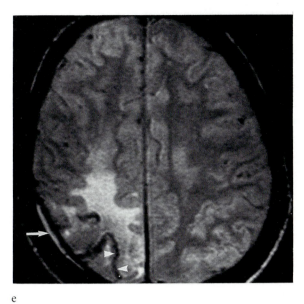

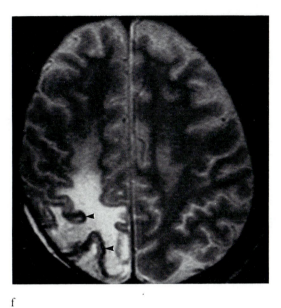

e

f

(**e**) Moderately
T$_2$-weighted high-axial section
demonstrates low-intensity,
superficial siderosis
(arrowheads). Note also small
post-operative epidural
hematoma (arrow) (SE 2500/
30). (**f**) Heavily T$_2$-weighted
image demonstrates superficial
siderosis (arrowheads) to
greater advantage (SE 2500/60).

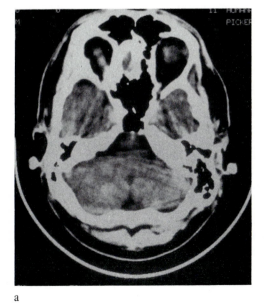

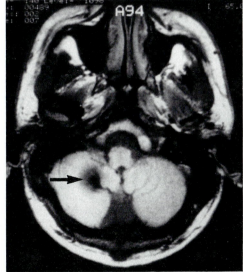

a

b

Figure 7.18

Asymptomatic cerebellar
hemosiderin deposit. (**a**) CT
through cerebellum is normal.
(**b**) Mildly T$_2$-weighted MR
image through the same level
demonstrates focal T$_2$-
shortening (arrow) (SE 2500/
20). This presumably reflects
hemosiderin deposition from
old hemorrhage from occult
AVM or venous angioma.

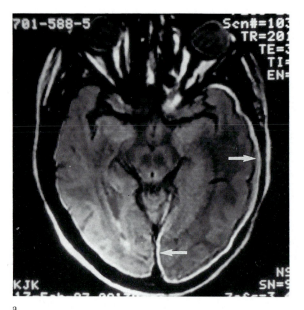

a

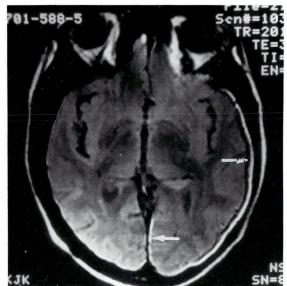

b

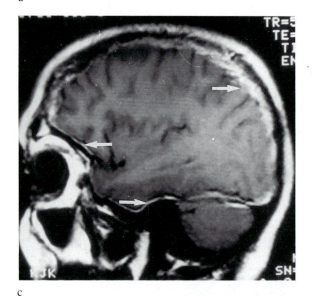

c

Figure 7.19

Subacute subdural hematoma. High-signal intensity (arrows) is noted over left hemisphere, extending into left posterior interhemispheric fissure.
(a) Mildly T_2-weighted axial section through the level of the midbrain (SE 2010/32).
(b) Mildly T_2-weighted section through level of the third ventricle (SE 2010/32). (c) T_1-weighted left parasagittal section demonstrates extra-axial high-signal intensity (arrows) subjacent to left frontal and temporal lobes and over the left parietal convexity (SE 506/32). (Courtesy of Meredith A Weinstein, MD, Cleveland, OH.)

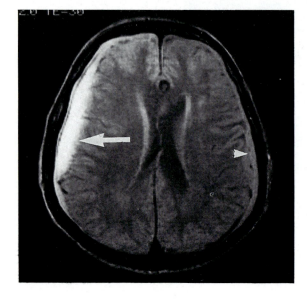

Figure 7.20

Bilateral subdural hematomas. On T_2-weighted image (SE 2000/30), subacute right subdural hematoma (arrow) appears bright due to methemoglobin. Smaller chronic left subdural hematoma (arrowhead) has lower signal intensity due to continued oxidative denaturation of methemoglobin to non-paramagnetic hemichromes. (Signal intensity is still greater than CSF due to T_1-shortening from the high protein content of the old hemorrhagic collection.)

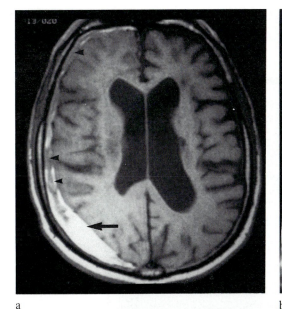

a

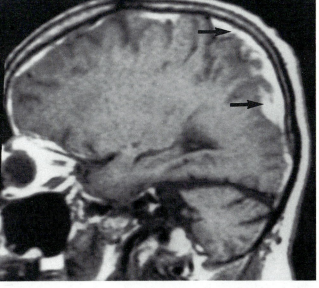

b

Figure 7.21

Subacute subdural hematoma.
(a) Five days after head trauma,
subdural hematoma is noted
over right parietal convexity.
On this T_1-weighted image,
high-intensity portion
posteriorly (arrow) represents
methemoglobin (either intra- or
extracellular) while lower-
intensity anterior component
(arrowheads) represents
intracellular deoxyhemoglobin
(SE 800/20). (b) T_1-weighted
right parasagittal section
demonstrates high intensity
(arrows) due to methemoglobin
(SE 600/20). (c) Coronal section
through parietal portion of
hematoma demonstrates
heterogeneous signal due to
recurrent bleeding. The high
signal (arrowhead) represents
free methemoglobin while the
lower signal (arrow) represents
intracellular methemoglobin
from a more recent bleed (SE
2800/30). (d) With additional
T_2-weighting, the intracellular
methemoglobin becomes
darker (arrow) and the
extracellular methemoglobin
remains bright (arrowhead) (SE
2800/70). (e) More anterior
coronal section demonstrates

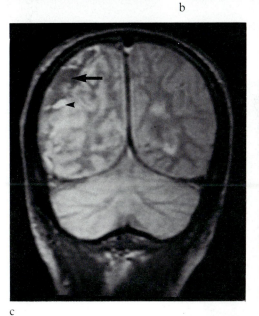

c

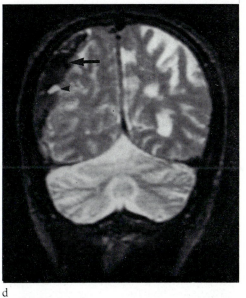

d

marked hypointensity
(arrowheads) in subdural
hematoma. Since this appeared
relatively dark on the T_1-
weighted image in (a), it
represents intracellular
deoxyhemoglobin. Incidentally
noted are multiple infarcts in
the basal ganglia (arrows) (SE
2800/70). (Courtesy of Michael
Brant-Zawadzki, MD,
Newport Beach, CA.)

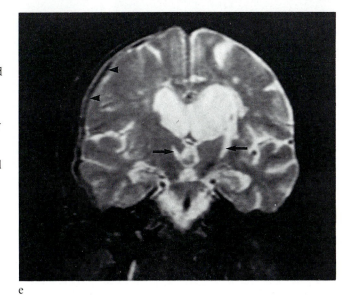

e

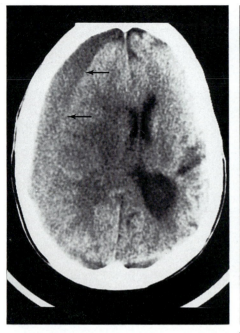

a

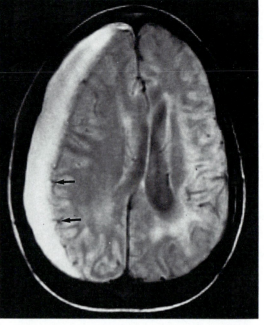

b

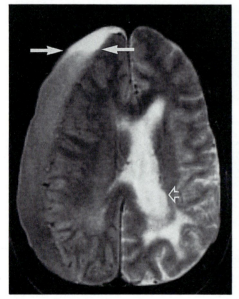

c

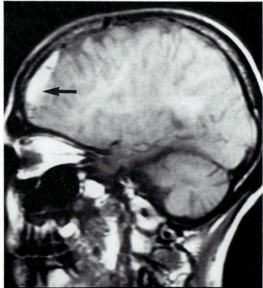

d

Figure 7.22

Subacute subdural hematoma with in vivo hematocrit. (**a**) Two weeks after minor trauma, non-enhanced CT demonstrates large right convexity subdural hematoma (arrows) which is hypodense anteriorly and isodense with subjacent brain posteriorly. (**b**) Mildly T_2-weighted axial image demonstrates large subdural hematoma with greater contrast than CT (SE 2500/20). Note position of cortical veins (arrows). (**c**) Heavily T_2-weighted image demonstrates fluid level within hematoma (arrows). The dependent low-intensity collection represents intact red cells containing methemoglobin. The higher-intensity non-dependent collection represents methemoglobin free in solution. Note also enlarged left lateral ventricle (open arrow) secondary to mass effect of subdural hematoma and entrapment at foramen of Monro (SE 2500/70). (**d**) T_1-weighted parasagittal section demonstrates T_1-shortening in anterior portion of subdural hematoma (arrow), confirming presence of free methemoglobin (SE 800/20). (Courtesy of Michael Brant-Zawadzki, MD, Newport Beach, CA.)

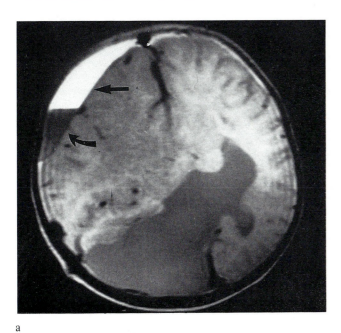

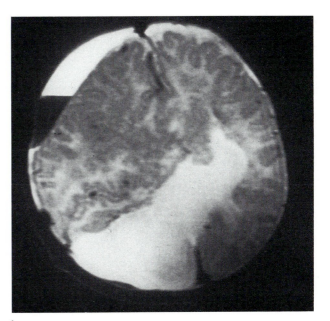

a

b

Figure 7.23

Subdural hematoma following ventricular shunting. (**a**) Mildly T$_2$-weighted axial image demonstrates in vivo hematocrit in right frontal subdural hematoma following shunting for holoprosencephaly. High signal is noted in non-dependent portion of hematoma due to free methemoglobin (straight arrow). Lower signal is noted in dependent posterior portion of hematoma due to intracellular methemoglobin or deoxyhemoglobin (curved arrow) (SE 2500/30). (**b**) On more heavily T$_2$-weighted image, non-dependent portion of subdural hematoma remains bright while dependent cellular fraction becomes darker due to magnetic susceptibility effects (SE 2500/80). (Courtesy of Jay S Tsuruda, MD, San Francisco, CA.)

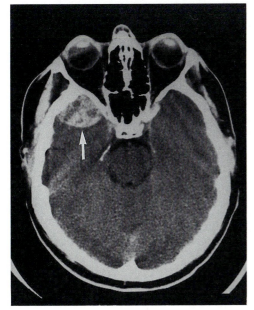

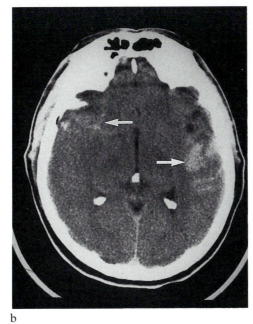

a

b

Figure 7.24

Evolving traumatic hematomas. (**a**) Several hours after trauma, unenhanced CT at the level of the upper pons demonstrates acute epidural hematoma (arrow) anterior to right temporal lobe. (**b**) Unenhanced CT through level of third ventricle demonstrates parenchymal hematomas (arrows) in both temporal lobes.

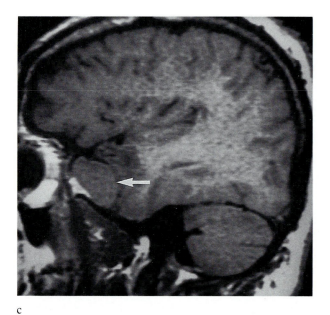

c

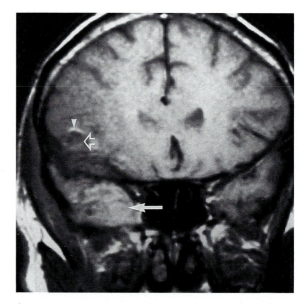

d

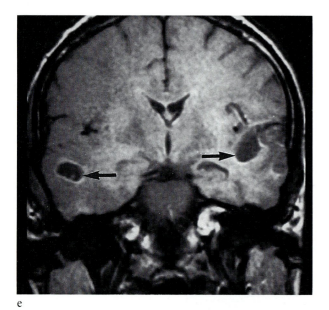

e

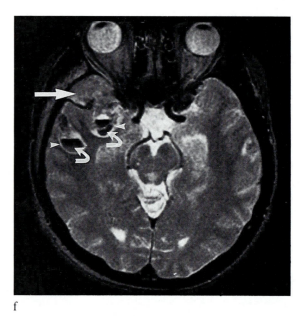

f

Figure 7.24 *continued*

(**c**) Thirty-six hours after
trauma, T_1-weighted
parasagittal section
demonstrates epidural
hematoma (arrow). Hematoma
is isointense with gray matter
due to persistence of
oxyhemoglobin (SE 600/20).
(**d**) Mildly T_1-weighted coronal
section demonstrates somewhat
higher signal intensity in
epidural hematoma (arrow)
than in contralateral normal left
temporal lobe. Parenchymal
right temporal hematoma has
high-intensity rim (arrowhead)

due to early methemoglobin
formation and low-intensity
center (open arrow) due to
intracellular deoxyhemoglobin
(SE 800/30). (**e**) More posterior
coronal section demonstrates
parenchymal hematomas in
both temporal lobes (arrows),
with similar high-intensity
outer rim and low-intensity
cores reflecting methemoglobin
and deoxyhemoglobin,
respectively (SE 800/30). (**f**)
Heavily T_2-weighted axial
section demonstrates
isointensity in epidural

hematoma (straight arrow) due
to persistence of
oxyhemoglobin 36 hours after
trauma. Parenchymal
hematomas, on the other hand,
have low-intensity cores
(curved arrows) due to
intracellular deoxyhemoglobin
with high-intensity rims
(arrowheads) due to
methemoglobin. Note in vivo
hematocrit effect within
hematomas, the non-dependent
collection containing free
methemoglobin (SE 2800/70).

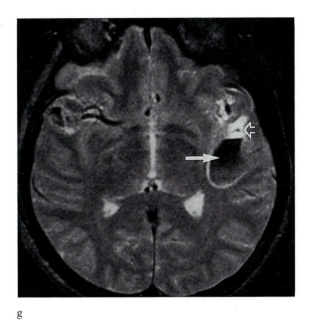

g

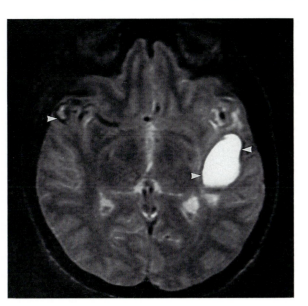

h

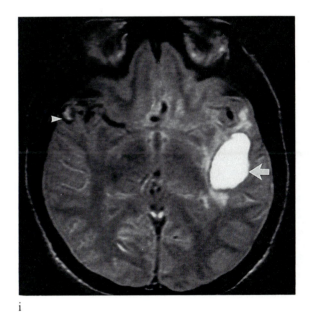

i

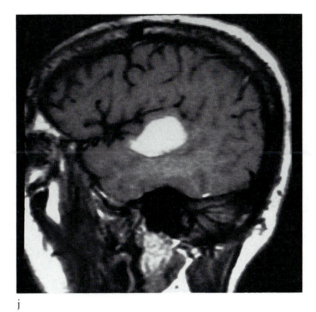

j

(**g**) Higher axial T$_2$-weighted section demonstrates left parenchymal hematoma. Note in vivo hematocrit effect with high-intensity free methemoglobin above (open arrow) and low-intensity intracellular deoxyhemoglobin below (straight arrow) (SE 2800/70). (**h**) One month after trauma, left temporal hematoma appears homogeneously hyperintense on mildly T$_2$-weighted image (arrow). Smaller right temporal hematoma has similar central hyperintensity with more prominent low-intensity rim (arrowhead) due to hemosiderin-laden macrophages (SE 2800/30). (**i**) Heavily T$_2$-weighted axial section through same level as (**h**) demonstrates even greater signal loss in hemosiderin rims (arrowheads) surrounding chronic parenchymal hematomas (SE 2800/70). (**j**) T$_1$-weighted left parasagittal section through parenchymal hematoma demonstrates homogeneous central high intensity due to free methemoglobin (SE 600/20). (Courtesy of Michael Brant-Zawadzki, MD, Newport Beach, CA.)

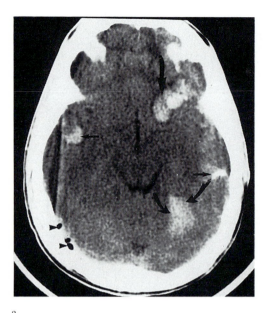

a

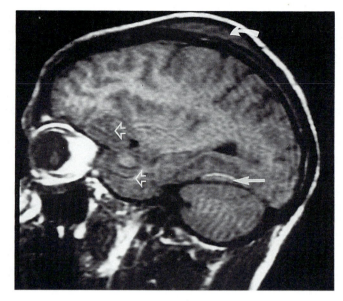

b

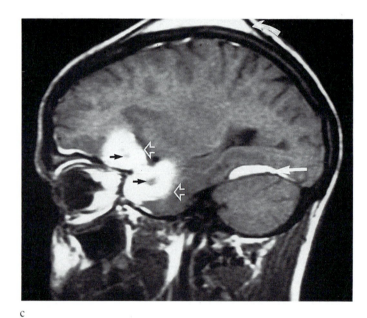

c

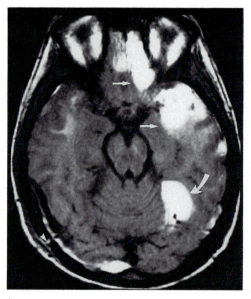

d

Figure 7.25

Evolving traumatic hematomas. (a) CT **several hours** after trauma demonstrates extra-axial air (arrowheads) subjacent to right occipital fracture (not shown). Contrecoup left frontal hematoma (large straight arrow) is noted as well as parenchymal hematomas in both temporal lobes (small arrows). High-density collection posteriorly suggests subdural hematoma adjacent to the left tentorial leaf (curved arrows). (b) Left parasagittal T_1-weighted MR study **one day** following trauma demonstrates isointense subdural hematoma above left tentorial leaf (straight arrow). Note also cephalohematoma (curved arrow) which is somewhat less intense than brain due to presence of oxyhemoglobin or deoxyhemoglobin. Subtle hypointensity in left subfrontal and anterior left temporal lobes (open arrows) is due to parenchymal hematomas containing either oxyhemoglobin or deoxyhemoglobin (SE 600/20).

(c) T_1-weighted left parasagittal section (same level as **b**) **10 days** following trauma demonstrates high-signal intensity in parenchymal hematomas (open arrows), left tentorial subdural hematoma (straight arrow), and cephalohematoma (curved arrow). These reflect the oxidative denaturation of deoxyhemoglobin to methemoglobin with secondary T_1-shortening. Hypointense centers of parenchymal hematomas (arrowheads) reflect continued presence of intracellular deoxyhemoglobin (SE 600/20). (d) T_1-weighted axial section through level of midbrain demonstrates right occipital skull fracture (arrowhead). High signal now seen in subfrontal and left temporal lobe hematomas (straight arrows) and in left tentorial subdural hematoma (curved arrow) is due to presence of methemoglobin (SE 600/20).

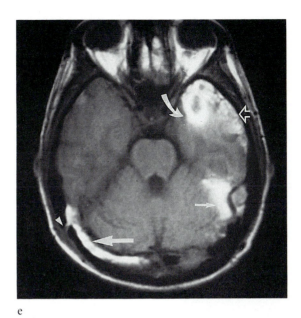

e

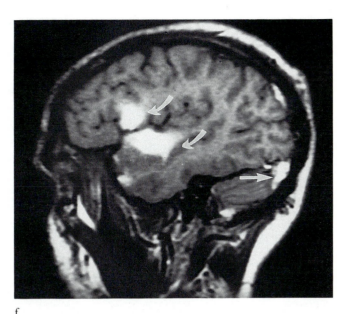

f

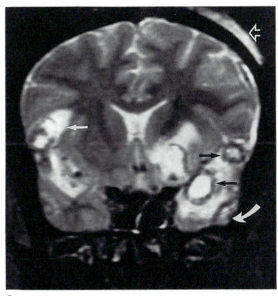

g

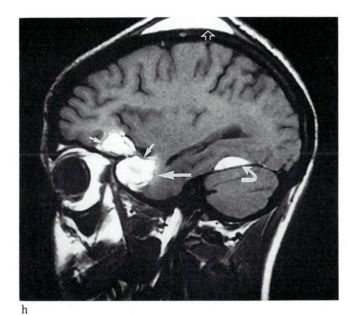

h

(e) T$_1$-weighted axial section through upper pons demonstrates subacute thrombosis of the right transverse sinus (large straight arrow) subjacent to right occipital skull fracture (arrowhead). Again noted is anterior left temporal hematoma (curved arrow) with peripheral hyperintensity secondary to methemoglobin formation and central hypointensity due to persistent deoxyhemoglobin. Loculated left temporal subdural hematoma is noted (open arrow), as well as lateral extent of subdural hematoma over left tentorial leaf (small arrow) (SE 800/20). (f) Right parasagittal T$_1$-weighted section demonstrates thrombosed right transverse sinus (straight arrow) as well as subacute parenchymal hematomas (curved arrows) (SE 600/20). (g) Heavily T$_2$-weighted coronal section demonstrates loculated left temporal subdural hematoma (curved arrow). Multiple parenchymal hematomas are noted with dark rims due to hemosiderin-laden macrophages (straight arrows). Left parietal cephalohematoma (open arrow) has somewhat less signal than parenchymal hematomas due to continued presence of intact red cells (SE 3000/70). (h) **Three weeks** after trauma, left parasagittal section demonstrates homogeneous high-signal intensity in parenchymal (straight arrow), subdural (curved arrow), and cephalo (open arrow) hematomas. Note presence of dark rim (arrowhead) surrounding parenchymal hematomas due to hemosiderin-laden macrophages which can be seen even on this T$_1$-weighted image (SE 800/20).

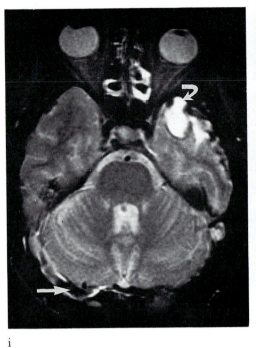

i

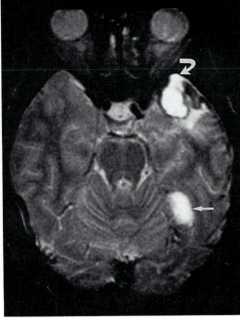

j

Figure 7.25 *continued*

(i) Heavily T$_2$-weighted axial section through same level as (e) now demonstrates recanalization of right transverse sinus (straight arrow). Homogeneous high-signal intensity is noted in left temporal hematoma (curved arrow) due to free methemoglobin. Surrounding rim of low intensity is due to hemosiderin-laden macrophages (SE 2800/70). (j) Heavily T$_2$-weighted image through level of upper pons demonstrates anterior left temporal hematoma (curved arrow) and lateral aspect of subdural hematoma over left tentorial leaf (straight arrow) (SE 2800/70). (Courtesy of Michael Brant-Zawadzki, MD, Newport Beach, CA.)

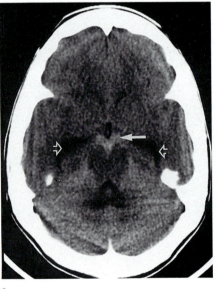

a

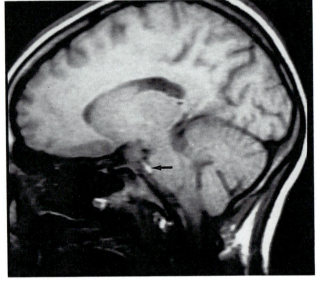

b

Figure 7.26

Evolving subarachnoid hemorrhage. (a) **Several days** after subarachnoid hemorrhage, CT demonstrates high density in the interpeduncular cistern (straight arrow). Enlarged temporal horns (open arrows) are due to communicating hydrocephalus. (b) **One week** after subarachnoid hemorrhage, high-signal intensity is noted in pontine cistern (arrow) due to early methemoglobin formation (SE 600/25).

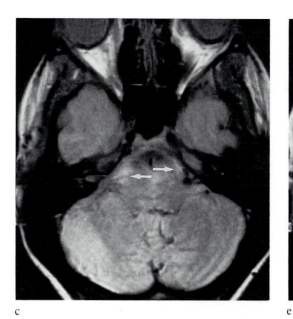

c

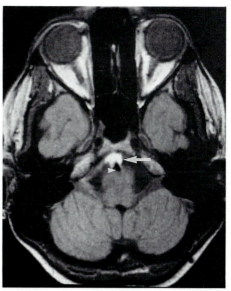

e

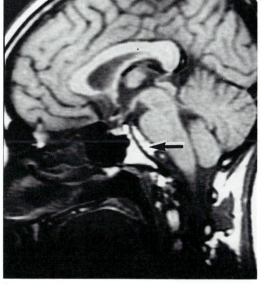

d

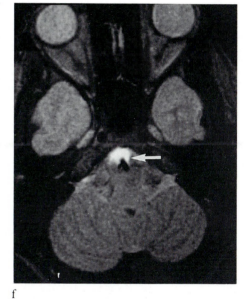

f

(**c**) Axial section through the medulla demonstrates minimal high-signal intensity in the medullary cisterns (arrows) due to early methemoglobin formation (SE 2000/20). (**d**) **One month** later, sagittal section now demonstrates high signal in pontine cistern (arrow) secondary to methemoglobin formation in subarachnoid hematoma (SE 600/25). (**e**) Axial section through the medulla demonstrates high-signal intensity (arrow) surrounding basilar artery (arrowhead) (SE 2000/20). (**f**) Heavily T$_2$-weighted image through same axial level as (**f**) demonstrates persistent high-signal intensity in subarachnoid thrombus (arrow), indicating presence of free methemoglobin (SE 2000/70). (Courtesy of Robert Jahnke, MD, Albuquerque, NM.)

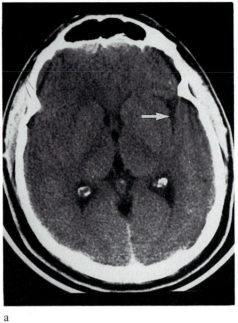

a

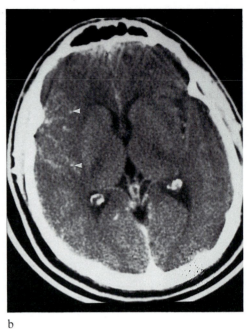

b

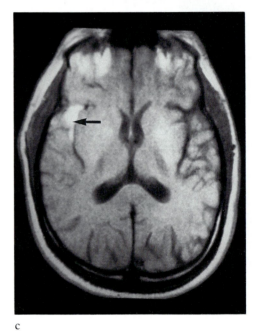

c

d

Figure 7.27

Subarachnoid hemorrhage. (**a**) Emergency unenhanced CT performed for worsening mental status demonstrates relatively high density in the right Sylvian cistern (making it isodense with surrounding brain) compared to the hypodense left Sylvian cistern (arrow). (**b**) Enhanced CT demonstrates many more right Sylvian vessels (arrowheads) compared to contralateral side. This suggests spasm in the right middle cerebral artery with secondary slow flow in its branches. (**c**) T_1-weighted axial MR image demonstrates T_1-shortening in the right Sylvian cistern (arrow), indicative of subarachnoid hemorrhage (SE 1000/26). (**d**) T_2-weighted axial section demonstrates high signal in right Sylvian cistern (arrow). This indicates that free methemoglobin is present, that is, the red cells have lysed (SE 2500/100).

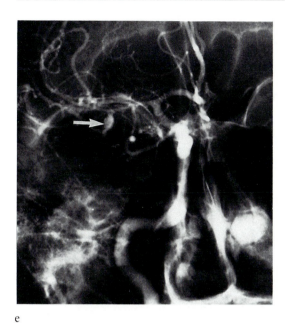

e

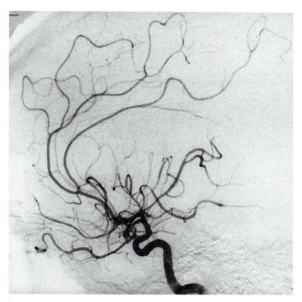

f

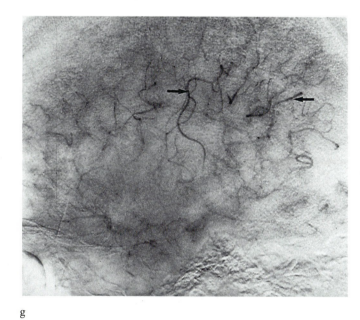

g

(**e**) AP projection of right internal carotid arteriogram performed on the next day demonstrates trifurcation aneurysm (arrow). (**f**) Lateral projection of right internal carotid arteriogram demonstrates filling of anterior cerebral branches with delayed filling of right middle cerebral artery branches suggesting right MCA spasm. (**g**) Later films from lateral projection demonstrate delayed filling of right Sylvian branches (arrow) secondary to spasm of the trifurcation of the middle cerebral artery. This corresponds to the increased vascularity noted in this region on the initial enhanced CT scan shown in (**b**). (Courtesy of Michael Brant-Zawadzki, MD, Newport Beach, CA.)

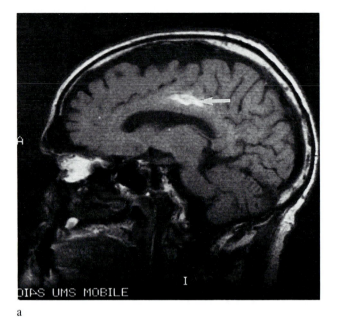

a

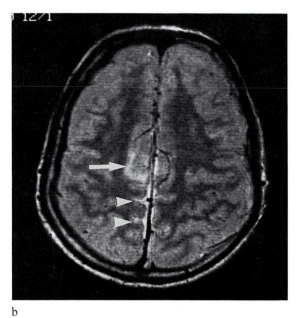

b

Figure 7.28

Subarachnoid hemorrhage
following bleeding from an
astrocytoma. (**a**) T_1-weighted
image demonstrates high-signal
intensity (arrow) in cingulate
sulcus due to methemoglobin
formation (SE 500/40).
(**b**) High-signal intensity is noted in
sulci of interhemispheric fissure
(arrowheads) confirming
subarachnoid (as opposed to
subdural) location. Source of
hemorrhage (astrocytoma) is
also noted (arrow) (SE 3000/
40). (**c**) Axial section through
roof of lateral ventricles
demonstrates tumor (arrow)
(SE 3000/40).

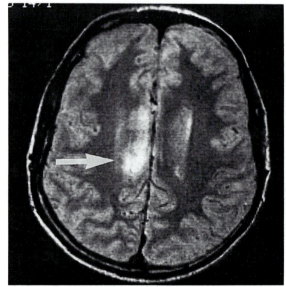

c

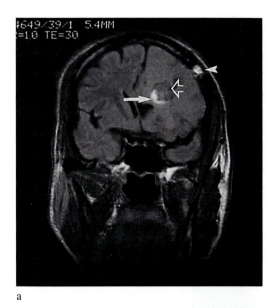

a

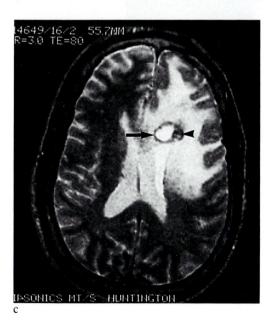

b

Figure 7.29

Metastatic melanoma
(**a**) T_1-weighted coronal section
demonstrates hemorrhage
along inferomedial aspect of
tumor (arrow). Isointense soft
tissue mass (open arrow)
suggests neoplastic origin. This
was confirmed by biopsy: (note
burr hole in left parietal region
(arrowhead)) (SE 1000/30).
(**b**) Moderately T_2-weighted
image demonstrates late
subacute hemorrhage medially
(arrow) with more acute
hemorrhage following biopsy
laterally (arrowhead). Note that
subacute hemorrhage is more
intense than surrounding
vasogenic edema, which
permits the diagnosis of
hemorrhage to be made on this
technique (SE 3000/40). (**c**) On
heavily T_2-weighted image,
subacute hemorrhage and
surrounding edema are of equal
maximum intensity, thus the
two cannot be distinguished.
Acute hemorrhage following
biopsy (arrowhead) and
hemosiderin rim (arrow) both
become relatively darker with
more T_2-weighting (SE 3000/
80).

c

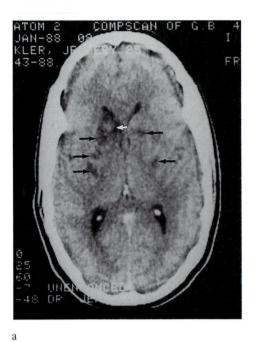

a

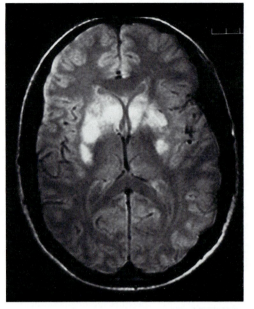

b

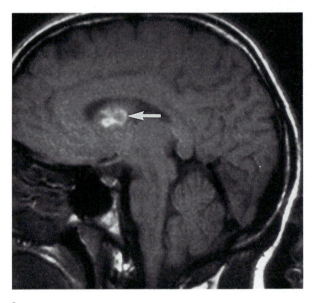

c

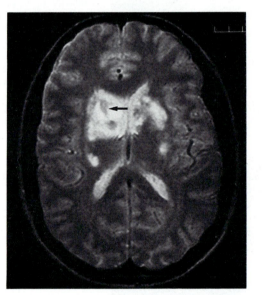

d

Figure 7.30

Hemorrhagic glioma.
(**a**) Unenhanced CT demonstrates low-density abnormalities in both basal ganglia (arrows) with central high density suggesting hemorrhage (arrowhead). While these abnormalities suggest the presence of lacunar infarcts, this would be somewhat unusual in this non-hypertensive 26-year-old male. (**b**) Mildly T_2-weighted axial MR section through same level as (**a**) demonstrates hyperintensity in region of previously noted abnormality (SE 2500/30). (**c**) Right parasagittal T_1-weighted image demonstrates high-signal intensity (arrow) in right caudate head, indicating methemoglobin formation (SE 600/30). (**d**) Heavily T_2-weighted axial section through same level as (**b**) demonstrates hypointensity in right caudate head (arrow), indicating that a portion of the methemoglobin is intracellular (SE 2500/60).

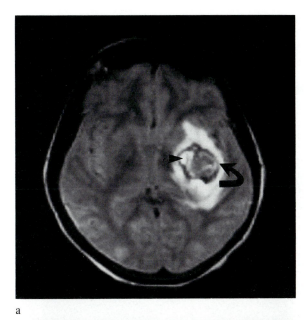

a

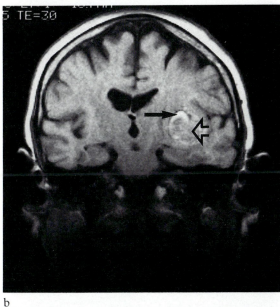

b

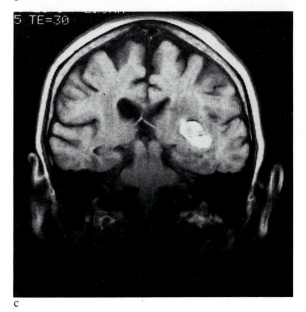

c

Figure 7.31

Hemorrhage glioma. (**a**) Axial T_2-weighted image demonstrates heterogeneous lesion with medial high signal (arrowhead) due to extracellular methemoglobin, while central and lateral portion are generally hypointense. Note surrounding rim of hemosiderin-laden macrophages which is incomplete laterally due to presumed tumor growth (curved arrow). Note also persistent vasogenic edema several months after initial presentation, suggesting neoplastic etiology (SE 2000/ 60). (**b**) T_1-weighted coronal section through the anterior portion of the tumor at the level of the foramen of Monro. Note medial position of methemoglobin (arrow) and isointense tumor (open arrow). (**c**) T_1-weighted coronal section through posterior portion of tumor demonstrating T_1-shortening due to presence of methemoglobin.

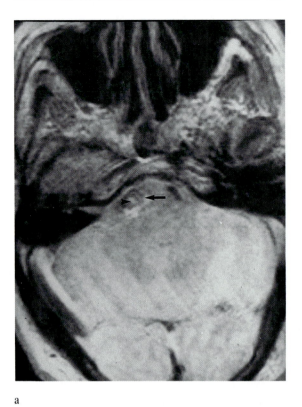

a

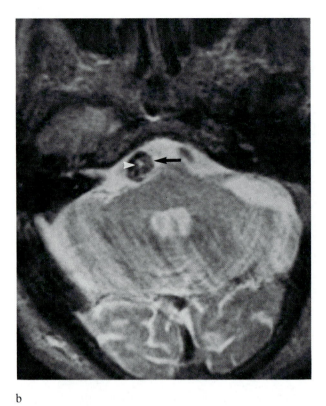

b

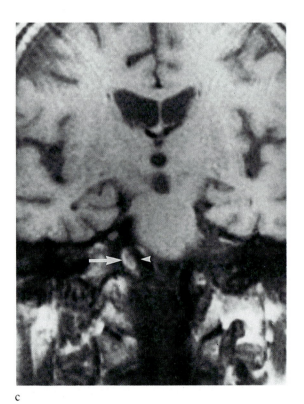

c

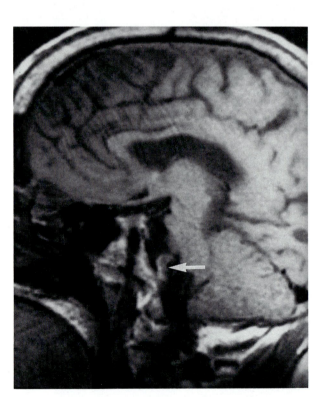

d

Figure 7.32

Aneurysm of right vertebral artery. (**a**) Mildly T_2-weighted axial section demonstrates abnormal low signal in enlarged right vertebral artery (arrow). Mural thrombus is hypointense to CSF due to intracellular methemoglobin. Central lumen (arrowhead) has higher signal than surrounding clot due to flow-related enhancement (SE 2700/30). (**b**) More heavily T_2-weighted axial image demonstrates marked hypointensity in thrombus (arrow) relative to surrounding CSF. This reflects the presence of intracellular methemoglobin (SE 2700/80). (**c**) T_1-weighted coronal section demonstrates high-intensity thrombus within aneurysm (arrow) due to methemoglobin formation. Note persistent flow void in central lumen due to inplane flow (arrowhead) (SE 600/20). (**d**) T_1-weighted parasagittal section through aneurysm (arrow) demonstrates high-signal intensity due to methemoglobin (SE 600/20).

Figure 7.33

Aneurysm of the right posterior communicating artery (arrow). Increase in central signal intensity is due to slow flow and even-echo rephasing in patent lumen. (**a**) First-echo image (SE 3000/40). (**b**) Second-echo image (SE 3000/80). (**c**) Angiogram demonstrates aneurysm of the posterior communicating artery (arrow).

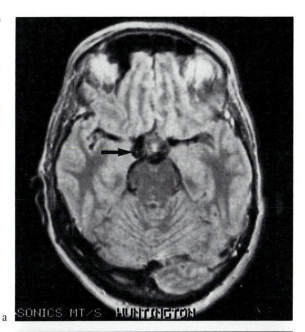
a

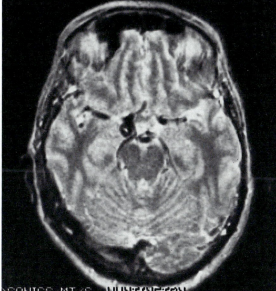
b

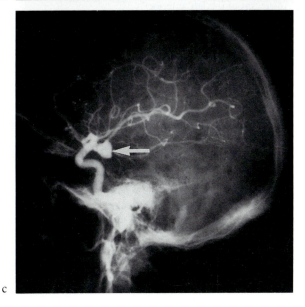
c

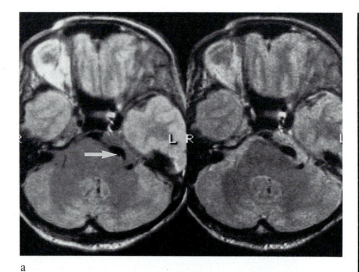

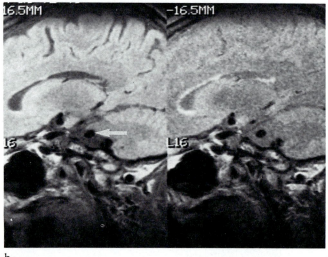

a

b

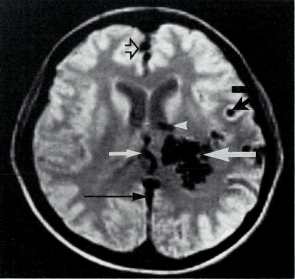

a

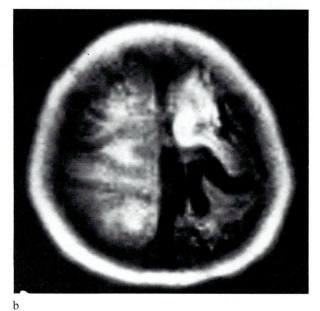

b

Figure 7.34

Aneurysm of the left anterior inferior cerebellar artery. Fusiform aneurysm of left AICA (arrow) is noted on axial and parasagittal views. (**a**) Axial views (SE 2000/40 and 80). (**b**) Left parasagittal section through left CP angle cistern (SE 1000/40 and 80).

Figure 7.35

Left hemispheric arteriovenous malformation. (**a**) Nidus of AVM is demonstrated by virtue of signal void (large straight arrow). Feeding branches of the anterior cerebral arteries (open arrow) are noted, as well as branches of the left middle cerebral artery (curved arrow). Drainage through the left thalamostriate vein (arrowhead) is noted, as well as enlargement of the left internal cerebral vein (small arrow) and straight sinus (long thin arrow). (**b**) Large draining vein noted over left vertex with drainage into the superior sagittal sinus (SE 2000/28).

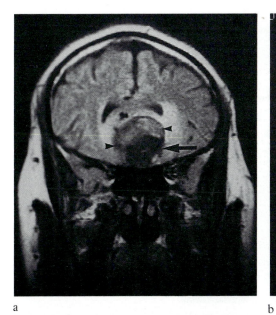

a

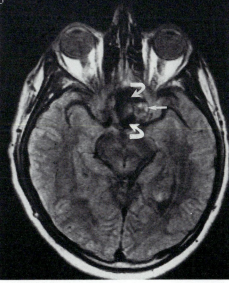

b

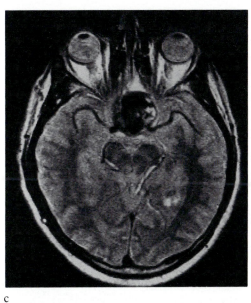

c

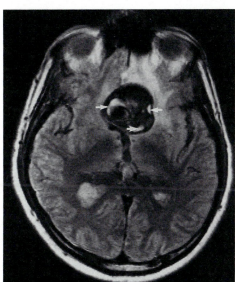

d

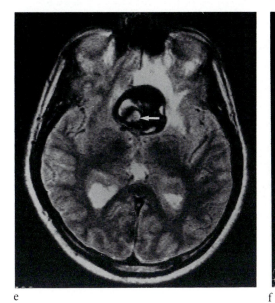

e

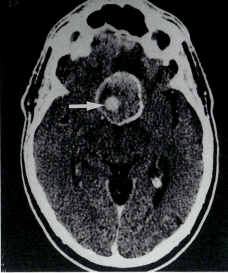

f

Figure 7.36

Giant intracranial aneurysm arising from the Circle of Willis. (**a**) Coronal section demonstrates mural thrombus (arrowheads) along dome and right lateral aspect of aneurysm, with signal loss inferiorly and to the left side suggesting the location of the patent lumen (arrow) on this coronal section (SE 1000/30). (**b**) Axial section at the level of the Circle of Willis demonstrating peripheral thrombus (arrow) and patent lumen (curved arrows). (**c**) Second echo at same level as (**b**) demonstrates additional signal loss in patent lumen due to time-of-flight losses and turbulence (SE 2000/60). (**d**) On a slightly higher axial section, peripheral methemoglobin is noted (arrowheads), with multiple areas of low signal scattered throughout. (**e**) On second-echo image at same level as (**d**) increased signal (arrow) is noted in rounded area of hypointensity in **d**, indicating the presence of slow flow with even-echo rephasing in patent lumen. (**f**) The position of the patent lumen (arrow) is confirmed on the contrast-enhanced CT at the same level

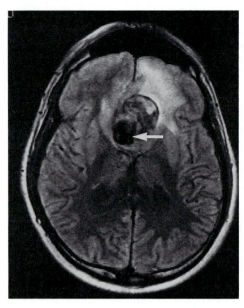

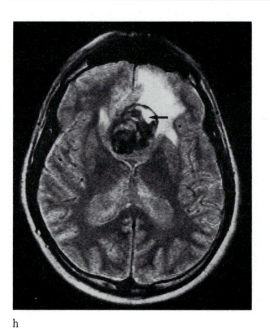

g

h

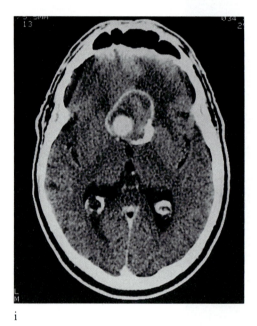

i

Figure 7.36 *continued*

as (**d**). (**g**). At a slightly higher
axial level, the patent lumen
(arrow) is noted along the right
posterior aspect of the lesion.
Heterogeneous high-signal
intensity is noted along the left
anterolateral aspect due to
methemoglobin in mural
thrombus (SE 2000/30).
(**h**) Second-echo image through
the same level as (**g**)
demonstrates persistent low
signal in the patent lumen due
to turbulence and time-of-flight
losses, with increasing signal in
mural thrombus containing
methemoglobin (arrow) (SE
2000/60). (**i**) Contrast-enhanced
CT through the same level as
(**g**) and (**h**) demonstrates
enhancement in the patent
lumen posteriorly and on the
right.

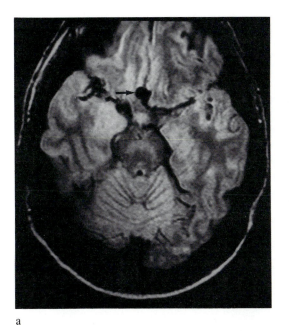

a

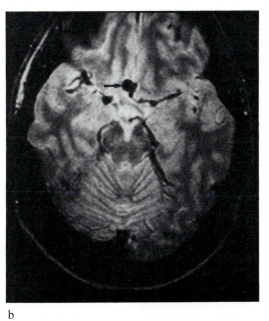

b

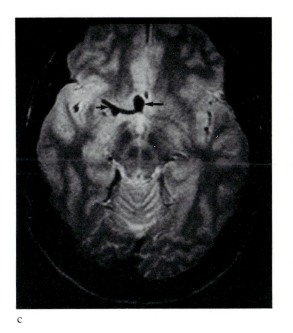

c

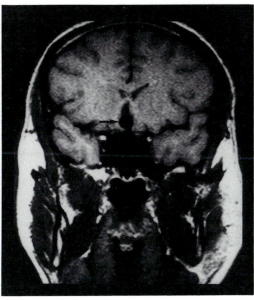

d

Figure 7.37

Anterior communicating artery aneurysm. (**a**) Low axial section through level of upper pons demonstrates small aneurysm (arrow) of the anterior communicating artery.
(**b**) On slightly higher axial section through midbrain, aneurysm is again seen (arrow).
(**c**) On higher section through upper midbrain, top of the aneurysm (arrow) and M1 segment of the right middle cerebral artery (arrowhead) are demonstrated. There is no evidence of mural thrombus in this small aneurysm. (**d**) Coronal section demonstrates craniocaudal extent of aneurysm (arrow).

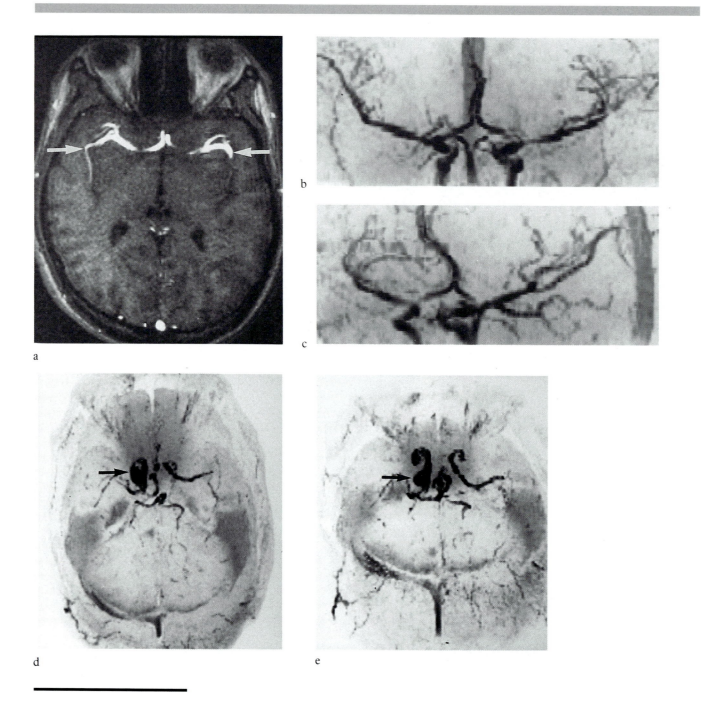

Figure 7.38

MR angiography. (**a**) Normal proximal middle cerebral arteries (arrows) imaged using FLASH technique with flip angle of 60° (to maximize flow-related enhancement). Spatial resolution of this three-dimensional acquisition is 1 mm along all three axes. This image is the sum of eight axial images (PS 40/10, θ = 60°).
(**b**) MR angiogram in frontal projection from three-dimensional FISP data set (PS 50/20, θ = 15°). (**c**) Off-lateral projection of normal intracranial arteries using same technique as (**b**). (**d**) Right middle cerebral artery aneurysm demonstrated by MR angiography. Aneurysm (arrow) demonstrated in axial plane using FISP-like technique (PS 40/13, θ = 15°). (**e**) Aneurysm (arrow) demonstrated in half-axial projection. (Courtesy of Mark Haake, PhD and Tom Masaryk, MD, Cleveland, OH.)

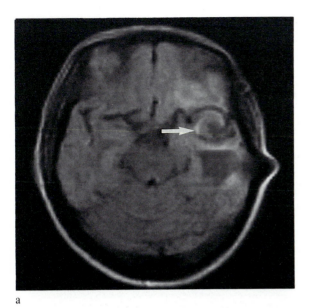

a

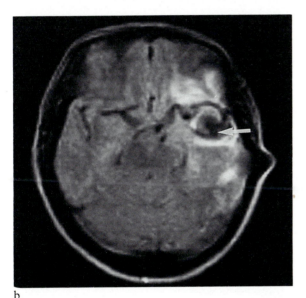

b

Figure 7.39

Hematoma resulting from aneurysmal rupture. Following rupture of aneurysm at trifurcation of left middle cerebral artery, hematoma is noted in left temporal and posterior frontal lobes (a) Mildly T_2-weighted axial section demonstrates peripheral methemoglobin (arrow) and central low signal (SE 2000/30). (b) On more T_2-weighted image (SE 2000/60), the core (arrow) has decreased significantly in intensity, indicating T_2-shortening due to the presence of intracellular methemoglobin or deoxyhemoglobin. (c) On coronal section, peripheral high signal is noted due to methemoglobin (arrow) with central isointensity on T_1-weighted image (SE 500/30). The combination of central isointensity on the T_1-weighted image with the hypointensity on the T_2-weighted image is consistent only with deoxyhemoglobin within intact red cells. The center cannot be a patent lumen (which would have appeared darker on the T_1-weighted image), nor can it represent intracellular methemoglobin (which would have appeared bright on the T_1-weighted image). Note also the presence of dilated ventricles despite shunting due to communicating hydrocephalus following subarachnoid hemorrhage. Metallic artifact from shunt reservoir also noted (open arrow).

c

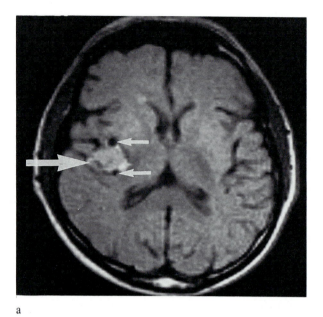

a

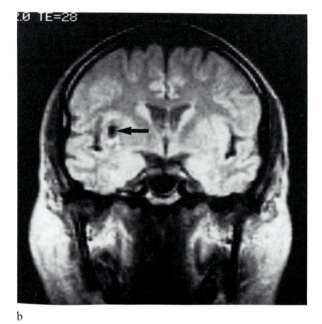

b

c

Figure 7.40

Chronic hematoma from right temporal AVM. (**a**) Mildly T_1-weighted image demonstrates old hematoma (large arrow) only slightly more intense than brain with surrounding vascular flow voids (small arrows) due to AVM (SE 1000/28). (**b**) Mildly T_2-weighted coronal section in front of AVM demonstrates abnormal vessel (arrow) (SE 2000/28).

(**c**) Mildly and moderately T_2-weighted coronal section through midportion of hematoma (arrow) demonstrates hyperintensity due to long T_2 of the chronic hemorrhage with surrounding rim (arrowhead) of hemosiderin-laden macrophages (SE 2000/28 and 56).

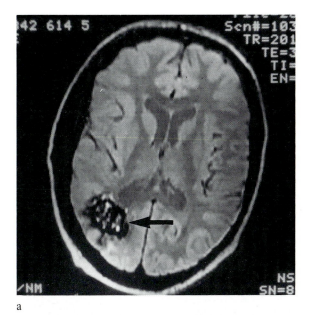

a

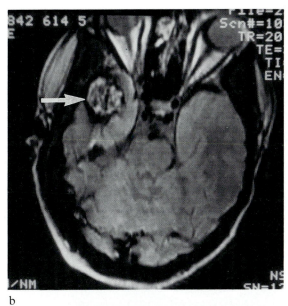

b

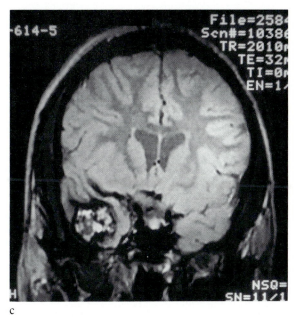

c

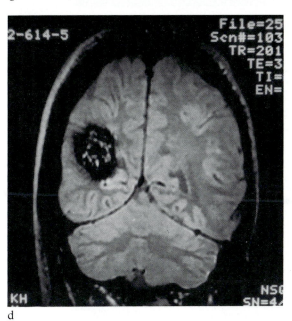

d

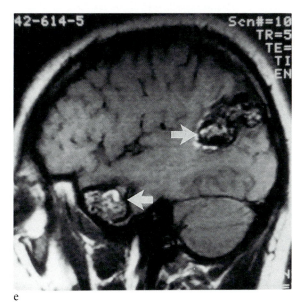

e

Figure 7.41

Chronic hemorrhage in multiple arteriovenous malformations. (**a**) Axial section through lateral ventricles demonstrates large lesion (arrow) in right occipital lobe, with surrounding rim of hypointensity due to chronic bleeding and hemosiderin deposition (SE 2010/32). (**b**) Lower axial section demonstrates similar lesion (arrow) in anterior right temporal lobe (SE 2010/32). (**c**) Coronal section demonstrates right anterior temporal lesion (SE 2010/32). (**d**) Coronal section posteriorly through the occipital lobes demonstrates right occipital hematoma with surrounding hemosiderin (SE 2010/32). (**e**) T_1-weighted right parasagittal section demonstrates both AVMs (arrows) in the same plane (SE 506/32).

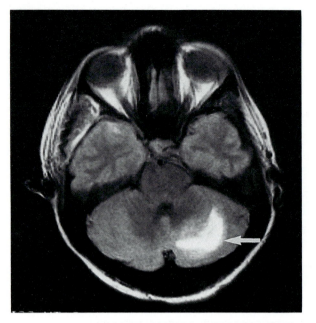

a

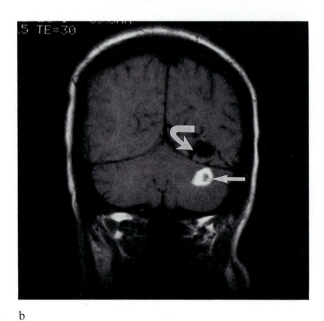

b

Figure 7.42

Subdural and intraparenchymal hematomas resulting from ruptured left tentorial AVM. (**a**) Axial section through pons demonstrates typical appearance of subdural hematoma beneath left tentorial leaf (arrow). High intensity indicates T_1-shortening due to methemoglobin formation (SE 2000/30). (**b**) Coronal section demonstrates parenchymal hematoma (straight arrow) beneath left tentorial leaf while AVM (curved arrow) is noted immediately above it in the left occipital lobe (SE 500/30).

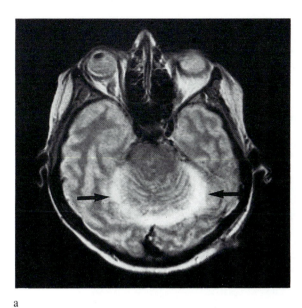

a

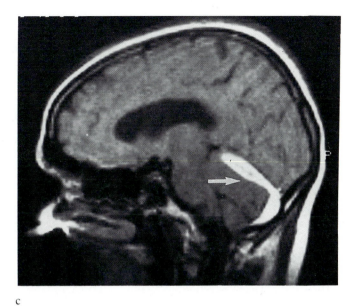

c

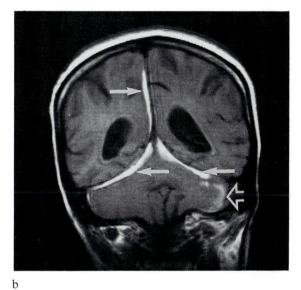

b

Figure 7.43

Subdural hemorrhage following resection of left cerebellar AVM. (**a**) Moderately T$_2$-weighted axial section demonstrates typical configuration of subdural hematoma (arrows) beneath both tentorial leaves. Note superior cerebellar vermis medially and occipital lobes laterally (SE 3000/40). (**b**) T$_1$-weighted coronal section demonstrates subdural hematoma in right interhemispheric fissure as well as beneath both tentorial leaves (arrows). Note parenchymal hematoma adjacent to side of surgical resection (open arrow). (**c**) Parasagittal section demonstrates posterior fossa subdural hematoma (arrow) (SE 500/40).

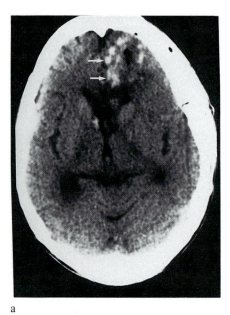

a

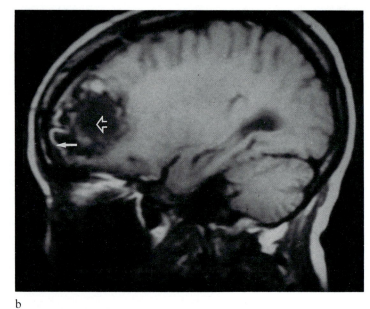

b

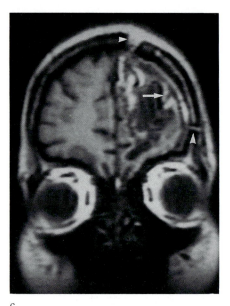

c

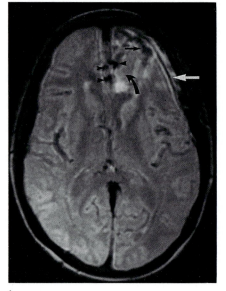

d

Figure 7.44

Chronic changes secondary to left frontal AVM. (**a**) Non-enhanced CT demonstrates foci of high density due to dystrophic calcification from prior bleeding (arrows). (**b**) T_1-weighted parasagittal section through left frontal lobe demonstrates central low signal due to encephalomalacia (open arrow) with peripheral high signal (arrow) due to methemoglobin (SE 600/20). (**c**) T_1-weighted coronal section demonstrates central low-intensity encephalomalacia following previous evacuation of hematoma. Note rim of high intensity due to residual methemoglobin (arrow). Note also craniectomy defects (arrowheads) in calvarium (SE 600/20). (**d**) Moderately T_2-weighted axial section demonstrates foci of low-signal intensity (arrowheads) which could represent flow voids from residual AVM or dystrophic calcification noted on CT. Encephalomalacic center (curved arrow) is only slightly more intense than intraventricular CSF. Rim surrounding encephalomalacia is now hypointense (small arrow), indicating that the methemoglobin noted in (**b**) and (**c**) is intracellular. Note also post-operative epidural hematoma (large arrow) (SE 2000/40). (**e**) Heavily T_2-weighted axial section through same level as (**d**) demonstrates hyperintensity in region of encephalomalacia (curved arrow), with persistent low-intensity foci secondary to either calcification or flow (arrowheads), low-intensity rim (small arrow), and epidural hematoma (large arrow)

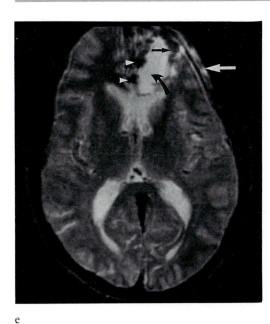

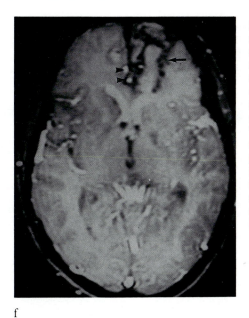

e

f

(SE 2000/80). (**f**) Flow-sensitive, single-slice GRASS image demonstrates high signal in several regions previously suspected of having either calcification or flowing blood (arrowheads). Remaining low signal represents calcification. The high signal confirms that these are vessels. Low signal in peripheral rim reflects sensitivity of GRASS technique to magnetic susceptibility effects of intracellular methemoglobin (arrow) (PS 50/15, θ = 50 degrees).

Figure 7.45

Hemorrhagic astrocytoma simulating giant intracranial aneurysm. (**a**) T_1-weighted coronal section demonstrates hemorrhagic mass (arrow) with central low intensity (arrowhead). The peripheral high intensity reflects methemoglobin formation in perfused outer portions of tumor, while hypoxic central portion remains in deoxyhemoglobin state. Note also surrounding edema with mass effect on right lateral ventricle (curved arrow) (SE 500/30). (**b**) T_2-weighted axial section through thalamus demonstrates tumor (arrow) with central calcification (arrowheads) and surrounding edema (SE 2000/80).

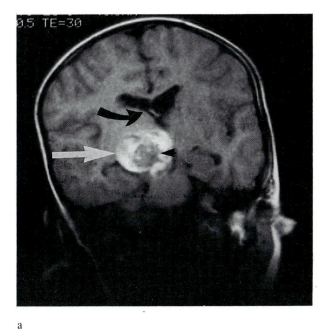

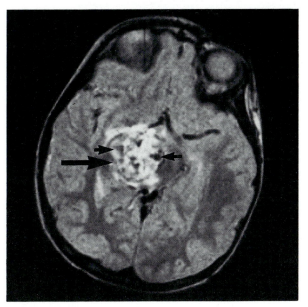

a

b

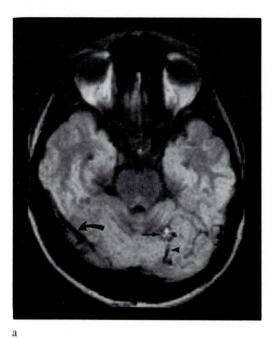

a

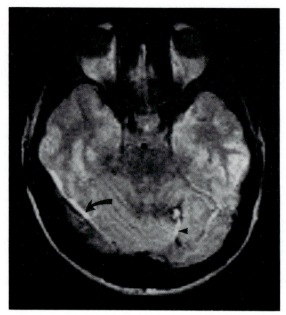

b

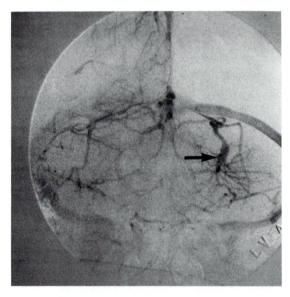

c

Figure 7.46

Cerebellar venous angioma.
(**a**) First-echo, mildly T$_2$-weighted image demonstrates high signal with surrounding dark rim (arrow) due to old hemorrhage with adjacent low-intensity linear structure (arrowhead) which represents venous angioma. Note also flow void in right tentorial vein (curved arrow) (SE 2000/28). (**b**) On second-echo, moderately T$_2$-weighted image, hematoma is essentially unchanged while both the venous angioma (arrowhead) and the right tentorial vein (curved arrow) have turned bright due to even-echo rephasing which indicates slow flow (SE 2000/56).
(**c**) Town view of left vertebral angiogram demonstrates classic appearance of venous angioma (arrow).

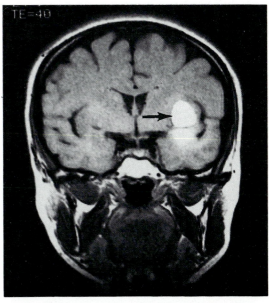

a

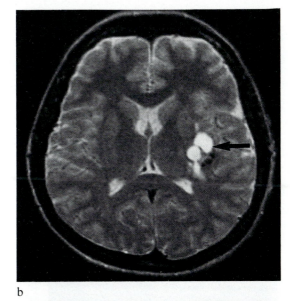

b

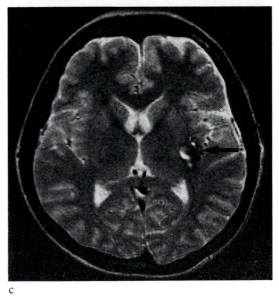

c

Figure 7.47

Capillary angioma with recurrent hemorrhage. Patient has had evidence of hemorrhage on CT since 1981 with two normal angiograms. (a) Coronal T_1-weighted section in September 1986 demonstrates mass effect in left Sylvian region due to subacute hemorrhage (arrow). High signal reflects methemoglobin formation (SE 500/40). (b) On follow-up examination one year later without clinical evidence of recurrent hemorrhage, axial T_2-weighted image demonstrates decreasing mass effect and partial resorption of hematoma noted previously (arrow) (SE 3000/80). (c) Moderately T_2-weighted axial section through left insular hematoma six months later still demonstrates increasing hemosiderin (arrow) (SE 3000/80).

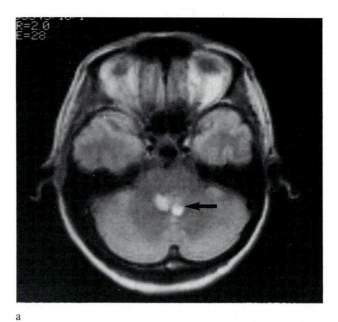

a

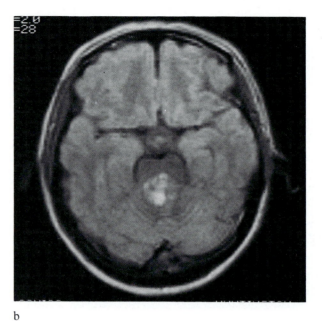

b

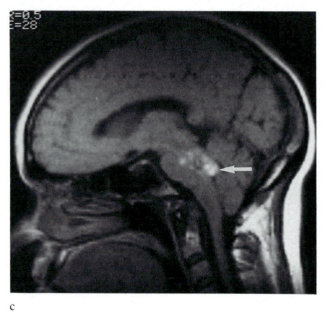

c

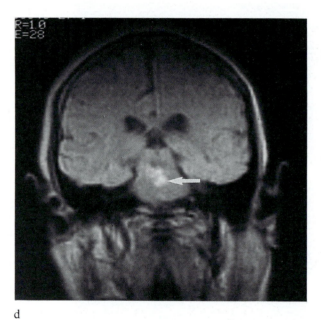

d

Figure 7.48

Idiopathic brainstem hemorrhage. Subacute hematoma is noted in pons and midbrain in non-hypertensive patient with negative angiogram in whom occult AVM is suspected. (**a**) Axial section through the pons demonstrates hematoma extending into fourth ventricle (arrow) (SE 2000/28). (**b**) On higher axial section, hematoma involves upper pons with extension into the upper fourth ventricle and aqueduct (SE 2000/28). (**c**) T_1-weighted sagittal section demonstrates hematoma involving pons with extension posteriorly into fourth ventricle (arrow) (SE 500/28). (**d**) Coronal section demonstrates pontine hemorrhage (arrow) (SE 1000/28).

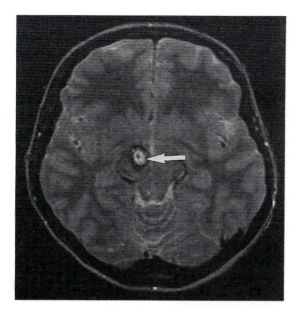

Figure 7.49

Idiopathic right midbrain hemorrhage. Hyperintense lesion (arrow) surrounded by hypointense rim in right midbrain in normotensive patient with normal angiogram. Angiographically occult AVM suspected as source of hemorrhage several weeks earlier (SE 3000/80).

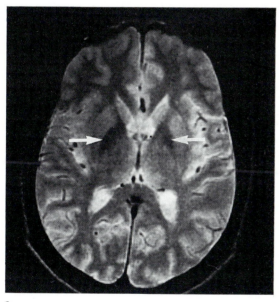

a

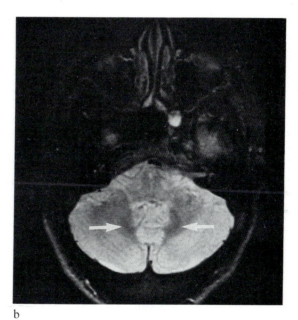

b

Figure 7.50

Normal iron deposition in the globus pallidus (arrows) demonstrated on high field (1.5 Tesla) T_2-weighted image (SE 2500/80). (**b**) Normal iron deposition in the dentate nuclei of the cerebellum (arrows) demonstrated on high-field, T_2-weighted image (SE 2500/80).

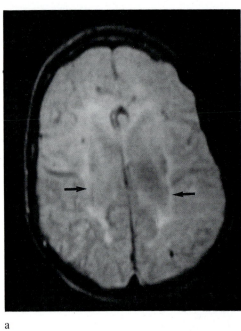

a

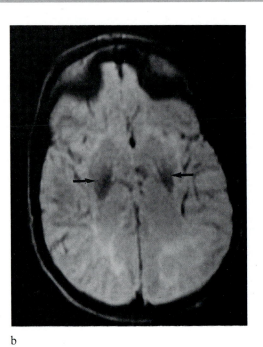

b

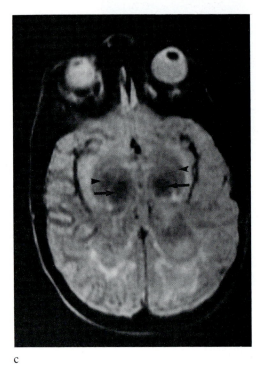

c

Figure 7.51

Abnormal iron deposition in the basal ganglia following ischemic-anoxic injury. Five-year-old boy had suffered severe anoxia as a result of traumatic birth. (a) Transaxial section through the lateral ventricles demonstrates periventricular hyperintensity (arrows) consistent with periventricular leukomalacia (SE 2000/84). (b) Lower transaxial section through the globus pallidus demonstrates abnormal low signal bilaterally (arrows), secondary to presumed iron deposition (SE 2000/84). (c) Transaxial section through pulvinar of thalami demonstrates short T_2, low-signal intensity in thalami medially (arrows) and inferior portions of globus pallidus laterally (arrowheads).

8

Hydrocephalus

William G Bradley

Introduction

From its Greek origin, 'hydrocephalus' literally means 'water on the brain'. By convention, the term usually refers to the water (CSF) which is within enlarged ventricles, although in the entity 'benign external hydrocephalus',[1] the child's head is enlarged primarily due to CSF outside the ventricles in the expanded subarachnoid space (although this has also been called 'benign subdural effusions'). Refinements in the usual nomenclature of hydrocephalus depend on the specific mechanism of ventricular enlargement. To most, the term hydrocephalus suggests a mechanism of elevated intraventricular pressure while the term atrophy implies ventricular enlargement through a loss of brain substance. An outmoded term for atrophy, 'hydrocephalus *ex vacuo*', illustrates the historical confusion in differentiating these entities.[2]

Hydrocephalus can be further divided on the basis of two possible mechanisms for elevation of the intraventricular pressure.[2,3] These mechanisms are (1) increased production of CSF and (2) decreased uptake (which results from obstruction of the normal outflow and reabsorption pathways for CSF). Increased production is much less common than obstruction and is due to a fairly rare intraventricular tumor, the choroid plexus papilloma. Obstructive forms of hydrocephalus can be further divided on the basis of the exact location of the obstruction. Blockage of flow can occur anywhere from the site of CSF production in the choroid plexus to the site of drainage into the arachnoid villi and ultimately the venous system. Common sites of obstruction include the foramen of Monro, illustrated in Figure 8.1, the aqueduct of Sylvius, the fourth

ventricular outlets, the basal cisterns, and the arachnoid villi. Obstruction proximal to the outlet foramina of the fourth ventricle is designated 'internal obstructive', 'intraventricular', or 'non-communicating' hydrocephalus. Obstruction distal to the foramina of Luschka and Magendie is termed 'communicating' or 'extraventricular' hydrocephalus. Since obstruction at a particular point usually causes only proximal dilatation, the site of obstruction can usually be inferred on either CT or MRI by the pattern of ventricular enlargement. Difficulties may arise, however, in differentiating aqueductal obstruction from communicating hydrocephalus, since the fourth ventricle may only enlarge minimally in the latter condition. It is also difficult to distinguish obstruction of the outlet foramina of the fourth ventricle (which is technically internal obstructive hydrocephalus) from communicating hydrocephalus, since both result in enlargement of the entire ventricular system. In such cases, nuclear cisternography may be useful in making this differentiation by demonstration of ventricular reflux in the communicating form.[4]

In benign external hydrocephalus, the increased pressure due to mild communicating hydrocephalus both increases ventricular size and increases the accumulation of fluid over the convexities in the subarachnoid space, shown in Figure 8.2 in a six-month-old child. Since the sutures can separate in this age group, the extra-axial space represents an additional site of CSF accumulation.[1]

Atrophy is generally distinguishable from hydrocephalus by either CT or MRI on the basis of associated enlargement of the cortical sulci. When both are enlarged, ventricular enlargement 'out of

265

proportion' to sulcal enlargement is considered indicative of hydrocephalus. This distribution is certainly true for diffuse causes of atrophy. However, diseases which primarily lead to 'central atrophy' (such as advanced multiple sclerosis or deep white matter infarction) may mimic hydrocephalus, particularly on CT. The relatively greater sensitivity of MRI to the presence of interstitial edema and periventricular parenchymal disease[3] generally allows central atrophy and hydrocephalus to be differentiated.[5]

Interstitial edema

Despite obstruction to CSF resorption, the choroid plexus continues to produce CSF, resulting in increased intraventricular pressure. When this occurs, CSF may be forced through gaps in the ependymal lining of the ventricles to be resorbed in the periventricular tissues.[6] Transependymal resorption of CSF is recognized on T_2-weighted MR images as a smooth border of increased intensity (Figure 8.1.) When associated with hydrocephalus, this is known as "interstitial edema" to distinguish it from the more common 'vasogenic' edema which is produced by blood-brain barrier breakdown.[6] While a smooth border of low attenuation may be appreciated on CT in advanced cases of hydrocephalus, mild to moderately T_2-weighted MR images are much more sensitive to the presence of interstitial edema in early cases.[5] This is due to the partial volume effects on CT which limit the differentiation of the low attenuation CSF from the low attenuation periventricular edema. On long TR/ intermediate TE, mild to moderately T_2-weighted MR images, the CSF is either hypointense or isointense with brain and edema is more intense than either.[5]

The increased intensity of CSF in the form of interstitial edema compared to that of intraventricular CSF reflects a change in the molecular environment of the CSF.[7] In the ventricles, CSF is essentially pure water. As such, it has a long T_1 relaxation time, reflecting the predominance of high natural motional frequencies of small water molecules in the bulk phase compared to the operating (Larmor) frequency of the MR imager. When forced into the periventricular tissues, the rapid motions of the CSF water molecules are slowed by attraction to the charged (hydrophilic) side groups of the myelin protein. This increases the component of motion in the hydration layer [8] water phase near the Larmor frequency, making T_1 relaxation more efficient. This in turn shortens the T_1 relaxation time and increases the intensity of the edema relative to CSF (which is bulk-phase water).[8] Since the long T_2 of the CSF water is only minimally decreased in its new periventricular environment, the interstitial edema has higher signal intensity than either the intraventricular CSF or the surrounding brain on mild to moderately T_2-weighted images, as in Figure 8.1a.

When the ventricles become dilated and are surrounded by a smooth border of high intensity, interstitial edema can be diagnosed. There are several other causes of smooth periventricular hyperintensity which can potentially be confused with interstitial edema. High signal is normally seen anterior to the frontal horns at the 'storm angles' of the lateral ventricles, shown in Figure 8.3. This has been called 'ependymitis granularis' and is a normal finding in patients over 40. The normally thin ependyma in this region allows more CSF to seep into the periventricular white matter. This tends to be symmetric and should not be confused with either early interstitial edema or focal processes such as multiple sclerosis or deep white matter infarction.

Linear high signal is normally present along the roofs of the lateral ventricles, illustrated in Figure 8.4. This represents the gray matter in the bodies of the caudate nuclei. While these can potentially be confused with interstitial edema (particularly if the ventricles are also enlarged), gray matter is not as bright as edema on more T_2-weighted images.

As the intraventricular pressure rises, interstitial edema and the smooth periventricular border are formed rapidly. In chronic obstruction (such as congenital aqueductal stenosis),. the ventricles continue to dilate and the pressure decreases to normal or near normal levels. Eventually, the smooth periventricular border of increased intensity is no longer seen, as in Figure 8.5, and the hydrocephalus is said to be 'compensated'. 'Partial' compensation can also be appreciated in chronic forms of hydrocephalus in which the thickness of the smooth periventricular border is decreased relative to the degree of ventricular enlargement, as shown in Figure 8.6. MRI is definitely superior to CT in the evaluation of partial or complete compensation, since the latter shows only enlarged ventricles. Clinically, of course, patients with elevated intraventricular pressure can usually be distinguished from those who are compensated on the basis of clinical findings, that is, papilledema, headaches, nausea, and vomiting. In certain cases, however, the clinical picture can be confusing and the MR finding of interstitial edema can be useful in the selection of patients for ventricular shunting.

While elevated intraventricular pressure always produces a smooth border of increased intensity on T_2-weighted images, the converse is, unfortunately, not true. A smooth border can also be seen in several conditions in which the intraventricular pressure is normal. If the obstruction goes untreated for a period of several weeks, the interstitial edema leaches out the lipid in the myelin and increases the relative water content of the periventricular tissues.[6] Thus, as Figures 8.7 and 8.8 illustrate, the smooth border of high intensity does not resolve immediately after ventricular shunting. Exactly how rapidly the periventricular signal returns to normal depends on how quickly the paracentral white matter is remyelinated. This probably depends on a number of factors, including the duration and severity of obstruction and the age of the patient. Younger patients appear to remyelinate more rapidly after obstruction. Thus, persistence of the smooth periventricular border on T_2-weighted images after shunting should not be considered synonymous with shunt malfunction.

Smooth periventricular hyperintensity may be totally unrelated to ventricular obstruction. Whenever there is blood-brain barrier breakdown and vasogenic edema is produced in the cerebral hemispheres, it tends to track centrally where it spreads out around the ependyma, eventually to be reabsorbed by the ventricles.[9] Thus, any cause of edema can produce a smooth border of increased intensity without ventricular obstruction. This includes primary or metastatic tumors (Figure 8.9), inflammation, demyelination, contusion (Figure 8.10), or infarction (Figure 8.11). Heterotopic gray matter can also give a periventricular border of high signal, although this is generally not as smooth as interstitial edema (Figure 8.12). If the ventricles are not enlarged in such cases, it should not be difficult to distinguish these causes of periventricular increased signal from interstitial edema. When atrophy is also present, however, it may be difficult to distinguish interstitial edema from centrally-tracking vasogenic edema (Figure 8.13).

Obstructive hydrocephalus

The ventricles can be obstructed anywhere from the foramen of Monro to the outlet foramina of the fourth ventricle, producing internal obstructive hydrocephalus.[2,3] Masses involving the anterior third ventricle can obstruct the foramen of Monro. These include gliomas, meningiomas, and other neoplasms arising from adjacent structures (Figure 8.1). Colloid (Figure 8.14) and cysticercotic cysts (Figure 8.15) can also obstruct the foramen of Monro. Cysticercotic cysts tend to be isointense with CSF (Figure 8.15),[10] while colloid cysts are more variable and can have signal greater than or less than CSF (Figure 8.14). Unilateral enlargement of a lateral ventricle with interstitial edema may be due to a small tumor obstructing one of the foramina of Monro, or to 'trapping' of the lateral ventricle by midline shift due to a large mass or extra-axial fluid collection (Figure 8.16). Unilateral enlargement of a lateral ventricle without associated interstitial edema is most often the result of benign constriction of the foramen.[2] In such congenital cases, the entire ventricular body is generally dilated, the septum pellucidum is bowed away from the site of obstruction and no lesion is evident near the foramen of Monro.

While most causes of obstruction near the foramen of Monro are of insidious onset, obstruction can also occur acutely, often with disastrous results. Acute obstruction due to migration of a cysticercotic cyst or positional change of a colloid cyst can lead to death.[11]

Obstruction of the aqueduct of Sylvius can be due to congenital, inflammatory, or neoplastic causes. Congenital aqueductal stenosis is associated with many other abnormalities including Chiari II malformation and dysgenesis of the corpus callosum.[12] Aqueductal stenosis can be subdivided into several forms including atresia, webs, and fenestration.[13] Although contrast will pass from the third ventricle into the fourth ventricle in such cases, the impedance to normal CSF flow is increased and the ventricles dilate as a result. Such patients (particularly young women) may remain compensated in childhood and not become symptomatic until CSF production increases during adolescence.[3]

Inflammatory lesions of the aqueduct can arise within the aqueduct proper or in the periaqueductal tissues (Figure 8.17). Cysticercotic cysts can migrate through the aqueduct producing acute obstruction.[11] Demyelinating plaques and brainstem encephalitis can inflame the periaqueductal tissues, leading to aqueductal obstruction.

In adults, the most common cause of acquired aqueductal obstruction is neoplasia.[14] Brainstem tumors, particularly gliomas involving the tectum of the midbrain, are a common cause of obstruction. Pineal region tumors, illustrated in Figure 8.18, may also cause obstruction because they eventually grow forward, compressing the tectum and the aqueduct.

Magnetic resonance imaging is superior to CT in the evaluation of aqueductal obstruction for several reasons. The ability to acquire thin slices directly in the sagittal plane is useful in the evaluation of aqueductal patency and periaqueductal masses. The high contrast between CSF in the aqueduct on heavily T_1- or T_2-weighted images facilitates this analysis by MRI. Moderately T_2-weighted axial MR images are also more sensitive than axial CT studies in the detection of small midbrain masses which may compress the aqueduct. The high contrast between the low-intensity flowing CSF in the aqueduct and the surrounding midbrain on thin-slice, heavily T_2-weighted images is a useful sign of aqueductal patency.[15–17] Single-slice GRASS images are also sensitive in the demonstration of aqueductal patency due to marked flow-related enhancement.[18] These signs are lost with aqueductal obstruction (but not with obstruction distal to the aqueduct).

Like obstruction elsewhere, blockage of the fourth ventricle can be congenital, inflammatory, or neoplastic. Congenital obstruction of the foramina of Luschka and Magendie results in marked enlargement of the fourth ventricle and is postulated as the cause of the Dandy Walker malformation.[19] When the outlet foramina of the fourth ventricle are obstructed after birth (for example, by ventriculitis), the fourth ventricle enlarges. In some cases, the fourth ventricle may become obstructed above and below, that is, at the level of the aqueduct as well as at the foramina of Luschka and Magendie. In such cases of 'isolated fourth ventricle', shunts must be placed in the lateral ventricles and in the fourth ventricle for proper decompression.[20] Cysticercosis can also produce inflammatory obstruction of the fourth ventricle.[10]

Tumors encroaching upon the fourth ventricle can lead to obstruction.[2] In children, these are most commonly medulloblastomas (arising from the posterior medullary velum) and cystic astrocytomas (arising in the cerebellum). Figure 8.19 shows an example of the latter case. Gliomas of the brainstem can grow posteriorly to occlude the fourth ventricle. Cerebellar tumors are less common in adults and include astrocytomas, ependymomas, and metastases. Hemgioblastomas are slowly growing vascular tumors of the cerebellum which can obtain large size before causing obstruction. Epidermoids can be located within the fourth ventricle and may also grow to a large size with minimal obstruction. Extra-axial tumors such as meningiomas and acoustic neuromas can attain a size sufficient to obstruct the fourth ventricle, as demonstrated in Figure 8.20.

Communicating hydrocephalus

Obstruction distal to the outlet foramina of the fourth ventricle produces 'extraventricular obstructive' or 'communicating' hydrocephalus, in which the ventricles (including the fourth) are all enlarged. Obstruction can occur at any point between the subarachnoid cisterns surrounding the brainstem at the skull base to the arachnoid villi at the vertex.

Causes of obstruction in the basal cisterns include carcinomatous (Figure 8.21) and infectious meningitis.[21] The inflammation and granulomatous reaction in the basal meninges produced by leptomeningeal carcinomatosis or by fungal or granulomatous meningitis may show enhancement following administration of Gd-DTPA.[22] In the basilar racemose form of cysticercosis, large cysts may be seen in the basal cisterns.[10,11]

If the CSF is able to flow through the basal cisterns to reach the cortical convexities, the next site of

potential obstruction is at the arachnoid villi. These parasagittal structures are located off-midline on both sides of the superior sagittal sinus. The arachnoid villi are normally responsible for the uptake of CSF, which is drained into the venous system via the superior sagittal sinus. The most common cause of obstruction of the arachnoid villi is subarachnoid hemorrhage following trauma (Figure 8.22), rupture of an aneurysm, or bleeding from an arteriovenous malformation. In such cases, obstruction tends to be acute due to the irritative affects of blood (producing a chemical meningitis) and due to physical obstruction of the arachnoid villi by red cells. Purulent meningitis (due to streptococci, staphylococci, and meningococci in adults and *Hemophilus influenza* and *E. coli* in children) may cause acute hydrocephalus through a high convexity block.[21] Carcinomatous meningitis produces a more insidious course of hydrocephalus.[21] In adults this is often due to an extracranial malignancy (such as breast carcinoma) while in children it is most often due to an intracranial malignancy (such as subarachnoid seeding of medulloblastoma). Myeloproliferative disorders such as leukemia and lymphoma may involve the meninges and cause communicating hydrocephalus.

Thrombosis of the cortical veins or the dural sinuses may produce hydrocephalus by impeding the drainage of CSF from the arachnoid villi. An older term 'otic hydrocephalus' reflects the ventricular enlargement which results from thrombosis of the sigmoid sinus in patients with destructive mastoiditis. In the past, dural sinus thrombosis has been diagnosed by angiography or by CT with bolus injection of contrast. Unfortunately, both of these techniques involve injection of hypertonic contrast in patients who may already be hypercoagulable. This may result in worsening of their clinical condition. For this reason, MRI has been advocated as the primary diagnostic imaging modality in the evaluation of patients with suspected dural sinus thrombosis,[23] although markedly slowed flow may mimic complete obstruction. In such cases, radionuclide angiography and blood pool imaging may be a more reliable indicator of dural sinus patency.

Normal pressure hydrocephalus

There is a chronic form of communicating hydrocephalus which has attracted much clinical attention and been the source of heated debate. The entity, known as 'normal pressure hydrocephalus' (NPH), is touted by its supporters as one of the few treatable causes of ataxia and dementia.[24,25] Its detractors, on the other hand, point to poor clinical results and have even questioned its existence.[26,27]

The term 'normal pressure hydrocephalus' is at first glance a misnomer. How can the ventricles be enlarged and the pressure still be 'normal'? Furthermore, why is ventricular shunting the treatment for NPH if the pressure is, in fact, normal?

Normal pressure hydrocephalus was first described in 1964 by Hakim and Adams in patients aged between 50 and 70, presenting with a clinical triad of gait disturbance, dementia, and urinary incontinence.[24,25] In properly selected patients, ventricular shunting may result in resolution of symptoms and slowing of an otherwise progressive deterioration. Radiologic diagnosis in the past has been based on the CT finding of ventricular dilatation out of proportion to cortical sulcal enlargement, that is, a pattern which is otherwise indistinguishable from other causes of communicating hydrocephalus or central atrophy. Nuclear cisternography in patients with NPH demonstrates ventricular reflux with slow convexity uptake of radionuclide.[4] While cisternography demonstrates alteration of CSF resorption pathways, it fails to demonstrate central parenchymal abnormalities (that is, deep white matter infarction) which may also result in ventricular enlargement and, in fact, may produce a similar symptom complex.

In the past, the patients who have had the best response to shunting have been those with a known cause of their chronic communicating hydrocephalus, such as subarachnoid hemorrhage or meningitis. Those patients in whom NPH is 'idiopathic' seem to have a less favorable response to ventricular shunting.[27]

Magnetic resonance imaging is useful in the selection of patients who are being considered for shunting for NPH. As with CT, the enlargement of the ventricles out of proportion to the cortical sulci can be visualized by MRI, as demonstrated in Figure 8.23. In addition, direct sagittal acquisition in patients with NPH (or any other form of communicating hydrocephalus) demonstrates upward bowing of the corpus callosum,[28] and flattening of the gyri against the inner table of the calvarium, shown in Figure 8.23b, which is more difficult to appreciate by CT. The loss of signal from the CSF flowing rapidly through the aqueduct ('CSF flow void sign') can also not be appreciated on CT.

Magnetic resonance imaging is sensitive to any interstitial edema which may be present and may indicate elevated intraventricular pressure. Generally, the interstitial edema is minimal to absent in such patients because of compensation and return of intraventricular pressure to 'normal'. While the mean intraventricular pressure is often normal in such patients, the pulse pressure may be six to eight times normal.[29] According to one theory,[30] it is this 'waterhammer' effect on the paracentral fibers which produces the symptoms of NPH. The objective of ventricular shunting is not to lower the mean pressure, but rather to dampen the pulse pressure by providing additional capacitance to the ventricular system.

In a recent study,[31] the magnitude of the CSF flow void was correlated with the response to ventricular shunting in 20 patients. Those who had a 'good' or 'excellent' response had marked loss of signal in the aqueduct and fourth ventricle. Those with a 'fair' or 'poor' response had minimal loss of signal. The results were quite significant ($P<.002$).[31] While deep white matter infarction and NPH have always been considered two separate diseases, in fact they may occur together more often than they occur separately,[32] suggesting a causal relationship, as shown in Figures 8.24 and 8.25. Deep white matter infarction may produce periventricular gliosis which decreases ventricular compliance. Decreased compliance and the resulting waterhammer pulse may cause ventricular enlargement and NPH.

Recent MR findings provide a basis for speculation of a relationship. Many infarcts previously considered bland by CT criteria, in fact, can be shown to be mildly hemorrhagic, probably reflecting small petechial bleeds (see Chapter 7). Should deep white matter infarcts be associated with mild hemorrhage and should the hemorrhage be able to enter the subarachnoid space via the Virchow-Robin spaces, then there would be a basis for communicating hydrocephalus. That all patients with deep white matter infarction do not develop communicating hydrocephalus may reflect variation in the handling of small subarachnoid bleeds by the arachnoid villi, or possibly, variations in the amount of bleeding at the time of infarction.

Regardless of the mechanisms, NPH and deep white matter infarction appear to be associated. Therefore, the presence of deep white matter infarction should not serve to discourage shunting of patients with prominent flow voids, as in Figure 8.25. The lack of a flow void, however, should discourage shunting of patients with presumed NPH as it would appear that the cause for CSF motion, ie, cerebral perfusion, has already decreased.

Atrophy

Atrophy is a pathologic diagnosis indicating an irreversible loss of brain substance. When atrophy is truly present, the ventricles and cortical sulci are prominent on either CT or MRI, as shown in Figure 8.26. Unfortunately, the converse may not be true, that is, the finding of enlarged ventricles on CT or MRI is not diagnostic of atrophy. Certain disease processes can mimic atrophy on the initial CT or MRI and yet, following treatment, the brain will return to a normal appearance. These include alcoholism,[32,33] starvation, anorexia nervosa,[34] and catabolic steroids.[35,36] Thus an attempt to form a definitive diagnosis of atrophy using only CT or MRI can lead to errors in these patients. It is also incorrect to equate the MR or CT finding of prominent ventricles and sulci with the clinical diagnosis of dementia.[37] Studies attempting correlation of dementia with ventricular size, brain volume, or other morphometric indices have been unsuccessful. Magnetic resonance imaging is performed on demented patients not to diagnose atrophy per se but to detect treatable causes of dementia such as hydrocephalus, subdural hematomas, or intracranial masses. At this time, Alzheimer's disease remains a diagnosis of exclusion by CT or MRI, although the finding of subcortical iron deposition may permit a more specific diagnosis of Alzheimer's by MRI in the future.[38]

Atrophy can result from multiple different insults which all lead to loss of brain parenchyma.[2] These processes include infarction, inflammation, demyelination, and hypoxia as well as certain insults which should be apparent by clinical history, such as trauma, radiation therapy, chemotherapy, or alcoholism.

The form of atrophy which is most likely to be confused with hydrocephalus on CT is that due to deep white matter infarction.[39,40] While CT is relatively insensitive to the presence of these periventricular, low-attenuation lesions (due to partial-volume averaging of the adjacent low-attenuation CSF), MRI is quite sensitive in the detection of these lesions.[39] On moderately T_2-weighted images,[41] in which the CSF and brain are isointense, such lesions stand out with positive contrast against a bland, relatively featureless background, as demonstrated in Figure 8.27b.

Clinically, it may also be difficult to distinguish deep white matter infarction from NPH. Both entities may present with dementia, gait disturbance, and incontinence. While classically described multi-infarct dementia has a stepwise progressive clinical course (as opposed to the more insidious onset of dementia in NPH), in practice, the two states may be difficult to distinguish. The similarity of resultant clinical symptoms is not surprising considering that both processes involve the same paracentral white matter tracts, either by vaso-occlusive disease or by 'barotrauma' from the 'waterhammer' pulsations of the intraventricular CSF in NPH. Presumably, it is the additional factor of decreasing cerebral perfusion to the deep white matter which explains why NPH is primarily a disease of the elderly.

Intracranial CSF motion in normal and hydrocephalic states

The signal intensity of CSF is variable throughout the ventricular system.[15–17] As discussed in Chapter 3,

signal loss can result from time-of-flight effects, turbulence, or dephasing. Time-of-flight effects are increased on thinner slices and on more heavily T_2-weighted (longer TE) images.[42] First-echo dephasing increases as the strength of the gradients increases (generally with thinner slices and higher spatial resolution) and as the velocity increases.[43,44] Turbulence is less commonly seen in CSF flow than in arterial flow, but can be observed in the upper portion of the fourth ventricle as the stream expands after coming through the narrow aqueduct, as in Figure 8.28.[45] Both high velocity and turbulence result in normal signal loss of the CSF in the foramen of Monro (Figure 8.29),[15–17] and in the aqueduct (Figure 8.30). At this point, it is useful to review the mechanisms responsible for CSF motion.

CSF is produced at a rate of approximately 500 ml/day, primarily in the choroid plexus of the lateral and third ventricles.[46] The bulk flow of CSF results in net movement from the choroid plexus within the ventricles to the arachnoid villi over the convexities. MR pixel intensity reflects the velocity of CSF at the moment of signal acquisition.[15] This velocity is expected to be greatest through the narrowest portion of the ventricular system, that is, through the aqueduct. This is due to the Bernoulli principle: for constant volumetric flow (in cc/sec), tubes with smaller cross-sectional areas have higher linear velocities (in cm/sec) than those with larger cross-sectional areas.[47]

Superimposed on the slow egress of CSF from the ventricles is a pulsatile motion due to transmitted cardiac pulsations.[48–50] This to-and-fro movement of CSF appears to reflect generalized systolic cerebral expansion,[49,50] expansion of the choroid plexus during cardiac systole,[30] and transmitted pulsations of the large arteries at the base of the brain. The velocity of CSF flowing through the aqueduct depends to a much greater degree on cardiac pulsations than on the rate of production of CSF.

In one study, the aqueductal CSF flow void was evaluated retrospectively in 60 subjects,[15] including normal volunteers, patients with acute and chronic communicating hydrocephalus, and patients with atrophy. The intensity of the CSF in the lateral ventricles and aqueduct was measured on mildly T_2-weighted axial images. The intensity of the CSF in the aqueduct was always lower than that in the lateral ventricles, reflecting the greater velocity through the aqueduct. In patients with chronic communicating hydrocephalus, the signal intensity in the aqueduct was decreased to an even greater degree compared to normals and compared to patients with acute communicating hydrocephalus or atrophy.[15] These data are summarized in Figure 3.50, page 107. The aqueductal CSF flow void sign is most marked in patients with chronic communicating hydrocephalus, whether or not they have clinical NPH. In such hyperdynamic CSF flow states, the flow void is seen in the adjacent enlarged third and fourth ventricles as well, as in Figures 8.25 and 8.31. The CSF flow void in chronic communicating hydrocephalus is typically more marked on high bandwidth, high field (Figure 8.31) than on low bandwidth, midfield (Figure 8.32) MR imagers due to the stronger gradients in the former. However, the CSF flow void may be quite marked on high bandwidth midfield units as shown in Figure 8.33. As discussed in Chapter 3, the same motion which produces a flow void on an inner slice can cause increased signal on an entry slice (due to flow-related enhancement), simulating a mass, as illustrated in Figure 8.32.

Postulated determinants of aqueductal CSF flow

While the above observations document a hyperdynamic CSF flow state in various disease states, the mechanism for such flow has not been specifically addressed. In an attempt to understand the mechanisms responsible for the hyperdynamic CSF flow state, a simple conceptual model was constructed.[51] Very simply, the brain is considered to be a balloon with another balloon inside (the ventricles). When the pressure inside either balloon increases, its volume increases proportionately. The proportionality constant is the 'capacitance'. The brain is further considered to be surrounded by CSF which can enter or leave the closed, rigid space of the cranial vault through the foramen magnum. When only the supratentorial compartment is considered, CSF can enter or leave through the aqueduct or the perimesencephalic cisterns. Arterial blood entering the brain increases its volume and venous blood exiting the brain decreases its volume. The brain, blood, and CSF are considered to be non-compressible liquids. When arterial blood enters the brain, venous blood or CSF have to be vented simultaneously or the intracranial pressure will rise, or a combination of both will occur, as shown in Figures 8.34 and 8.35.

In this simple conceptual model of the brain, the factors which seemed responsible for aqueductal CSF flow were varied. These included resistance to CSF flow through the aqueduct, resistance to flow through the perimesencephalic cistern, and resistance to venous outflow. To perform a semiquantitative analysis, the mechanical properties of a balloon were considered equivalent to the properties of an electrical circuit, as characterized by Ohm's law. In this analogy, the volume in the balloon is considered equivalent to electrical current, the driving force for expansion (the pressure) is considered equivalent to the driving force for current (the voltage), and the constant of proportionality is considered to be the resistance. For a simple sinusoidal arterial pulse wave, these assumptions in the electrical analog model lead to a relatively simple set of equations, which can be solved by use of a personal computer.

The results of the computer analysis indicated that aqueductal diameter was the single greatest determinant of the hyperdynamic CSF flow state. Increasing aqueductal diameter decreases the resistance to flow and increases the volume of the CSF pulsing back and forth during the cardiac cycle. Resistance to CSF flow through the aqueduct is actually proportional to the fourth power of the inverse of the radius, this means there is a marked increase in aqueductal flow for a relatively small increase in aqueductal diameter. The cause of aqueductal dilatation in most of our cases is communicating hydrocephalus, which increases the size of all of the ventricles as well as the aqueduct. On the other hand, increased CSF flow has also been documented in the aqueduct in patients with brainstem atrophy. If the perimesencephalic cisterns are blocked after arterial inflow to the supratentorial brain, then systolic outflow through the aqueduct must necessarily increase.

When the resistance to venous outflow from the supratentorial space is increased, this too increases outflow through the aqueduct. After normal arterial inflow, there is a phase lag as the blood passes through the capillaries of the brain and into the veins for drainage. As a result, the brain swells during systole and CSF is forced out of the supratentorial space through both the aqueduct and the perimesencephalic cistern. This primary cause of aqueductal CSF flow has been documented recently by cine MR techniques.[18] When the resistance to venous outflow increases (for example, secondary to sclerosis of cortical veins following meningitis or hemorrhage), the phase delay between arterial inflow and venous drainage increases, as does the requisite outflow of CSF through the aqueduct. While it is difficult to find clinical examples of sclerosis of cortical veins distinct from obstruction of the arachnoid villi due to communicating hydrocephalus, both factors may be operative in the setting of communicating hydrocephalus leading to increased aqueductal CSF flow.

References

1 KENDALL B, HOLLAND I, Benign communicating hydrocephalus in children, *Neuroradiology* (1981) **21**:93–6.

2 TerBRUGGE KG, RAO KCVG, LEE SH, Hydrocephalus and atrophy. In: Lee SH, Rao KCVG, eds. *Cranial computed tomography and MRI.* (McGraw-Hill: New York 1987) Chapter 5.

3   HAUGHTON VM, Hydrocephalus and atrophy. In: Williams AL, Haughton VM, eds. *Cranial computed tomography a comprehensive text.* (CV Mosby and Co: St Louis 1985) Chapter 6.

4   TATOR CH, FLEMING JFR, SHEPARD RD et al, A radioscopic test for communicating hydrocephalus, *J Neurosurg* (1968) **28**:327–40.

5   BRADLEY WG, Magnetic resonance imaging of the central nervous system, *Neurol Res* (1984) **6**:91–106.

6   FISHMAN RA, Brain edema, *N Engl J Med* (1975) **293**:706.

7   BRADLEY WG, Magnetic resonance imaging in the central nervous system: comparison to computed tomography. In: Kressel HY, ed. *Magnetic resonance annual.* (Raven Press: New York 1985).

8   FULLERTON GD, CAMERON IL, ORD VA, Frequency dependence of magnetic resonance spin-lattice relaxation of protons in biological materials, *Radiology* (1984) **151**:135–8.

9   ZIMMERMAN RD, FLEMING CA, LEE BCP et al, Periventricular hyperintensity as seen by magnetic resonance: prevalence and significance, *AJNR* (1986) **7**(1):13–20.

10 TEITELBAUM GP, OTTO RJ, LINN MCW et al, MR imaging of neurocysticercosis *AJNR* (in press).

11 ZEE CS, SEGALL HD, APUZZO MLJ, Intraventricular cysticercal cysts: further neuroradiologic observations and neurosurgical implications, *AJNR* (1984) **5**:727.

12 FITZ CR, The ventricles and subarachnoid spaces in children. In: Lee SH, Rao KCVG, eds. *Cranial computed tomography and MRI.* (McGraw-Hill: New York 1987) 266–72.

13 MCMILLAN JJ, WILLIAMS B, Aqueduct stenosis, *J Neurol Neurosurg Psychiatry* (1977) **40**:521–32.

14 RUSSEL DS, RUBINSTEIN LJ, eds, *Pathology of tumours of the nervous system,* (Edward Arnold: London 1963).

15 BRADLEY WG, KORTMAN KE, BURGOYNE B, Flowing cerebrospinal fluid in normal and hydrocephalic states: appearance on MR images, *Radiology* (1986) **159**:611–16.

16 CITRIN CM, SHERMAN JL, GANGAROSA RE et al, Physiology of the CSF flow-void sign: modification by cardiac gating, *AJNR* (1986) **7**:1021–4.

17 SHERMAN JL, CITRIN CM, Magnetic resonance demonstration of normal CSF flow, *AJNR* (1986) **7**:3–6.

18 ATLAS SW, MARK AS, FRAM EK, Aqueductal stenosis: evaluation with gradient-echo rapid MR imaging, *Radiology* (1988) **169**:449–56.

19 RAO KCVG, HARWOOD-NASH DC, Craniocerebral anomalies. In: Lee SH, Rao KCVG, eds. *Cranial computed tomography and MRI.* (McGraw-Hill: New York 1987) 178–82.

20 ZIMMERMAN RA, BILANIUK LA, GALLO E, Computed tomography of the trapped fourth ventricle, *AJR* (1978) **130**:503–6.

21 WILLIAMS AL, Infectious disease. In: Williams AL, Haughton VM, eds. *Cranial computed tomography a comprehensive text.* (CV Mosby and Co: St Louis 1985) 288–300.

22 FRANK JA, GIRTON ME, DWYER AJ et al, Meningeal carcinomatosis in the VX2 rabbit tumor model: detection with Gd-DTPA-enhanced MR imaging, *Radiology* (1988) **167**:825–30.

23 MCMURDO SK Jr, BRANT-ZAWADSKI M, BRADLEY WG et al, Dural sinus thrombosis: study using intermediate field strength MR imaging, *Radiology* (1986) **161**:83.

24 HAKIM S, Some observations on CSF pressure: hydrocephalic syndrome in adults with 'normal' CSF pressure, Thesis No 957, Javerian University, School of Medicine, Bogota, Colombia, 1964.

25 ADAMS RD, FISHER CM, HAKIM S et al, Symptomatic occult hydrocephalus with 'normal' cerebrospinal fluid pressure: a treatable syndrome, *N Engl J Med* (1965) **273**:117–26.

26 JACOBS L, CONTI D, KINKEL WR et al, Normal pressure hydrocephalus, *JAMA* (1976) **235**:510–12.

27 GREENBERG JO, SHENKIN HA, ADAM R, Idiopathic normal pressure hydrocephalus: a report of 73 patients, *J Neurol Neurosurg Psychiatry* (1977) **40**:336–41.

28 EL GAMMAL T, ALLEN MB Jr, BROOKS BS et al, MR evaluation of hydrocephalus, *AJNR* (1987) **8**:591.

29 EKSTEDT J, FRIDEN H, CSF hydrodynamics of the study of the adult hydrocephalus syndrome. In: Shapiro K, Marmarou A, Portnoy H, eds. *Hydrocephalus.* (Raven: New York 1984).

30 BERING BA Jr, Choroid plexus and arterial pulsations of cerebrospinal fluid: demonstration of the choroid plexus as a cerebrospinal fluid pump, *Arch Neurol Psychiatry* (1955) **73**:165–72.

31 BRADLEY WG, KORTMAN KE, WHITTEMORE AR, et al, The significance of the aqueductal CSF flow void as an indicator for favorable response to shunting of patients with suspected NPH, *Radiology* (submitted).

32 BRADLEY WG, Association of deep white matter infarction with chronic communicating hydrocephalus: implications regarding the possible etiology of NPH, presented at SMRM, Amsterdam, Aug 11-18, 1989.

33 CARLEN PL, WORTZMAN G, HOLGATE RC et al, Reversible cerebral atrophy in recently abstinent chronic alcoholics measured by computed tomography scans, *Science* (1987) **200**:1076–8.

34 ENZMANN DR, LANE B, Cranial computed tomography findings in anorexia nervosa, *J Comput Assist Tomogr* (1977) **1**:410–14.

35 HEINZ E, MARTINEX J, HAWNGGELI A, Reversibility of cerebral atrophy in anorexia nervosa and Cushing's syndrome, *J Comput Assist Tomogr* (1977) **1**:415–8.

36 BENTSON J, REZA M, WINTER J et al, Steroids and apparent cerebral atrophy on computed tomography scans, *J Comput Assist Tomogr* (1978) **2**:16–23.

37 FOX JK, KASZNIAK AW, HUCKMAN M, Computerized tomographic scanning not very helpful in dementia—nor in craniopharyngioma, *N Engl J Med* (1979) **300**:437.

38 DRAYER B, BURGER P, DARWIN R et al, Magnetic resonance imaging of brain iron, *AJNR* (1986) **7**:373–80.

39 BRADLEY WG, WALUCH V, BRANT-ZAWADSKI M et al, Patchy, periventricular white matter lesions in the elderly: a common observation during NMR imaging, *Noninvasive Med Imaging* (1984) **1**(1):35–41.

40 BRANT-ZAWADSKI M, FEIN G, VAN DYKE C et al, MR imaging of the aging brain: patchy white matter lesions and dementia, *AJNR* (1985) **6**(5):675–82.

41 BRADLEY WG, Fundamentals of MR image interpretation. In: Wong WS, Tsuruda JS, Kortman KE, Bradley WG, eds. *Practical MRI a case study approach.* (Aspen: Rockville MD 1986).

42 BRADLEY WG, WALUCH V, Blood flow: magnetic resonance imaging, *Radiology* (1985) **154**:443–50.

43 VALK PE, HALE JD, CROOKS LE et al, MRI of blood flow: correlation of image appearance with spin-echo phase shift and signal intensity, *AJR* (1981) **146**:931–9.

44 VAN SCHULTHESS GK, HIGGINS CB, Blood flow imaging with MR: spin-phase phenomena, *Radiology* (1985) **157**:687–95.

45 WHITE DN, WILSON KC, CURRY GR et al, The limitation of pulsatile flow through the aqueduct of Sylvius as a cause of hydrocephalus, *J Neurol Sci* (1979) **42**:11–51.

46 LORENZO AV, PAGE LK, WATTERS GV, Relationship betwen cerebrospinal fluid formation, absorption and pressure in human hydrocephalus, *Brain* (1970) **93**:679–92.

47 BIRD RB, STEWARD WE, LIGHTFOOT EN, *Transport phenomena*, (Wiley: New York 1960) 153–8.

48 LAITENEN L, Origin of arterial pulsation of cerebrospinal fluid, *Acta Neurol Scand* (1968) **44**:168–76.

49 DU BOULAY GH, Specialization broadens the view: the significance of CSF pulse, *Clin Radiol* (1972) **23**:401–9.

50 DU BOULAY GH, Pulsatile movements in the CSF pathways, *Br J Radiol* (1966) **39**:255–62.

51 BRADLEY WG, WHITTEMORE A, JINKINS JR et al, Cerebrospinal fluid flow patterns in hydrocephalus: correlation of clinical and phantom studies using MR imaging, *Radiology* (1987) **78**(**p**):165.

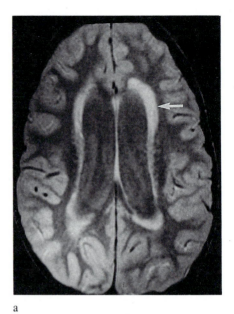

a

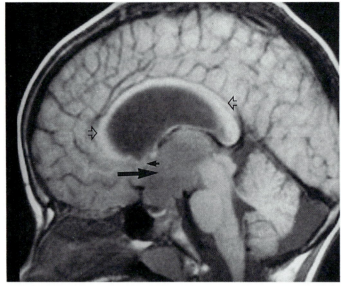

c

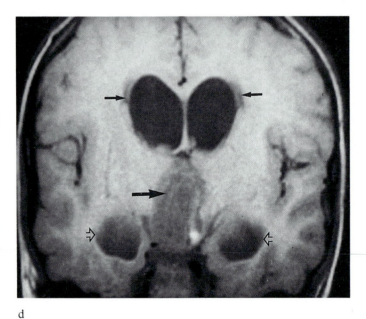

b

d

Figure 8.1

Obstructive hydrocephalus.
(**a**) Moderately T$_2$-weighted axial section through the lateral ventricles demonstrates smooth border of high-signal intensity (arrow) surrounding enlarged ventricles (SE 2800/30).
(**b**) Lower axial section through the third ventricle demonstrates smooth border of interstitial edema (large arrow). Interstitial edema tracks between the ependyma (smaller arrows) and the genu and splenium of the corpus callosum (curved arrows) which are darker (SE 2800/30). (**c**) T$_1$-weighted sagittal section demonstrates suprasellar-hypothalamic tumor (large arrow), obstructing foramen of Monro (arrowhead). Note upward bowing of corpus callosum (open arrows) due to enlargement of lateral ventricles (SE 600/20). (**d**) Coronal section demonstrates enlarged bodies of the lateral ventricles including the temporal horns (open arrows) due to large tumor (large arrow) obstructing the foramen of Monro. Note hypointense appearance of interstitial edema (small arrows) on T$_1$-weighted images (SE 800/20).

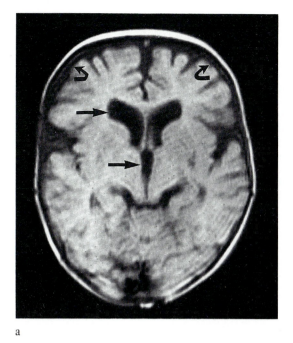

a

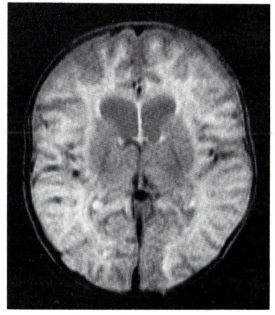

b

Figure 8.2

Benign external hydrocephalus. Six-month-old child presents with enlarged head. (**a**) T_1-weighted axial image demonstrates mild enlargement of the third and lateral ventricles (arrows) as well as small extra-axial fluid collection over the frontal convexities (curved arrows) (SE 500/30). (**b**) T_2-weighted image is less sensitive in demonstration of small frontal CSF collections. The high intensity of the white matter on this T_2-weighted image is normal in this age group due to the higher water content of the myelin (SE 2000/84). (Courtesy Rosalind Dietrich, MD, Los Angeles, CA.)

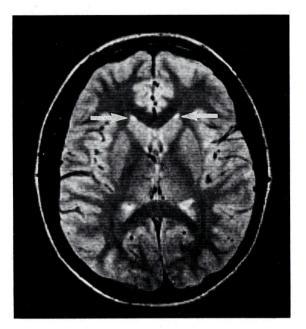

Figure 8.3

Ependymitis granularis. High signal is normally present anterior to the frontal horns of the lateral ventricles in patients over 40 years of age (arrows). This represents a more loosely integrated portion of the white matter with a higher water content and, therefore, increased signal intensity on T_2-weighted images. This region is known as the 'storm angles' by pathologists, since it is also the earliest area of CSF accumulation due to transependymal resorption in early obstructive hydrocephalus (SE 2000/40).

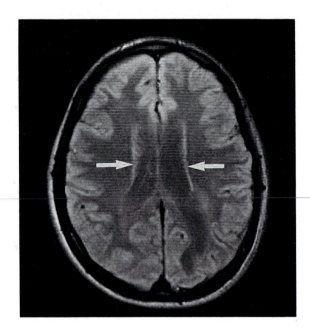

Figure 8.4

Caudate body simulating interstitial edema. High-signal intensity is noted along the superolateral margins of the lateral ventricles (arrows) which could conceivably be mistaken for the smooth border of interstitial edema due to obstructive hydrocephalus. This represents the gray matter in the body of the caudate nuclei and is a normal finding (SE 2000/30).

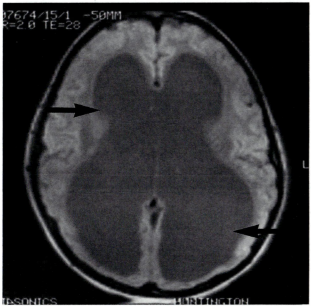

a

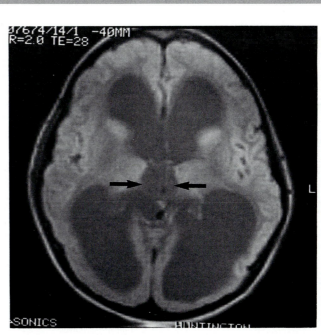

b

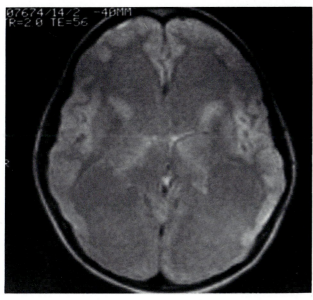

c

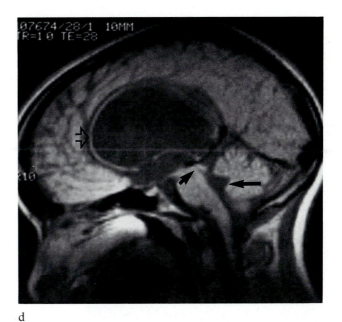

d

Figure 8.5

Compensated hydrocephalus. (a) Mildly T_2-weighted axial section through the lateral ventricles demonstrates ventricular enlargement (arrows) without evidence of interstitial edema (SE 2000/28). (b) Lower axial section demonstrates outward bowing of walls of the third ventricle (arrows) as well as dilated lateral ventricles. There is no evidence of surrounding border of high-signal intensity to indicate elevation of intraventricular pressure (SE 2000/28). (c) Moderately T_2-weighted axial section demonstrates isointensity between intraventricular CSF and surrounding white matter. Although this is the most sensitive technique for the detection of edema, there is no evidence of periventricular high intensity (SE 2000/56). (d) T_1-weighted sagittal section demonstrates upward bowing of the thinned corpus callosum (open arrow). The anticipated CSF flow void is not seen in the aqueduct (arrowhead) due to stenosis. Note the only minimally enlarged fourth ventricle (straight arrow) (SE 1000/28).

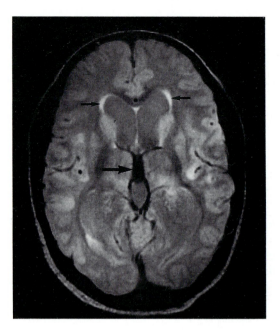

Figure 8.6

Partial compensation. Thin rim of high-signal intensity (small arrows) is noted surrounding frontal horns in this case of partially compensated communicating hydrocephalus. The ventricles are dilated to the same degree as noted in the case of more acute obstruction shown in Figure 8.1. Note presence of hyperdynamic flow state indicated by prominent CSF flow void in third ventricles (larger arrow) (SE 2500/30).

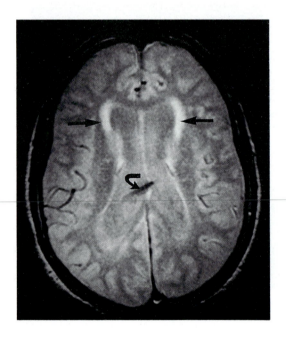

Figure 8.7

Persistence of 'edema' after ventricular shunting. Ventricles remain dilated with a smooth border of surrounding edema (arrows), despite presence of ventricular shunt tube (curved arrow) and absence of clinical signs of elevated intraventricular pressure. If the ventricles remain unshunted for as little as three weeks following elevation of intraventricular pressure, myelin lipids are leached out by the interstitial edema and are not immediately replaced upon successful shunting. The smooth border of high intensity will resolve more slowly as remyelination occurs (SE 2800/30).

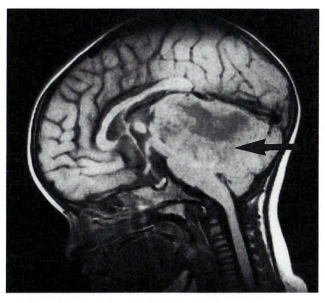

a

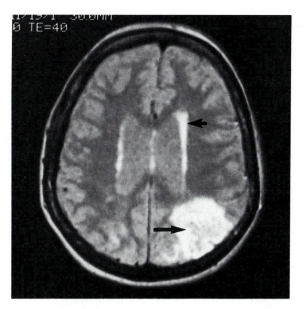

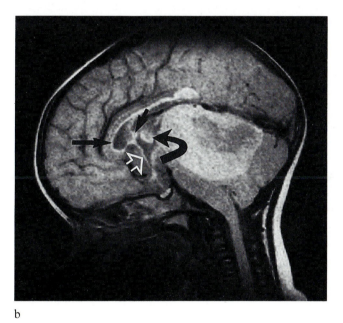

b

Figure 8.9

Edema from tumor simulating interstitial edema. Vasogenic edema tracking centrally from left temporo-occipital tumor (arrow) causes periventricular hyperintensity (arrowhead), greater on the side of the tumor than contralateral to it (SE 3000/40).

Figure 8.8

Persistence of interstitial edema despite ventricular shunting.
(a) Large cystic astrocytoma (arrow) noted in one-year-old girl with obvious compression of the fourth ventricle and aqueduct (SE 1000/40).
(b) Despite shunting and return of ventricles to normal size, interstitial edema remains between ependyma and corpus callosum (straight arrow). Edema also noted in anterior commissure (arrowhead), massa intermedia (curved arrow), and columns of fornix (open arrow) (SE 1000/80).

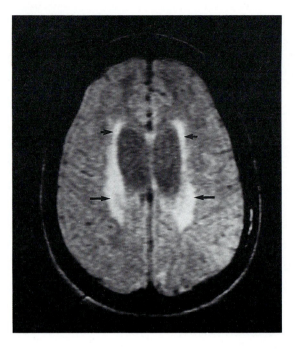

Figure 8.10

Edema from contusion simulating interstitial edema. After severe head trauma, periventricular hyperintensity is noted in this young man. The smooth border (arrowheads) represents centrally-tracking vasogenic edema following severe contusion. The focal high signal more posteriorly (arrows) represents shearing injury from the severe rotatory head trauma (SE 2550/60). (Courtesy Charles Seibert, MD, Denver, CO.)

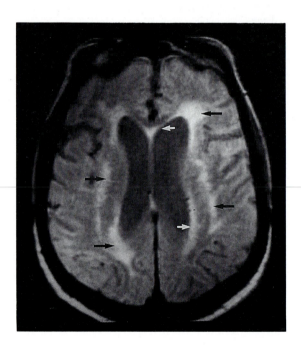

Figure 8.11

Edema from deep white matter infarction simulating interstitial edema. Vasogenic edema produced by deep white matter infarction (arrows) tracks centrally to simulate interstitial edema (arrowheads) (SE 2000/30).

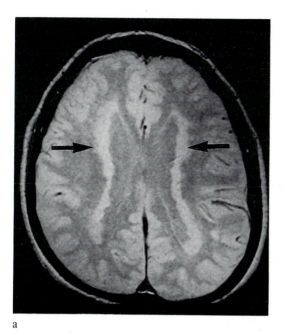

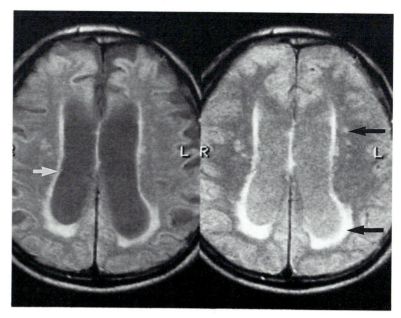

a

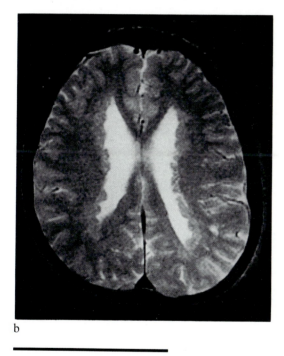

b

Figure 8.13

Atrophy and infarct edema simulating ventricular obstruction. Mildly T_2-weighted axial section (left image) demonstrates enlarged ventricles and cortical sulci due to diffuse cortical atrophy. Periventricular hyperintensity is noted, despite the fact that the ventricles are not dilated out of proportion to the enlarged cortical sulci. On the moderately T_2-weighted image (right image), deep white matter infarcts are noted (black arrows), which have produced centrally tracking vasogenic edema (white arrow on left image), which is simulating interstitial edema and ventricular obstruction (SE 2000/30 and 60).

Figure 8.12

Heterotopic gray matter simulating interstitial edema. (a) High signal (arrows) surrounds the ventricles on mildly T_2-weighted image. Note this pattern is 'bumpy' rather than smooth as seen with interstitial edema (SE 3000/40). (b) With greater T_2-weighting, heterotopic periventricular gray matter remains isointense with cortical gray matter rather than becoming hyperintense as interstitial edema would be (SE 3000/80).

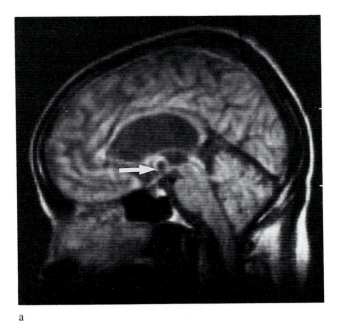

a

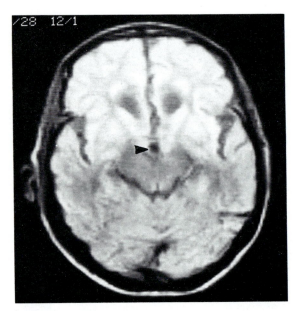

b

Figure 8.14

Colloid cyst obstructing
foramen of Monro. (**a**) T$_1$-
weighted sagittal image
demonstrates 1 cm anterior
third ventricular abnormality
with signal similar to that of
CSF (arrow) (SE 500/28).
(**b**) Mildly T$_2$-weighted axial
section through the third
ventricle demonstrates 1 cm
mass in anterior third ventricle
which is less intense than CSF
(arrowhead) (SE 2000/28).
(**c**) Moderately T$_2$-weighted
axial section through the same
level as (**b**) demonstrates
definite hypointensity of the
colloid cyst due to much shorter
T$_2$ than that of CSF
(arrowhead) (SE 2000/56).

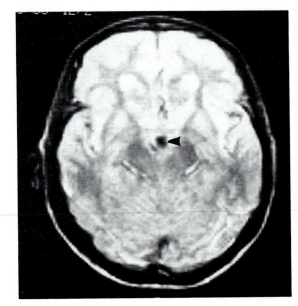

c

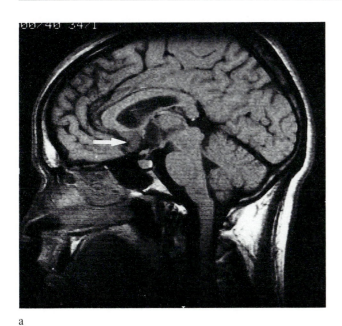

a

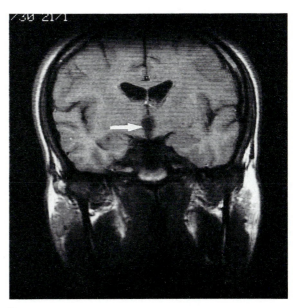

b

Figure 8.15

Cysticercotic cyst obstructing foramen of Monro. (**a**) T_1-weighted sagittal section demonstrates 1.5 cm cyst in anterior third ventricle (arrow), with signal intensity slightly greater than that of free CSF within the ventricles and subarachnoid spaces (SE 500/40). (**b**) T_1-weighted coronal section demonstrates cyst with slightly higher signal intensity than CSF (arrow) bowing the walls of the anterior third ventricle. Note also mild enlargement of the lateral ventricles (SE 500/30). (**c**) Mildly T_2-weighted axial section through the third ventricle demonstrates cyst which is isointense to slightly hypointense relative to CSF (arrow) with surrounding edema secondary to inflammation (SE 2000/30).

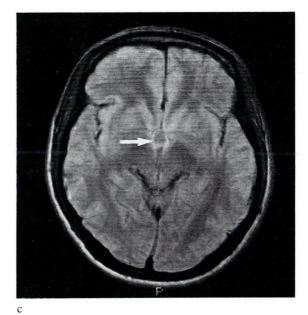

c

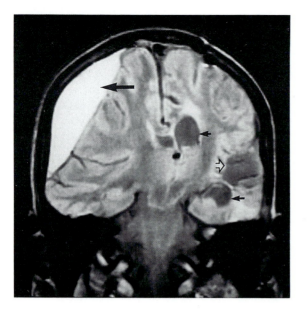

Figure 8.16

Trapped lateral ventricle. Mildly T_2-weighted coronal section demonstrates mass effect and midline shift secondary to large right subdural hematoma (arrow). There is secondary entrapment of the left lateral ventricle (arrowheads) at the foramen of Monro. Incidentally noted is left Sylvian encephalomalacia from prior surgical resection (open arrow) (SE 2500/30). (Courtesy Michael Brant-Zawadzki, MD, Newport Beach, CA.)

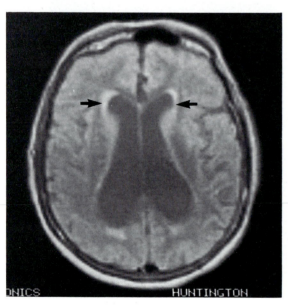

a

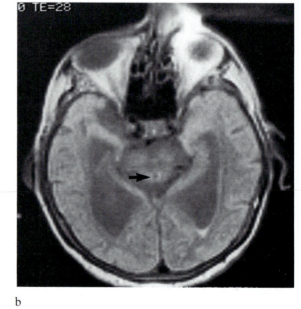

b

Figure 8.17

Obstructive hydrocephalus due to inflammatory aqueductal stenosis. (**a**) Mildly T_2-weighted axial section demonstrates moderate ventricular enlargement with thin rim of interstitial edema (arrowheads) indicating partial compensation. (**b**) Lower axial section through the aqueduct fails to demonstrate a significant flow void (arrowhead) indicating absent or very slow flow of CSF through stenotic aqueduct following meningitis (SE 2000/28).

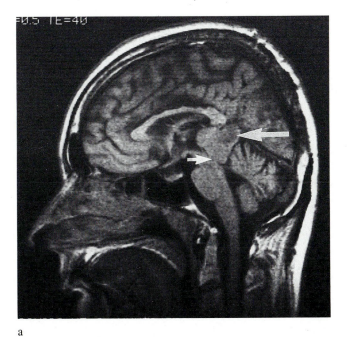

a

Figure 8.18

Pineal-region tumor obstructing aqueduct. (**a**) T_1-weighted midsagittal section demonstrates pineal-region mass (arrow) compressing aqueduct (arrowhead). There is no bowing of the corpus callosum, indicating successful shunting (SE 500/40). (**b**) Mildly and moderately T_2-weighted axial sections demonstrate pineal-region tumor in quadrigeminal plate cistern (arrow) (SE 2000/30 and 60).

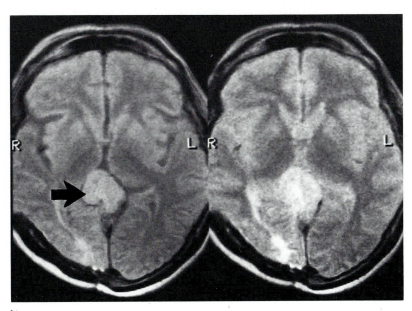

b

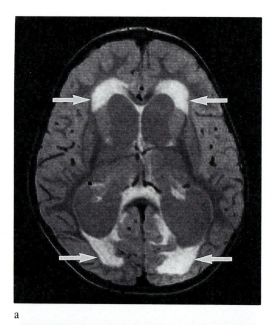

a

b

c

Figure 8.19

Cystic astrocytoma obstructing
fourth ventricle. (**a**) Moderately
T_2-weighted axial section
through the lateral ventricles
demonstrates ventricular
enlargement with marked
surrounding interstitial edema
(arrows) (SE 3000/40). (**b**) On
lower axial section through the
Circle of Willis, enlargement of
the anterior recesses of the third
ventricle (arrowheads) is noted,
as well as enlarged temporal
horns (arrows). Note high
signal of obstructing cystic
astrocytoma involving the
superior cerebellar vermis
(curved arrow) (SE 3000/40).
(**c**) T_1-weighted sagittal section
demonstrates cystic
astrocytoma (curved arrow)
compressing fourth ventricle
(straight arrow) and aqueduct
(arrowhead). Note also upward
bowing of corpus callosum
(open arrow) and foramen of
Monro (small thin arrow) (SE
500/40).

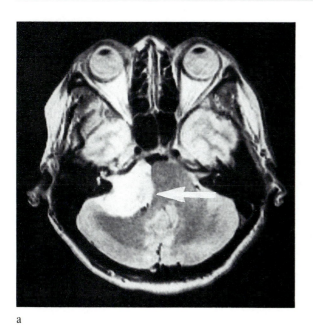

a

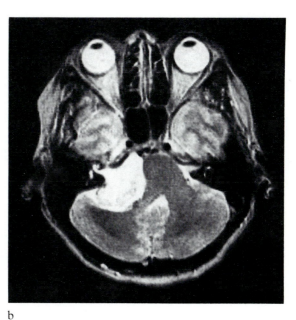

b

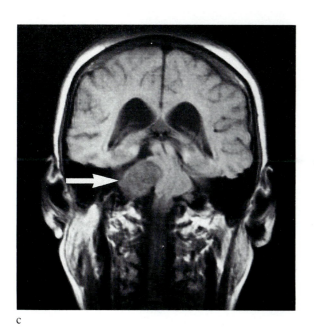

c

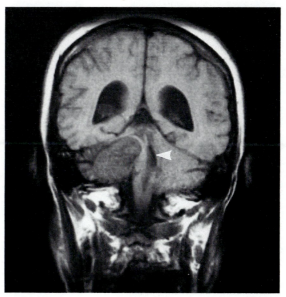

d

Figure 8.20

Obstruction of fourth ventricle by acoustic neuroma. (**a**) Axial section through the fourth ventricle demonstrates a large mass (arrow) in the right cerebellopontine angle cistern with extension into the right internal auditory canal. This mass displaces the pons and compresses the fourth ventricle (SE 3000/40). (**b**) Heavily T_2-weighted image through the same level as (**a**) demonstrates high-signal intensity in acoustic neuroma (SE 3000/80). (**c**) T_1-weighted coronal section through the pons demonstrates right CP angle mass (arrow) distorting the brain stem. Note enlarged lateral ventricles due to obstruction at the level of the fourth ventricle (SE 500/30). (**d**) Coronal section slightly posterior to (**c**) demonstrates right CP angle mass distorting fourth ventricle with obstruction along its superior margin (arrowhead) (SE 500/30).

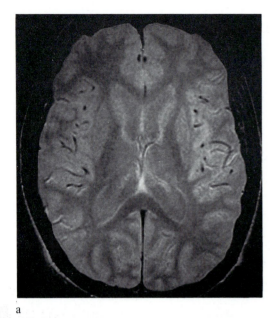
a

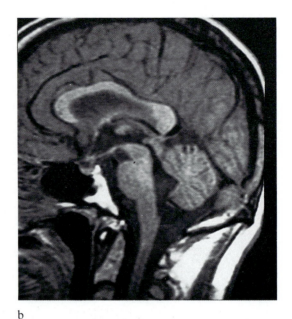
b

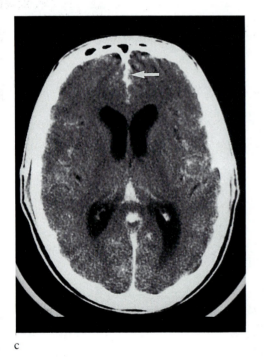
c

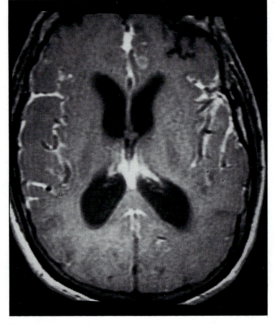
d

Figure 8.21

Communicating hydrocephalus secondary to leptomeningeal carcinomatosis. Thirty-four-year-old male who had spinal ependymoma resected previously now presents with decreasing mental status. (a) T$_2$-weighted axial MR image demonstrates mild ventricular dilatation (SE 2800/30). (b) T$_1$-weighted sagittal image at the same time is apparently normal (SE 600/20). (c) Two weeks later, contrast-enhanced CT is suspicious for abnormal enhancement of the anterior falx (arrow). (d) One month after the CT scan, T$_1$-weighted, gadolinium-enhanced, axial section through the lateral ventricles demonstrates diffuse leptomeningeal enhancement secondary to carcinomatosis. Notice that the ventricles have not increased significantly in size since the study shown in (a) six weeks earlier (SE 800/20).

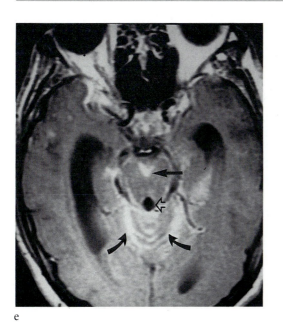

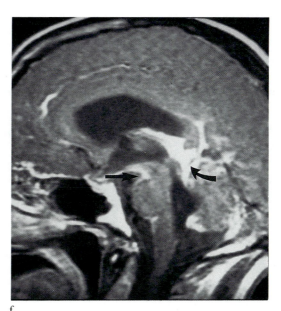

e   f

(e) In a lower axial section through the midbrain, leptomeningeal enhancement is noted in the interpeduncular cistern (arrow) as well as over the superior cerebellar vermis (curved arrows). Note hyperdynamic CSF flow state in aqueduct (open arrow) due to communicating hydrocephalus (SE 800/20).
(f) Midline T_1-weighted sagittal section demonstrates marked leptomeningeal enhancement in the interpeduncular cistern (arrow) as well as in the CSF spaces contiguous with the quadrigeminal plate cistern (curved arrow) (SE 600/20). (Courtesy Michael Brant-Zawadzki, MD, Newport Beach, CA.)

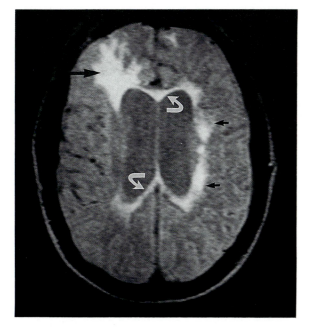

Figure 8.22

Communicating hydrocephalus following subarachnoid hemorrhage. After severe head trauma and subarachnoid hemorrhage, lateral ventricles are dilated due to communicating hydrocephalus. Interstitial edema (curved arrows) surrounds enlarged lateral ventricles. Note also right frontal encephalomalacia (arrow) from previous contusion and left periventricular shearing injury (arrowheads) (SE 2550/60). (Courtesy Charles Seibert, MD, Denver, CO.)

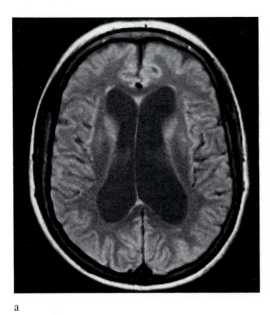

a

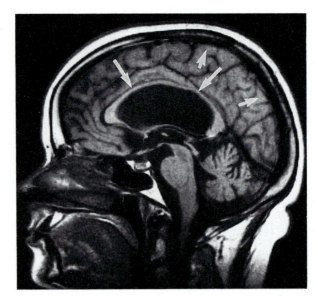

b

Figure 8.23

Normal pressure
hydrocephalus. (**a**) Axial
section demonstrates
enlargement of the lateral
ventricles without concomitant
enlargement of the cortical sulci
(SE 2000/30). (**b**) T_1-weighted
sagittal section demonstrates
upward bowing of the corpus
callosum (arrows) and
flattening of the cortical gyri
against the inner table of the
calvarium (arrowheads) (SE
500/40).

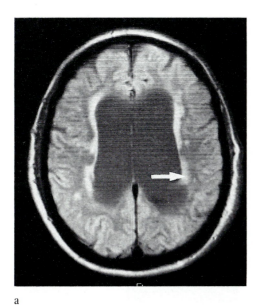

a

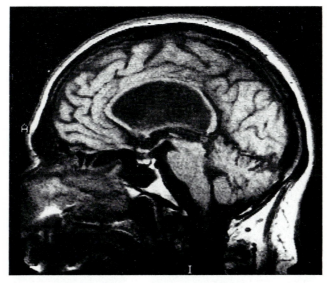

d

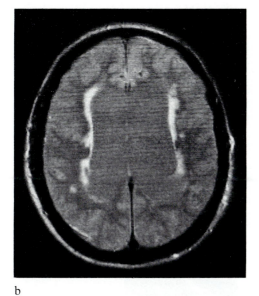

b

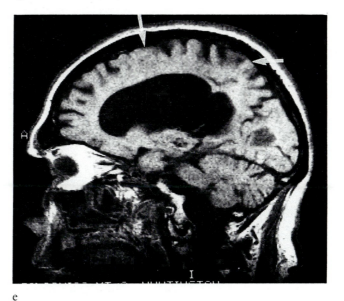

e

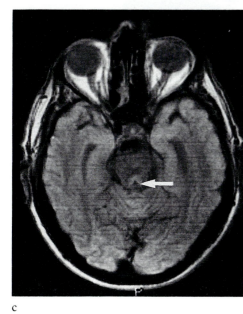

c

Figure 8.24

Combined communicating hydrocephalus and deep white matter infarction in 68-year-old man with difficulty walking. (**a**) Mildly T_2-weighted axial section demonstrates ventricular enlargement out of proportion to enlargement of the cortical sulci. Mild deep white matter infarction is also noted (arrow) (SE 2000/30). (**b**) Moderately T_2-weighted axial section demonstrates deep white matter infarcts to greater advantage since the CSF is now isointense with gray matter (SE 2000/60). (**c**) Axial section through the aqueduct demonstrates no evidence of a significant flow void (arrow) as would be expected in active communicating hydrocephalus (SE 2000/30). (**d**) Midline sagittal section demonstrates upward bowing of the corpus callosum due to communicating hydrocephalus (SE 500/40). (**e**) Parasagittal section demonstrates flattening of the cortical gyri (arrows) against the inner table of the cavarium secondary to communicating hydrocephalus (SE 500/40).

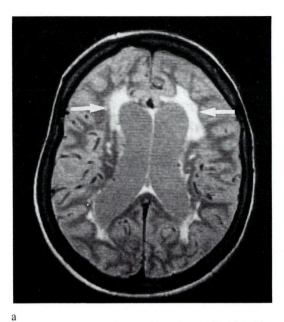

a

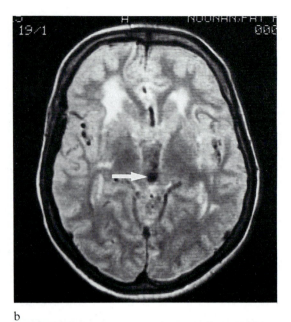

b

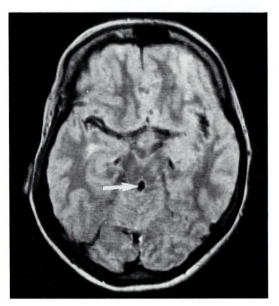

c

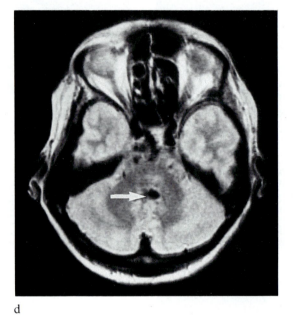

d

Figure 8.25

Combined communicating
hydrocephalus and deep white
matter infarction in 55-year-old
woman with worsening
memory loss. (**a**) Moderately
T_2-weighted axial section
through the lateral ventricles
demonstrates ventricular
dilatation and moderately
severe deep white matter
infarction (arrows) (SE 3000/
40). (**b**) Lower axial section

through the third ventricle
demonstrates prominent flow
void (arrow) and dilated third
ventricle due to hyperdynamic
CSF flow state (SE 3000/40).
(**c**) Axial section through
aqueduct demonstrates
prominent flow void (arrow)
(SE 3000/40). (**d**) Axial section
through the pons demonstrates
prominent flow void in fourth
ventricle (arrow) (SE 3000/40).

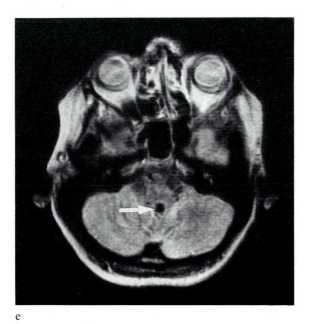

e

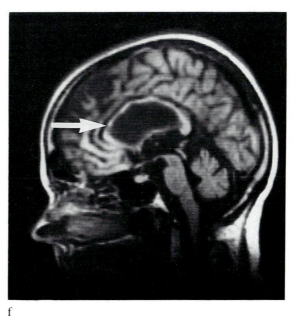

f

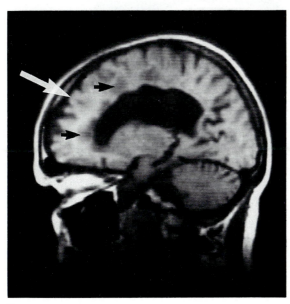

g

(**e**) Axial section through the medulla demonstrates prominent flow void in the inferior fourth ventricle due to hyperdynamic CSF flow (arrow) (SE 3000/40).
(**f**) Midline sagittal section demonstrates upward bowing and focal thinning of the corpus callosum (arrow). The upward bowing is due to communicating hydrocephalus. The focal thinning is due to the presence of bilateral deep white matter infarcts (SE 500/40).
(**g**) Parasagittal section demonstrates deep white matter infarcts (arrowheads) and flattening of the cortical gyri against the inner table of the calvarium (arrow) which is secondary evidence of communicating hydrocephalus (SE 500/40).

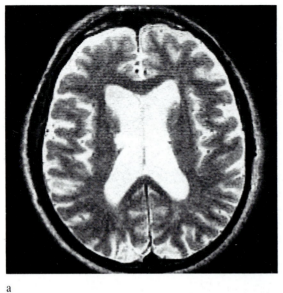

a

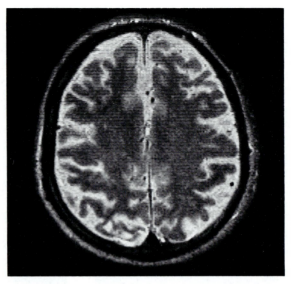

b

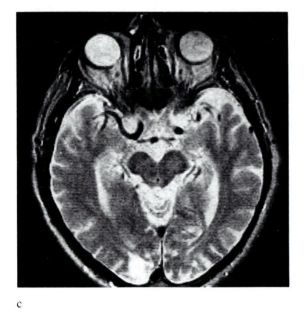

c

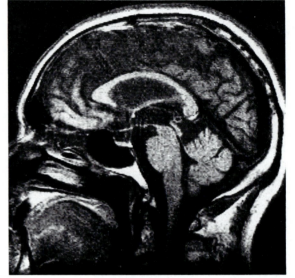

d

Figure 8.26

Diffuse cortical atrophy in 76-year-old man. (**a**) Heavily T_2-weighted transverse axial section through the lateral ventricles demonstrates both ventricular enlargement and prominence of the cortical sulci (SE 3000/80). (**b**) Higher axial section demonstrates prominence of the subarachnoid spaces over the convexities with enlarged sulci (SE 3000/80). (**c**) Lower axial section through the midbrain demonstrates prominence of the temporal sulci (SE 3000/80). (**d**) T_1-weighted midsagittal section does not show upward bowing of the corpus callosum which would be seen in communicating hydrocephalus. Note apparent lack of brain substance rostral to the corpus callosum due to image plane within the inner hemispheric fissure (SE 500/40).

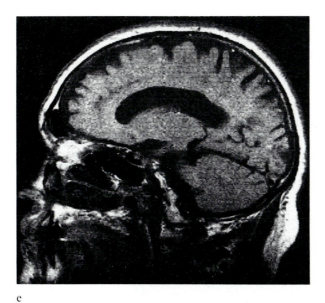

e

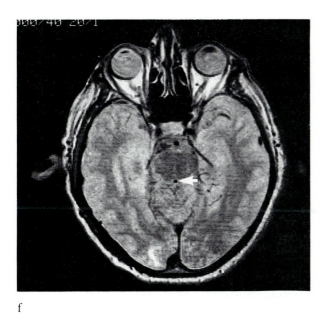

f

(**e**) Parasagittal section through the body of the right lateral ventricle demonstrates enlargement of the subarachnoid space without evidence of flattening of the cortical gyri against the inner table of the calvarium (SE 500/40). (**f**) Mildly T_2-weighted axial section through the aqueduct demonstrates no evidence of aqueductal enlargement or particular prominence of the CSF flow void (arrow) (SE 3000/40).

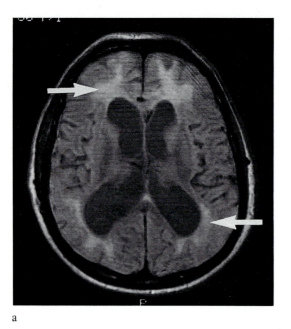

a

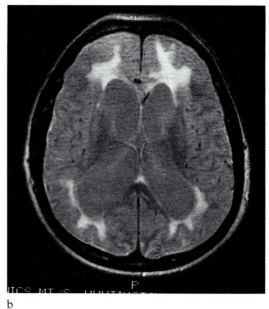

b

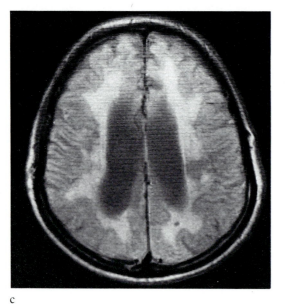

c

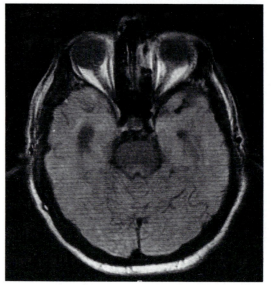

d

Figure 8.27

Central atrophy due to deep white matter infarction. (**a**) The lateral ventricles are enlarged out of proportion to the mildly enlarged cortical sulci with surrounding high signal (arrows) due to deep white matter infarction (SE 2000/30). (**b**) On more T$_2$-weighted image, the isomorphic gliosis surrounding the deep white matter infarcts becomes more prominent due to the prolonged T$_2$ value (SE 2000/60). (**c**) Higher axial section through the bodies of the lateral ventricles demonstrates extensive deep white matter infarction (SE 2000/30). (**d**) Lower axial section through the aqueduct demonstrates no evidence of a significant CSF flow void (SE 2000/30).

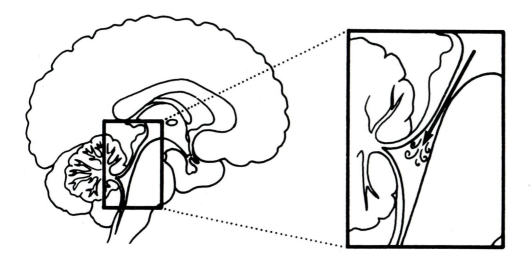

Figure 8.28

CSF flow through aqueduct and upper fourth ventricle. Since the aqueduct is the narrowest part of the ventricular system, the velocity of CSF is greatest through it. This alone can result in signal loss due to time-of-flight effects. As the CSF flows down into the fourth ventricle during cardiac systole, the stream expands and may become turbulent due to a venturi or nozzle effect. Turbulence is an additional cause of signal loss.

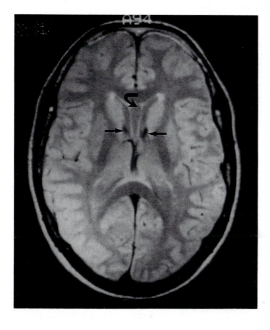

Figure 8.29

Normal CSF flow void in foramen of Monro. Mildly T$_2$-weighted axial section through the foramen of Monro demonstrates bilateral flow voids (arrows) due to regurgitant jet of CSF returning to frontal horns during diastole. Incidentally noted is cavum septum pellucidum (curved arrow) (SE 2000/30).

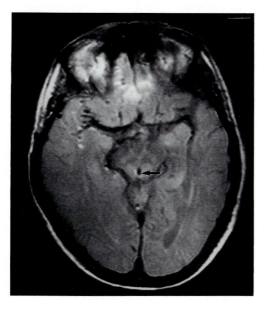

Figure 8.30

Normal CSF flow void in aqueduct. Low signal is noted in aqueduct (arrow) due to rapid to-and-fro motion of CSF (SE 2000/30).

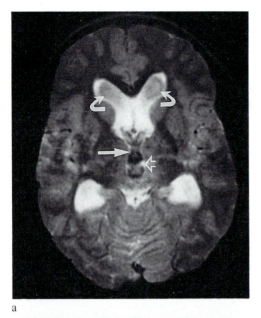

a

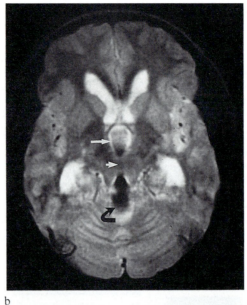

b

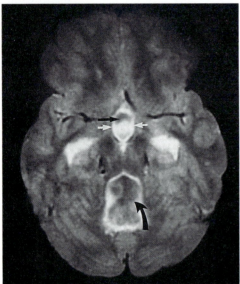

c

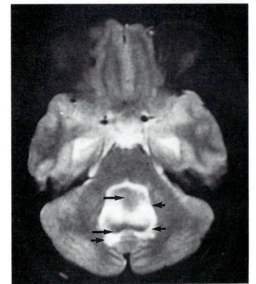

d

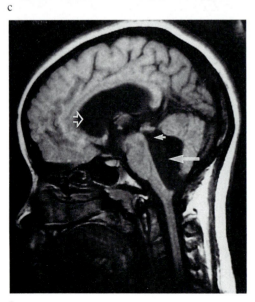

e

Figure 8.31

CSF flow void from chronic communicating hydrocephalus at high field. (**a**) Axial section through the foramen of Monro (arrow) demonstrates CSF flow void due to turbulence on this symmetric second-echo image. Note also flow void in third ventricle (open arrow) and in frontal horns (curved arrows) due to hyperdynamic CSF flow state (SE 2500/60). (**b**) Angled axial section through the third ventricle (straight arrow), aqueduct (arrowhead), and fourth ventricle (curved arrow) demonstrates marked flow void due to turbulent jet in third and fourth ventricles with even-echo rephasing noted in aqueduct (SE 2500/60). (**c**) Lower axial section demonstrates outward bowing of third ventricular walls (arrowheads) with flow void in fourth ventricle (curved arrow) due to turbulent jet (SE 2500/60). (**d**) Lower axial section through fourth ventricle demonstrates intraventricular flow voids (arrows) and interstitial edema (arrowheads) in markedly enlarged fourth ventricle (SE 2500/60). (**e**) T$_1$-weighted sagittal section demonstrates marked enlargement of fourth ventricle (straight arrow) with moderate enlargement of lateral ventricles (open arrow). CSF flow void in upper fourth ventricle (arrowhead) is subtle but can be seen (SE 600/20).

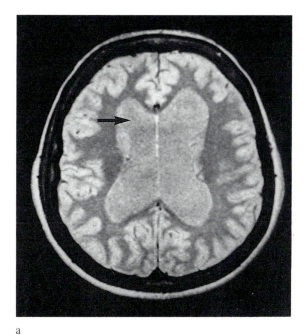

a

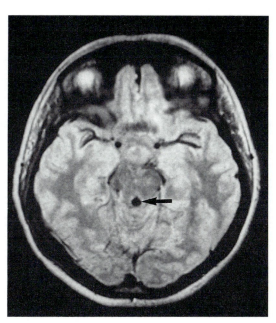

b

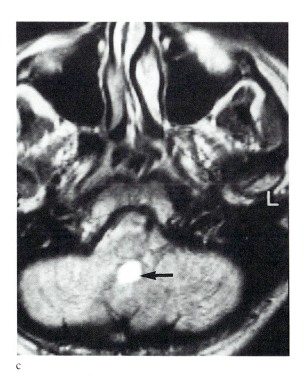

c

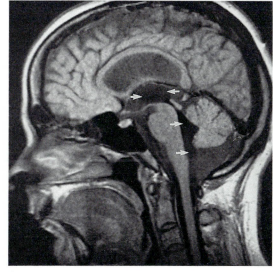

d

Figure 8.32

CSF flow void in chronic communicating hydrocephalus on low bandwidth, midfield system. (**a**) Axial section demonstrates lateral ventricular enlargement (arrow) without enlargement of the cortical sulci indicating hydrocephalus instead of atrophy (SE 3000/40). (**b**) Axial section through aqueduct demonstrates flow void in aqueduct (arrow) (SE 3000/40). (**c**) Section through inferior fourth ventricle demonstrates high signal (arrow) suspicious for mass. Since this is the lowest slice in the acquisition, the possibility of flow-related enhancement was raised. (**d**) T$_1$-weighted sagittal section shows no evidence of mass in the inferior fourth ventricle. Instead there is a prominent CSF flow void (arrowheads) due to turbulent jets in both the fourth ventricle and third ventricle (SE 500/40). (Courtesy Michael Trombello, MD, Abilene, TX.)

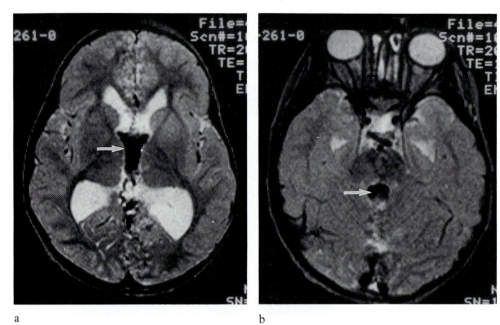

a   b

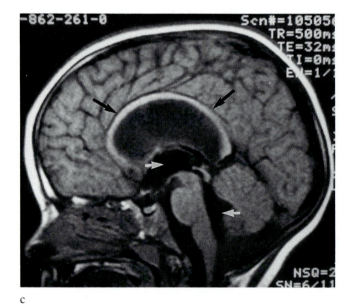

c

Figure 8.33

Chronic communicating hydrocephalus on high bandwidth, midfield system. (**a**) Heavily T_2-weighted axial section through the third ventricle demonstrates prominent flow void (arrow). This is due to stronger gradients and long echo-delay time, both of which increase dephasing and signal loss (SE 2010/120). (**b**) Axial section through the upper fourth ventricle demonstrates marked flow void (arrow) (SE 2010/120). (**c**) T_1-weighted sagittal section demonstrates upward bowing of corpus callosum (arrows) and relative signal loss in third and fourth ventricles (arrowheads) (SE 500/32). (Courtesy Meredith A Weinstein, MD, Cleveland, OH.)

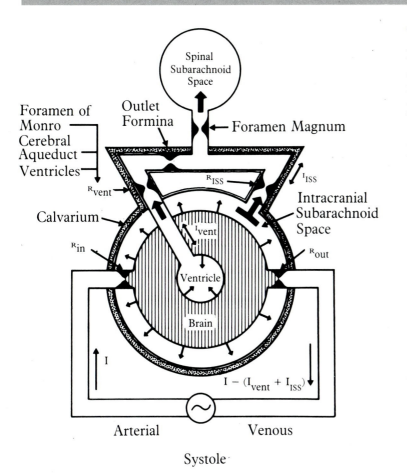

Systole

Figure 8.34

Computer (electrical analog) model of brain. Following arterial inflow, the brain swells within the rigid intracranial space. This will lead to an increase in pressure unless non-compressible blood or CSF can be simultaneously vented from the intracranial space. CSF can leave the supratentorial space through the aqueduct at flow rate I_{vent} or through the perimesencephalic cisterns at flow rate I_{iss} and it can leave the intracranial space through the foramen magnum into the spinal subarachnoid space. When venous resistance R_{out} increases, there is a greater tendency for CSF to be vented through both the aqueduct and subarachnoid space. When the aqueductal diameter increases, a lower resistance pathway R_{vent} is provided for the outflow of CSF during systole.

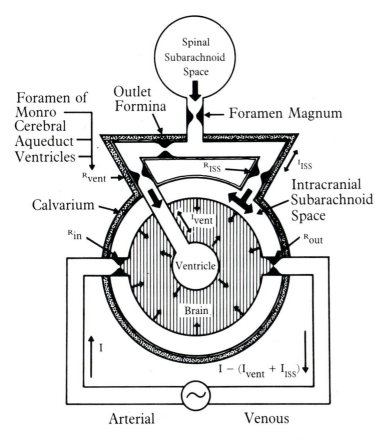

Diastole

Figure 8.35

During diastole, venous blood is vented from the intracranial space, allowing the brain to decrease in size. This leads to a consequent enlargement of both the intracranial subarachnoid space and the ventricles, with retrograde flow of CSF through the aqueduct into the third ventricle.

9

Use of Gadolinium-DTPA

Graeme Bydder

Introduction

Early in the development of magnetic resonance imaging (MRI) it was apparent that a high level of soft tissue contrast was available *de novo* and it was thought that the need for externally administered contrast agents might be small. This observation was tempered by the fact that separation of tumor from edema was frequently better with contrast-enhanced X-ray computed tomography (CT) than with unenhanced MRI. It was therefore felt that a contrast agent might be needed for MRI.[1]

At the end of 1983 the first parenteral agent, gadolinium diethylene triamine pentaacetic acid (Gd-DTPA) was used in volunteers, and clinical studies began in 1984. At present, Gd-DTPA, oral, and intravenous iron compounds are in clinical use. There are a number of other agents which have been used in animals and some of these may become available for clinical use in the foreseeable future.

Types of contrast agent

Paramagnetic agents

Paramagnetic agents form the commonest group of contrast agents and metallic ions form the basis for the majority of these agents.[2,3] Iron, chromium, manganese, and gadolinium have all been used in the free form in animals, but in this state these ions are toxic and they are complexed to common chelating agents such as EDTP, DTPA, DOTA, and EHPG to render them less hazardous. Studies on the relative merits of these agents depend on many factors and a general discussion of these has been published by several groups.[4-6] These factors include the number of unpaired electrons available, molecular size, and mobility, as well as the number of binding sites available for water. In human studies, pharmacological aspects are of basic importance and the choice of Gd-DTPA for clinical studies has been discussed.[7] The reasons include its low toxicity, which is less than that of Gd-EDTA, possibly as a result of its higher association constant.

Another group of paramagnetic agents of interest is the nitroxide-stable free radicals and some of the earliest animal studies were performed with these agents.[2] There has been some concern about the potential toxicity of these compounds and to date they have not been used in clinical studies, although they may well have some novel pharmacological properties when compared with Gd-DTPA.

Monoclonal antibodies have also been linked to paramagnetic complexes in the form of antimyosin antibodies,[8] as well as anti-tumor antibodies.[9] While the former agents have been effective in vivo on 60 to 80 per cent of occasions, no consistent results have been achieved with the latter agents. This result has been predicted from considerations of the number of available binding sites and the known effectiveness of paramagnetic agents in producing relaxation enhancement.

Paramagnetic agents have also been administered to animals in the form of liposomes and polymers designed to enhance the reticulo-endothelial system.

Susceptibility agents

The second major class of contrast agents is the susceptibility group, of which the most important agent is the superparamagnetic form of magnetite, Fe_3O_4. Particles of micron size are coated with inert materials and these have been administered to patients both orally and intravenously. These agents produce a striking decrease in T_2, with a relatively small change in T_1.[10,11]

Other agents

A further group of contrast agents is worth mentioning, although as yet they have not been used in clinical studies. These include fluorinated compounds such as the fluorinated hydrocarbons which are inhaled, as well as fluorinated blood substitutes. Some of the latter group of compounds may provide additional information since their T_1 varies with the level of tissue oxygenation.

There is no doubt that more agents will be developed, either as variants within the above groups, or as new classes of agents in their own right. However, there are many problems to be overcome before an agent is approved for human usage.

General effects of Gd-DTPA

There have been two general approaches to understanding the effect of Gd-DTPA in clinical practice. The first has been a straightforward comparison with the iodinated contrast agents used in X-ray CT, and the second has been an analytical approach relating the dosage, rate of excretion, pulse sequence, and other factors to the change in tissue signal intensity on the image. Both approaches are helpful. The first approach notes that the molecular weight of Gd-DTPA is similar to that of the common iodinated contrast agents and that its general pharmacological properties are similar. Hence in both physiological and pathological situations, where contrast enhancement is seen with X-ray CT, a similar result might be expected with MRI. Whilst this is true in general, there are major differences with MRI according to the pulse sequence which is used. Highly T_1-dependent pulse sequences show greatest enhancement and highly T_2-dependent pulse sequences show least enhancement. There are also other differences which reflect the general differences between X-ray CT and MRI. These include differences in flow effects and the display of calcified tissue as well as differences in examination of the posterior fossa, spinal cord, etc.

The analytic approach is considered in more detail in subsequent sections.

Distribution and excretion of Gd-DTPA (normal and abnormal)

The basic pharmacology of Gd-DTPA has been studied by Weinmann et al.[7] After intravenous injection, Gd-DTPA circulates within the vascular and extracellular compartment, after which it is concentrated within the kidney and excreted unchanged within the urine. A few per cent at most may be excreted through the gastrointestinal tract.

Gadolinium-DTPA does not cross the normal blood-brain barrier, but is present in higher concentration in gray matter as compared to white matter, reflecting the different vascularity of these tissues. Areas of the brain without a blood-brain barrier, such as the choroid plexus, show enhancement. The normal dura displays variable enhancement just posterior to C1 and C2. This is probably a reflection of changes in the venous plexus in this area.

Within the soft tissues of the body outside the central nervous system, Gd-DTPA is distributed within the vascular and extracellular compartments and the distribution follows a two-compartment model.

In pathological circumstances we can consider first changes in blood vessels, the most obvious of which is occlusion leading to failure of Gd-DTPA to reach the dependent tissue. Increased blood flow may lead to more rapid delivery of Gd-DTPA on a focal basis, but in addition the flow effects may produce changes in their own right, depending on the particular sequence which is used (see later).

The next consideration is vascular permeability. Whilst the blood-brain barrier is generally impermeable to Gd-DTPA, in a variety of pathological circumstances, including tumors, infections, and demyelinating disease, it becomes permeable and Gd-DTPA accumulates in an extravascular location. Outside the central nervous system, capillaries may also be abnormally permeable allowing accumulation of Gd-DTPA. The kidney is a special case as the only organ system which concentrates Gd-DTPA. Failure to concentrate the Gd-DTPA may be a feature of renal insufficiency.

Simple pharmacodynamic models are appropriate for the description of both the normal and pathological accumulation of Gd-DTPA, but unlike iodinated agents in conventional radiography and X-ray CT, there is no direct relationship between the concentration of Gd-DTPA and the observed signal intensity. To understand the effect of Gd-DTPA on image signal intensity we must first consider the effect of Gd-DTPA in producing changes in tissue T_1 and T_2, and then consider the effect of these changes on signal intensity with different pulse sequences.

Effect of Gd-DTPA on tissue T_1 and T_2

In solution Gd-DTPA produces a change in relaxation *rate* which is proportional to concentration. The relaxation rate is the reciprocal of T_1 or T_2 so that

$$\frac{1}{T_1} \quad \alpha \quad [Gd\text{-}DTPA]$$

and

$$\frac{1}{T_2} \quad \alpha \quad [Gd\text{-}DTPA]$$

Thus an increase in Gd-DTPA concentration produces a decrease in both T_1 and T_2. From the above equations the absolute decrease in T_1 is larger for fluids with longer values of T_1 or T_2 than it is for fluids with shorter values. The above results seem applicable to soft tissues as well as fluids, and in this situation T_1 is always less than T_2 so that the absolute decrease in T_1 is greater than that for T_2. Protons within fat are not as accessible to Gd-DTPA as protons in free water so the changes to protons in fat would be expected to be less than that for protons in water. The essential features described from equations (9.1) and (9.2) for CSF, muscle, and fat are illustrated in Figure 9.1. The decrease in relaxation time depends on the initial value of T_1 and T_2 as well as the tissue concentration of Gd-DTPA.

Effects of changes in T_1 and T_2 on tissue signal intensity—the effect of different pulse sequences

From the above section we can expect that Gd-DTPA will decrease both T_1 and T_2 and that this reduction will be greater in absolute terms for T_1 than for T_2. To predict what will happen to the tissue signal intensity, standard equations for signal intensity are used.[12] The important features of these equations are that for the common forms of the pulse sequences, partial saturation (PS), inversion recovery (IR) and spin echo (SE), a decrease in T_1 produces a net *increase* in signal intensity, but a decrease in T_2 produces a net *decrease* in signal intensity. Thus these two effects are opposed. With highly T_1-dependent sequences (such as IR) the

first effect dominates, whereas with highly T_2-dependent sequences the second effect dominates. In addition, there is a limit to the increase in signal intensity that may be obtained by decreasing T_1 and beyond this point increasing Gd-DTPA concentration produces a net decrease in signal intensity. The term 'negative enhancement' is used to describe the situation where tissue signal intensity is decreased by a contrast agent.

The most T_1-dependent sequence is the IR sequence, and usually the greatest contrast enhancement is seen when the TI of the IR sequence is intermediate between the T_1 of the tissue before and that after enhancement with Gd-DTPA. T_1-dependent forms of the SE and PS sequence display moderate contrast enhancement, which is generally greatest when TR is between the values of tissue T_1 before and after contrast enhancement. Spin-echo sequences with high values of TR and TE are generally insensitive to contrast enhancement. These points are illustrated in Figure 9.2.

The net effect of Gd-DTPA

The overall effect of Gd-DTPA depends on the dosage of contrast agent. To date, dosages of 0.1 and 0.2 mmol/kg have been used. The next factor of importance is the duration of administration and the time following injection of the drug. For example, transport of Gd-DTPA across the blood-brain barrier may take time and delayed examinations may show a greater effect than immediate examinations. The reverse may be true with very vascular lesions.

The concentration of Gd-DTPA in the lesion and the pulse sequence are also of critical importance.

For the clinician deciding what new information has been derived (if any) after use of Gd-DTPA, it is necessary to consider normal tissue signal intensities before and after Gd-DTPA with the different pulse sequences as well as abnormal tissue signal intensities before and after Gd-DTPA with the different pulse sequences. Not surprisingly, when several different tissues (normal and abnormal) are studied with several different pulse sequences at different times before and after use of Gd-DTPA, the results may be complex with no single pulse sequence providing all the available information. For example, with malignant tumors, IR sequences usually display maximal contrast enhancement whilst highly T_2-dependent sequences usually display the greatest extent of disease.

It is also important to remember that whereas many pathological processes *increase* T_1 and T_2, Gd-DTPA *decreases* T_1 and T_2. Thus there is considerable potential for isointense behavior whereby the contrast agent reduces tissue T_1 and T_2 values back to those of the adjacent normal tissue, producing a net loss of tissue conspicuity.

From another point of view, it is possible to regard Gd-DTPA as providing physiological or pathophysiological data, for example about the integrity of the blood-brain barrier, the vascularity of tumors, and the state of renal excretory function. This is not directly obtainable with conventional MRI pulse sequences.

A further feature of note is the fact that so far the effects of Gd-DTPA have been considered only in terms of changes in T_1 and T_2, but there are other image parameters of potential importance including flow effects, chemical shift effects, and susceptibility changes, and these may affect tissue signal intensity.

The appearance of flowing blood on MR images has been described in detail[13–15] and, in general, the changes in the appearance of blood due to Gd-DTPA can be predicted by noting the effect of a change in T_1 and T_2. With some processes, such as entry of unsaturated blood into the slice, the T_1 of the inflowing blood is of little importance and minimal change is seen. Little change may also be seen with rapidly flowing blood where dephasing occurs quickly. In other circumstances, such as slow flowing blood, the decrease in T_1 may produce a marked increase in signal intensity. Detailed knowledge of the pulse sequence is necessary to predict the effect, together with a knowledge of the rate of blood flow, its direction, the phase of the cardiac cycle, and other factors.

Chemical-shift effects using proton phase-contrast techniques of the Dixon type can readily be produced with asymmetrical SE[16] or PS sequences.[17] Since Gd-DTPA affects protons in water more than those in fat, the relaxation time of the water component may be relatively shortened, thus changing the balance in signal between the two components. While effects attributable to this mechanism have been observed, their clinical significance has been limited.

Paramagnetic contrast agents may also change tissue susceptibility and this may be demonstrated by field mapping techniques. To date, this has been seen most obviously with the naturally occurring paramagnetic compounds associated with hematoma (deoxyhemoglobin, methemoglobin, free Fe^{3+}, and hemosiderin) but it may also be seen with Gd-DTPA.

Among the more recent imaging approaches is the use of fast field echo (PS) imaging with a reduced flip angle. This enables reasonable quality images to be obtained in a few seconds and thus the time course of enhancement can be studied in a manner analagous to dynamic X-ray CT. This technique uses field-echo techniques pioneered in Aberdeen,[18] but has been used since under a variety of different names such as FLASH, GRASS, and FISP.

Notwithstanding the well established theoretical basis for understanding contrast enhancement, exceptions to the above general rules occur. In some cases enhancement is observed with a highly T_2-dependent sequence and not with the T_1-dependent sequence, and the explanation may not be clear. Patient movement, flow effects, delayed enhancement, artifacts, and other mechanisms are usually invoked with varying degrees of conviction in order to try and explain these effects.

In the next sections clinical results are reviewed, beginning with the commonest application to date—tumors of the brain.[19–30]

Meningiomas

Meningiomas are relatively common and amongst the most treatable tumors within the cranium. They usually display a high level of contrast enhancement on X-ray CT and the combinations of extracerebral location, preferred sites, generally uniform appearance, high level of contrast enhancement, as well as calcification and/or bone involvement generally allows a high degree of sensitivity and specificity with X-ray CT.

The situation with MRI is not so clear. Whilst many meningiomas display an increase in T_1 and T_2 relative to brain, a significant number only display a slight increase in T_1 compared with white matter and have values of T_2 within the normal range for brain. As a consequence, if heavily T_2-weighted sequences are used, some meningiomas may only be detected as a result of their indirect signs, such as by their mass effect or as a result of edema in the adjacent brain. This can result in a lack of sensitivity and a lack of specificity.

In the clinical context the situation is complicated by the fact that meningiomas may present with a wide range of symptoms and signs which are not particularly specific, so that prediction of a meningioma in advance may be difficult. On the other hand, a certain proportion of meningiomas are asymptomatic and failure to detect these may not be of any particular significance. Whilst in general, bigger meningiomas are clinically more significant, small tumors at vulnerable sites may also be important. Magnetic resonance imaging has the disadvantage that it displays calcification and bony change poorly, but on the other hand meningiomas en-plaque are not obscured by the presence of artifact or partial-volume effects from bone as they may be with CT.

Particular problems arise with the design of a screening examination for MRI. The most common approach is the use of highly T_2-weighted SE sequences, which are insensitive to some meningiomas and are also insensitive to contrast enhancement. The alternative is to add a T_1-weighted sequence (either IR or SE) which will reveal better anatomical detail and provide sensitivity to contrast enhancement. If this sequence is repeated after administration of Gd-DTPA, it provides a useful means of detecting meningiomas. However, the effect of adding this procedure to the basic T_2-weighted SE sequence on a routine basis is a decrease in patient throughput, in addition to the discomfort of an intravenous injection and the extra expense of Gd-DTPA. The proposition has therefore been put forward that it is very unusual for significant meningiomas to be present and show no sign on a T_2-weighted SE sequence, exceptions to this rule have also been presented and the issue is not really resolved at the present time.

Apart from the wider issues, meningiomas provide a useful test situation for Gd-DTPA, and features common to enhancement in general can be demonstrated using examples of this tumor. For example, signal intensities before and after Gd-DTPA are shown in Figure 9.3, which summarizes results in six cases.[19] Maximal enhancement is seen with the IR image. Figure 9.4 shows a convexity meningioma which can be seen on the IR image, but is really only detectable as a result of the associated edema with the T_2-weighted SE images (Figure 9.4b). The tumor displays no evidence of an increase in T_2. Following enhancement the tumor is highlighted (Figure 9.4c), but note that this tumor enhancement is *not* demonstrated on the SE image (Figure 9.4d). Additional areas of abnormality are seen on Figure 9.4c and these probably represent vascular changes.

Another aspect of MRI of meningiomas is seen in Figure 9.5, where the IR images display enhancement of the tumor as well as the adjacent dura and the lining of the right frontal sinus. At surgery the associated changes in the sinus were due to increased vascularity rather than tumor invasion. Demonstration of involvement of the dura may be of particular value in planning surgery when the tumor is adjacent to the superior sagittal sinus.

Separation between tumor and edema is demonstrated in Figure 9.6. The meningioma-en-plaque is not separated from the adjacent brain without contrast enhancement, but demarcation is clear following Gd-DTPA. Magnetic resonance imaging thus has the potential to demonstrate this variant of meningioma with greater clarity than does CT.

The rationale for the use of contrast in meningioma in various clinical situations and the alternative strategies for the detection of meningioma are worth thinking through in detail, for whatever approach is taken the clinician responsible for the examination needs to be able to defend his or her own approach.

Acoustic neuroma

This type of tumor has been of particular interest in MRI studies. The tumor occurs in a limited range of sites and the various possibilities can be analyzed systematically. As with meningiomas, the tumor usually shows an increase in T_1 and T_2, but variants may also be found when T_1 and T_2 are within the normal range.

The three basic sites in which the tumor may be found are within the internal auditory canal (IAC), within the cerebellar pontine angle (CPA), and within the posterior fossa as a whole. In the first situation (IAC), contrast between tumor and CSF is the important determinant, whereas within the CPA the contrast with brain as well as fatty bone marrow is also important. With larger tumors, contrast between brain and cerebral edema is important. Sequences with varying degrees of T_1 and T_2-weighting have been used. T_2-weighted sequences are useful to demonstrate the cochlear and semicircular canals, but may obscure tumors which have no significant increase in T_2. T_1-weighted SE sequences usually display these tumors well.

The pattern of contrast enhancement in acoustic neuroma is predictable from CT experience and consideration of the pulse sequence. Figure 9.7 demonstrates bilateral acoustic neuromas and well-defined enhancement is seen. In the strictest sense, Gd-DTPA has been essential in only two situations to date. One was very small tumors, where it was unclear whether or not the lesion was an artifact. The other situation was after surgery, where postoperative changes and the loss of tissue planes made interpretation difficult. Contrast enhancement was of value in both these situations, although in the majority of cases studied to date it has not been essential for diagnosis.[20]

Other benign tumors

Enhancement has been seen with pituitary tumors, chordomas, glomus jugular tumors, and epidermoid tumors. Some of the considerations relevant to meningiomas and acoustic neuromas also apply to this group of tumors. Some tumors display only a small increase in T_2 relative to brain, but the fact that these tumors often show contrast enhancement provides a useful approach to their detection.

Malignant tumors

Problems in the separation of edema from tumor were identified early in the clinical development of MRI. Both processes produce an increase in T_1 and T_2, and the relative differences in degree between these changes must be exploited for the processes to be distinguished. When more imaging sequences are used, tumor and edema are more likely to be separated, although microscopic spread is difficult to identify and it is probably only the bulk of the tumor which is generally differentiated from edema.

Malignant tumors of the brain have been studied with Gd-DTPA to a greater extent than any other disease, and in fact many of the basic pharmacological properties of Gd-DTPA have been established in patients with malignant tumors.[21-28]

In general, highly malignant tumors display greatest enhancement and a variety of patterns are seen, including patchy, linear, ring, and central forms. The enhancement increases with dosage (at least up to 0.2 mmol/kg) and has been demonstrated for at least an hour in many cases.

An astrocytoma grade IV is shown in Figure 9.8. The high level of enhancement is shown on the IR and T_1-dependent SE images.

Enhancement within cystic components of tumors has also been seen. One of the interesting findings with Gd-DTPA has been enhancement of areas of apparent edema. The enhancement seen in these circumstances probably represents tumor infiltration.

There has been some argument as to whether the same level of separation of tumor from edema achieved with Gd-DTPA may also be obtained by use of a selection of T_1- and T_2-weighted pulse sequences. Although this issue is not resolved to date, our own experience has certainly favored the use of Gd-DTPA.

Cerebrovascular disease

Although cerebrovascular disease represents a limited application of contrast agents with CT, some interesting results have already been noted with MRI.

So-called 'luxury perfusion' has been identified in cases of cerebral infarction. Arteriovenous malformation displays a variable pattern. With slow-flowing blood, enhancement has been seen. With fast-flowing blood no enhancement at all may be seen. Enhancement of the membrane associated with subdural hematomas may be visualized, as in Figure 9.9. The lateral aspect of this enhancement is displayed better with MRI than with CT. No particular difficulty has so far been encountered with MRI in the detection of subdural hematomas so that contrast enhancement will probably not be necessary in this disease.

Ring enhancement has been identified at the margin of giant aneurysms, probably reflecting proliferation of the vasa vasorum, as shown in Figure 9.10.

Demyelinating disease

Multiple sclerosis was the first disease in which MRI was demonstrated to have a significant advantage over X-ray CT, and it has remained a major indication for MRI since that time. The results of imaging with CT have been improved by doubling the standard dose of contrast agent and delaying the examination by a period of about one hour. As a result, the possibility has been raised that the sensitivity of MRI might be increased by use of Gd-DTPA and by delayed examination.

Studies addressing this question are now in progress. Preliminary results indicate that the sensitivity of MRI is probably not improved by Gd-DTPA, although an assessment of the activity of specific lesions may be possible. Enhancement of a single lesion is demonstrated in Figure 9.11.

The suggestion has been made that the majority of lesions are already being detected down to the spatial resolution limit of the MRI system, and there is thus little hope for improvement in sensitivity with Gd-DTPA.

Infections of the CNS

Ring enhancement is a well known feature of cerebral abscess and other patterns of enhancement may also be seen with both abscesses and other forms of CNS infection.

As might be expected, some of these signs have already been identified in the first cases studied with MRI. No features have yet been identified which clearly separate focal CNS infection from other space-occupying lesions, but the presence of enhancement may certainly improve localization and Gd-DTPA may also be of value in indicating that an active process is involved in cases where this is not clinically obvious.

Orbit

Although contrast enhancement has only a limited range of application with X-ray CT, the situation may be a little different with MRI. Enhancement of tumor, including an extra-conal component, is illustrated in Figure 9.12. Advantages of MRI over CT include the lack of radiation to the lens and the high soft-tissue contrast, as well as visualization of the optic nerve within the optic canal. It may be possible to visualize enhancement in the orbit where it has not been previously seen.

Nasopharynx and soft tissue of the neck

The normal nasal mucosa displays a moderately high level of enhancement with Gd-DTPA. This is not surprising considering its high level of vascularity and its high water content. In the visualization of tumors and other pathology within the nasopharynx it is therefore important to be aware of the differential enhancement between the lesion and normal mucosa, as in Figure 9.13, for example. A limited amount of work has now been done on the enhancement of the soft tissues of the neck, but more work will be required before clear indications are established.

Spinal cord

In conventional radiology, intrathecal contrast agents are required to outline the subarachnoid space surrounding the spinal cord in order to visualize the cord as a filling defect. This may produce minor and major side effects. With MRI it is possible to visualize the spinal cord directly without recourse to intrathecal contrast agents. In addition, parenchymal changes within the cord can also be visualized directly. Thus the spinal cord is similar to the brain (in technical terms) when MRI is used.

These considerations extend to Gd-DTPA, which can be used in a manner similar to that within the brain.[30,31] It has been of value in the definition of extramedullary lesions (Figure 9.14), as well as in the separation of tumor from edema and definition of the extent of metastatic spread (Figure 9.15) in the cervical cord. Results in the thoracic cord have also been useful, as in Figure 9.16.

There are also other applications of MRI within the spinal column, including differentiation of scar from recurrent disc following surgery.

With MRI it may be difficult to distinguish a complicated syrinx from a cyst associated with a tumor or a syrinx associated with a tumor. The presence of contrast enhancement in this situation is of considerable diagnostic value.

Overall, this has been one of the most useful areas for Gd-DTPA.

Remainder of body

In general, the impact of Gd-DTPA has been less in the body than within the CNS. This parallels the pattern with contrast agents used with CT. In addition, the flow properties of MRI enable differentiation between masses and vascular structures to be achieved without contrast agents (unlike CT), so that the indications in MRI might be expected to be less for MRI than for CT.

Mediastinal masses have displayed enhancement and the pattern of the proximal pulmonary vasculature can be demonstrated with them. Contrast enhancement has been seen at the margin of areas of myocardial infarction, but the effect has not been consistently reproduced as yet. It depends on the time since the infarction, the perfusion of the surrounding myocardium, and the performance of the affected muscle. Results in animal models have been more consistent and follow the pattern expected by analogy with [201]Thallium studies.

Gadolinium-DTPA has been of value in the separation of neoplastic from fibrotic lesions within the breast, although it remains difficult to distinguish benign and malignant tumors.[32]

The liver has been the principal focus of study within the abdomen and the general features of contrast enhancement have been published.[33]

The normal liver parenchyma shows quite marked enhancement soon after intravenous injection of Gd-DTPA, but this decreases with redistribution and excretion of Gd-DTPA.

Tumors show variable enhancement, but not infrequently they show greater enhancement than the normal liver and so produce a net loss of contrast between normal and abnormal tissues, as illustrated in Figure 9.17. This isointense situation is commonly seen with X-ray CT, but it has meant that relatively little additional information has been provided with Gd-DTPA. The improvements include better definition between necrotic and other areas of tumor, more precision in tumor definition, and separation between portal veins and dilated bile ducts.

Another approach to liver imaging is the use of rapid imaging techniques which normally show little soft-tissue lesion contrast, combined with contrast enhancement to provide lesion definition. This might have the advantage of permitting imaging in times less than that required for breath-holding, but so far success with this approach has been limited.

A variety of retroperitoneal lesions have displayed enhancement and this may certainly produce better definition of the extent of particular lesions.

Within the kidney, Gd-DTPA is concentrated and sharp differentiation between cortex and medulla can be produced. The concentration of Gd-DTPA in the collecting system is usually sufficient to produce a zero signal with all sequences using the conventional doses. However, if a low dose is given and the patient is scanned quickly, increased signal may be seen in the collecting system.

General considerations applicable to imaging of soft tissue outside the CNS apply also to the pelvis. As with the thorax, some of the indications for contrast agents in CT, such as distinguishing between small nodes and vascular structures, do not apply with MRI.

Tumors display enhancement and similar parallels have been seen with other pathological processes.

The bladder displays concentration phenomena,

whereby signal from the posterior bladder (concentrated Gd-DTPA) may be zero, with a zone of enhancement between lower and upper zones where the concentration is optimal, with essentially normal urine above. This graphically illustrates the potential problems with excessive concentrations of Gd-DTPA. There may possibly be some clinical use of this phenomenon in order to reduce signal from the urine and visualize the bladder wall more clearly.

To date, the use of Gd-DTPA has been restricted in the musculo-skeletal system although it is clear that it may be effective in lesions such as osteosarcomas, as in Figure 9.18. This may be useful to define active areas of tumor for biopsy purposes, as opposed to necrotic and cystic areas, but the extent of the disease is usually well defined with conventional techniques. In cases of infection the extent of disease has been better defined with Gd-DTPA, but the choice of sequence may be particularly important in this group of diseases where phase-contrast chemical-shift methods are very helpful.

Toxicity of Gd-DTPA

The early studies of Gd-DTPA were principally concerned with dosage, sequence choice, duration of enhancement, and toxicity, with clinical efficacy as a relatively low priority. As a result, much of the information on efficacy has been extrapolated from studies designed for other purposes, or has been accumulated almost as an incidental byproduct. While this has been a problem in some respects, it has meant that information on side-effects has been accumulated fairly quickly. Immediate short-term side-effects have not been a problem, for example, blood pressure and pulse rate have been stable. Variable findings on hematological screening testing have been found with apparent increases or decreases in some parameters. In our experience, the only marked change has been seen in two cases, where the clotting profiles were abnormal, but on immediate rechecking these were normal.

One consistent finding has been a 15 to 30 per cent incidence of transient increase in serum iron concentration. This has generally persisted for less than 24 hours and has returned to normal in each case. There have been no recognized clinical sequelae. As a result of studies by Schering (Niendorf HP, personal communication), the proposed mechanism is an increased rate of sequestration of aging red cells within the spleen. There has been no evidence of dissociation of the Gd-DTPA complex, and further trials have been planned on the assumption that this side-effect is not of major clinical importance.

A transient rise in serum bilirubin has also been observed in a small proportion of cases, although there have been no significant clinical sequelae.

Conclusions

Whether or not it is possible to obtain all the information available from use of Gd-DTPA by appropriate manipulation of sequences is still debated, but there are circumstances, such as the diagnosis of meningiomas, where there is general agreement that Gd-DTPA has a major advantage. This has meant that MRI is no longer non-invasive in the strict sense, and the duration of the examinations may also be increased. However, the extensive use of contrast agents in radiological practice as a whole has meant that their introduction into clinical MRI has been expected and their acceptance has been relatively straightforward. Once these agents have been accepted, the next question concerns their strict clinical indications. Here the issues related to use in screening examinations (including the detection of meningiomas) have been central, since if Gd-DTPA became part of a screening examination its usage would increase radically.

Apart from screening examinations, it is possible that Gd-DTPA may be used on a fairly widespread basis when the initial MRI examination is positive in order to characterize lesions, although the hope is that contrast agents in MRI will be used more sparingly than they are in CT. With the higher soft-tissue contrast available with MRI this seems reasonable.

As with other aspects of MRI the options are wide, and the principal agent in use at the present time, Gd-DTPA, is one of the most obvious choices. Much more effort will undoubtedly be expended on developing other contrast agents and undoubtedly some of these will enter clinical practice, although this process may be both blocked and facilitated by the successful introduction of Gd-DTPA.

References

1 BYDDER GM, STEINER RE, YOUNG IR et al, Clinical NMR imaging of the brain: 140 cases, *AJR* (1982) **139**:215–36.

2 BRASCH RC, Methods of contrast enhancement for NMR imaging and potential applications, *Radiology* (1983) **147**: 781–8.

3 RUNGE VM, Paramagnetic agents for contrast enhanced NMR imaging: a review, *AJR* (1983) **141**:1209.

4 GADIAN DG, PAYNE JA, BRYANT DR et al, Gadolinium-DTPA as a contrast agent in MRI – theoretical projections and practical observations, *J Comput Assist Tomogr* (1985) **9**(2):242–51.

5 KOENIG SH, BAGLIN C, BROWN RD III, Magnetic field dependence of solvent proton relaxation in aqueous solutions of Fe^{3+} complexes, *Magn Reson Med* (1985) **2**(3):283–8.

6 KOENIG SH, BROWN RD III, Relaxation of solvent protons by paramagnetic ions and its dependence on magnetic field and

chemical environment: implications for NMR imaging, *Magn Reson Med* (1984) **1**:478.

7 WEINMANN H-J, BRASCH RC, PRESS WR et al, Characteristics of gadolinium-DTPA complex: a potential NMR contrast agent, *AJR* (1984) **142**:619–24.

8 BRADY TJ, Selective decrease in T_1 relaxation times of infarcted myocardium with the use of a manganese labelled monoclonal antibody Antimyosin. Society of Magnetic Resonance in Medicine, works-in-progress, San Francisco Meeting, 19 August 1983.

9 UNGER EC, TOTTY WG, NEUFIELD DM, Magnetic resonance imaging using gadolinium labelled monoclonal antibody, *Invest Radiol* (1985) **20**:693.

10 MENDONCA-DIAS MH, BERNARDO ML, MULLER RN et al, Ferromagnetic particles as contrast agents for magnetic resonance imaging, *Book of abstracts Society of Magnetic Resonance in Medicine*, Vol 2, fourth annual meeting, 19–23 August 1985, London UK, 887–8.

11 STARK DD, WEISSLEDER R, ELIZONDO G et al, Magnetic iron oxide clinical studies, *Magn Reson Imaging* (1988) **6**(S1):79.

12 YOUNG IR, BAILES DR, BURL M et al, Initial clinical evaluation of a while body NMR tomography, *J Comput Assist Tomogr* (1982) **6**(1):1–18.

13 AXEL L, Blood flow effects in magnetic resonance imaging, *AJR* (1984) **143**:1157–66.

14 BRADLEY WG, NEWTON TH, CROOKS L, Physical principles of NMR. In: Newton TH, Potts DG, eds. *Advanced Imaging Techniques*, Vol 2. (Clavadel Press: San Anselmo 1983) 15–61.

15 BRADLEY WG, WALUCH V, LAI, KS et al, The appearance of rapidly flowing blood in magnetic resonance imaging, *AJR* (1984) **143**:1167–74.

16 DIXON WT, Simple proton spectroscopic imaging, *Radiology* (1984) **153**:189–94.

17 BYDDER GM, YOUNG IR, Clinical use of the partial saturation and saturation recovery sequences in MR imaging, *J Comput Assist Tomogr* (1985) **9**:1020–32.

18 HUTCHISON JMS, EDELSTEIN WA, JOHNSON G, A whole body NMR imaging machine, *J Phys (B)* (1980) **13**:947–62.

19 BYDDER GM, KINGSLEY DPE, BROWN J et al, MRI of meningiomas (including studies with and without gadolinium-DTPA), *J Comput Assist Tomogr* (1985) **9**(4):690–97.

20 CURATI WL, GRAIF M, KINGSLEY DPE et al, Acoustic neuromas: Gd-DTPA enhancement in MR imaging, *Radiology* (1986) **158**:447–51.

21 BRADLEY WG, BRANT-ZAWADZKI M, BRASCH RC et al, Initial clinical experience with Gd-DTPA in North America: MR contrast enhancement of brain tumors, *Radiology* (1985) **157**(P):125.

22 FELIX R, SCHORNER W, LANIADO M et al, Brain tumors: MR imaging with gadolinium-DTPA, *Radiology* (1985) **156**: 681–8.

23 BRANT-ZAWADZKI M, BERRY I, OSAKI L et al, Gd-DTPA in clinical MR imaging of the brain I: intraaxial lesions, *AJNR* (1987) **7**:781–6.

24 BERRY I, BRANT-ZAWADZKI M, OSAKI L et al, Gd-DTPA in clinical MR of the brain II: extraaxial lesions and normal studies, *AJNR* (1986) **7**:789–96.

25 VALK J, Gadolinium-DTPA in magnetic resonance imaging of the brain, *Acta Radiol [Diagn] (Stockh)* (1987) **28**:430–36.

26 RUSSELL EJ, GEREMIA GK, JOHNSON CE et al, Multiple cerebral metastases: Detectability with Gd-DTPA enhanced MR imaging, *Radiology* (1987) **165**:609–17.

27 HEALY ME, HESSELINK JR, PRESS GA et al, Increased detection of intracranial metastases with intravenous Gd-DTPA, *Radiology* (1987) **165**(3):619–24.

28 GRAIF M, BYDDER GM, STEINER RE et al, Contrast enhanced MRI of malignant brain tumors, *AJNR* (1985) **6**:855–62.

29 DWYER J, FRANK JA, DOPPMAN JL, Pituitary adenomas in patients with Cushing Disease: Initial experience with Gd-DTPA-enhanced MR imaging, *Radiology* (1987) **163**:421–6.

30 BYDDER GM, BROWN J, NIENDORF HP et al, Enhancement of cervical intraspinal tumors with intravenous gadolinium-DTPA, *J Comput Assist Tomogr* (1985) **9**(5):847–51.

31 VALK J, Gd-DTPA in MR of spinal lesions, *AJNR* (1988) **9**:345–50.

32 HEYWANG SH, HAHN D, SCHMIDT H et al, MR imaging of the breast using Gd-DTPA, *J Comput Assist Tomogr* (1986) **10**(2):199–204.

33 CARR DH, GRAIF M, NIENDORF HP et al, Gadolinium-DTPA in the assessment of liver tumors by MRI, *Clin Radiol* (1986) **37**(4):347–53.

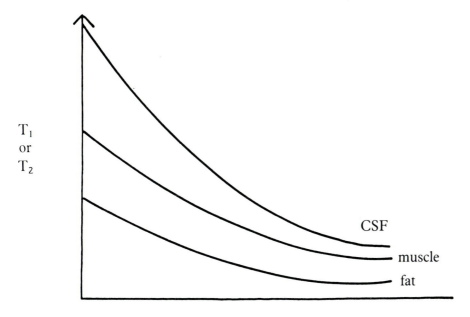

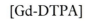

[Gd-DTPA]

Figure 9.1

Change in T_1 or T_2 with increasing concentration of Gd-DTPA. The absolute decrease is greatest for tissues or fluids with high values of T_1 or T_2.

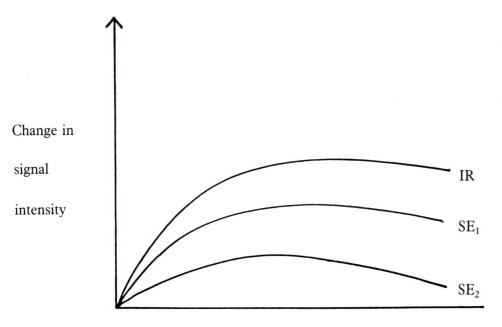

[Gd-DTPA]

Figure 9.2

Change in signal intensity with increasing concentration of Gd-DTPA. The change is maximal for the IR sequence, followed by the T_1-dependent spin-echo (SE_1) sequence and then by the T_2-dependent spin echo (SE_2) sequence.

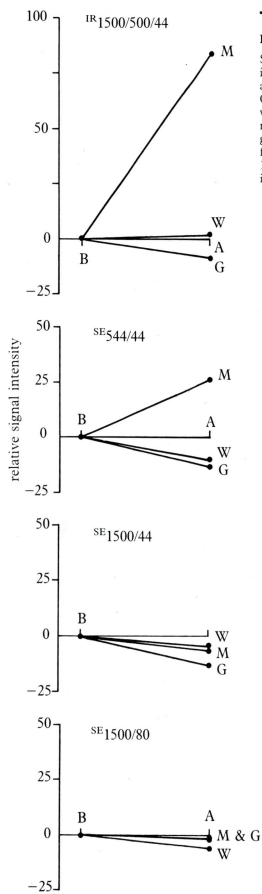

Figure 9.3

Six meningiomas (M). change in signal intensity before (B) and after (A) Gd-DTPA. Changes are compared with white matter (W) and gray matter (G). The change is greatest for IR 1500/44/500 followed by SE 544/44, SE 1500/44, and SE 1500/80 images.

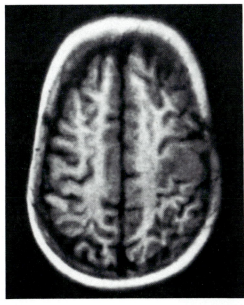

a

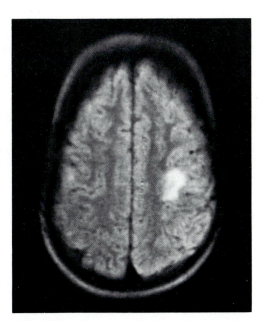

b

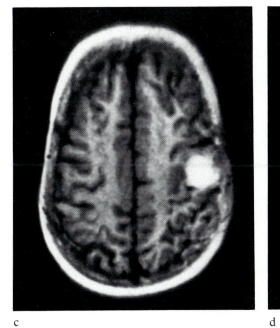

c

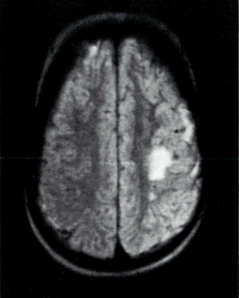

d

Figure 9.4

Meningioma. IR 1500/44/500 (**a**) and SE 1500/40 (**b**) images before Gd-DTPA compared with IR 1500/44/500 (**c**) and SE 1500/80 (**d**) images after Gd-DTPA. The tumor shows obvious enhancement between (**a**) and (**c**) but not between (**b**) and (**d**). The tumor is not defined on (**b**) and (**d**) although associated edema is seen. Slight enhancement remote from the tumor is seen on (**d**) but not on (**c**).

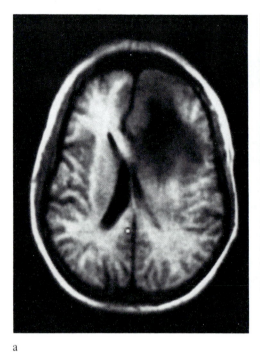

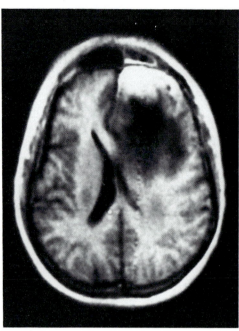

a   b

Figure 9.5

Meningioma. IR 1500/44/500 images before (**a**) and after (**b**) Gd-DTPA. Enhancement of the tumor, adjacent dura, and mucosa in the frontal sinus is seen in (**b**).

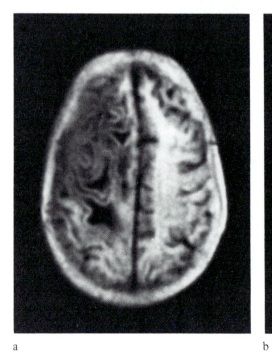

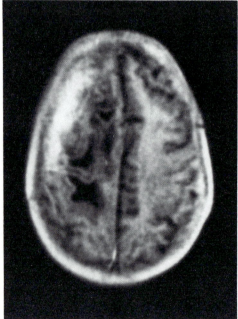

a   b

Figure 9.6

Meningioma-en-plaque. IR 1500/44/500 images before (**a**) and after (**b**) Gd-DTPA. Clearer separation between tumor and edema is seen on (**b**).

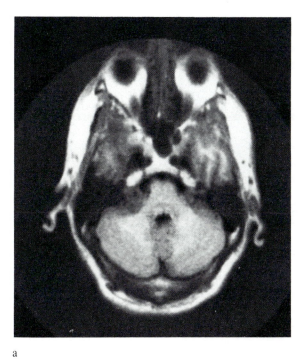

a

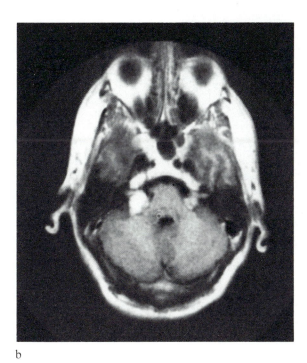

b

Figure 9.7

Bilateral acoustic neuromas. IR 1500/44/500 images before (**a**) and after (**b**) Gd-DTPA. Enhancement of both tumors is seen in (**b**).

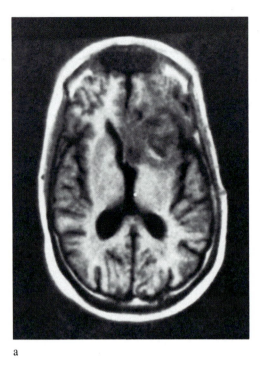

a

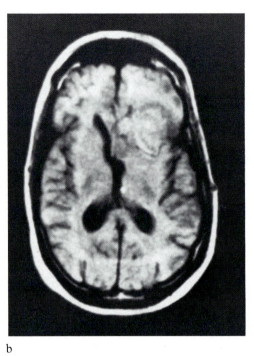

b

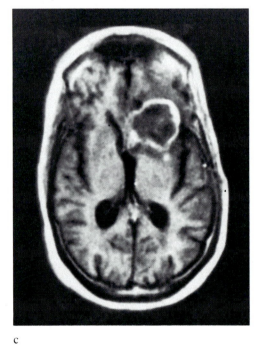

c

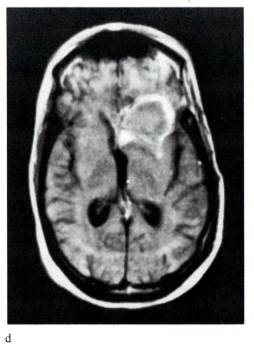

d

Figure 9.8

Astrocytoma grade IV. IR 1500/44/500 (**a**) and SE 544/44 (**b**) images before Gd-DTPA, compared with IR 1500/44/500 (**c**) and SE 544/44 (**d**) images after Gd-DTPA. Ring enhancement is seen.

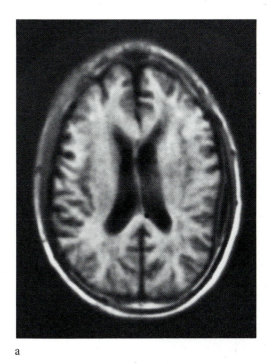

a

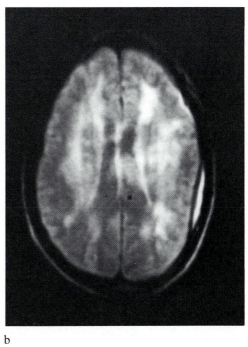

b

Figure 9.9

Subdural hematoma. IR 1500/44/500 (**a**) and SE 1500/80 (**b**) images before iv Gd-DTPA, and IR 1500/44/500 (**c**) and SE 1500/80 (**d**) images after iv Gd-DTPA. Enhancement of the membrane around the hematoma is seen in (**b**). Several areas of enhancement are seen in (**d**) (arrows), but not in (**c**).

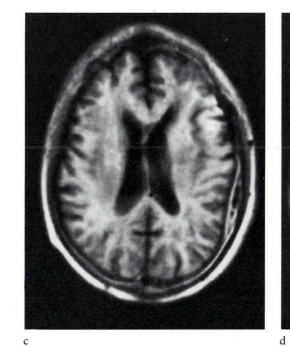

c

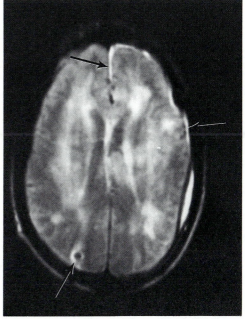

d

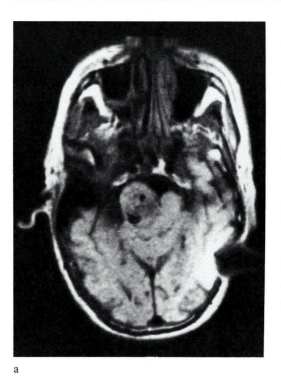

a

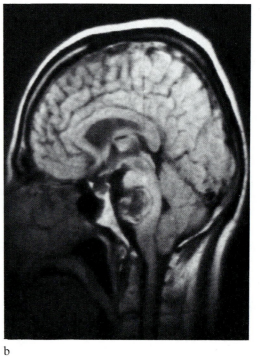

b

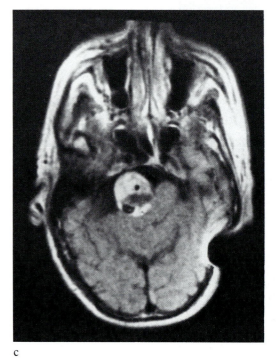

c

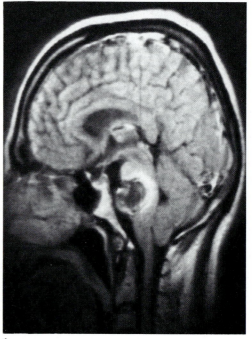

d

Figure 9.10

Giant aneurysm. SE 544/44 images before (**a–b**) and after (**c–d**) Gd-DTPA. Some of the blood within the aneurysm displays enhancement. There is also ring enhancement around the lesion.

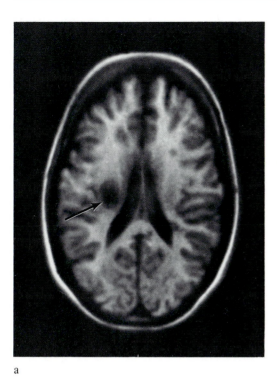

a

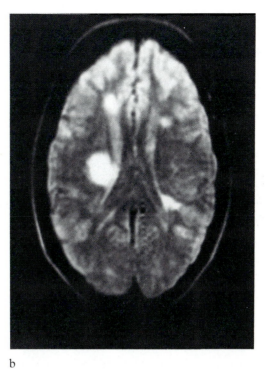

b

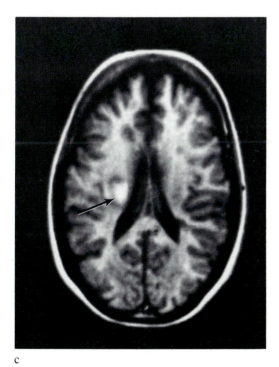

c

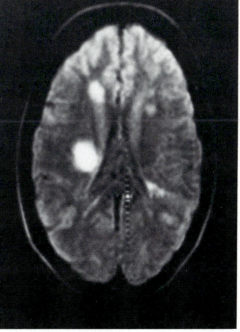

d

Figure 9.11

Multiple sclerosis IR 1500/44/
500 (**a**) and SE 1500/80 (**b**)
images before Gd-DTPA
compared with IR 1500/44/500
(**c**) and SE 1500/80 (**d**) scans
after Gd-DTPA.

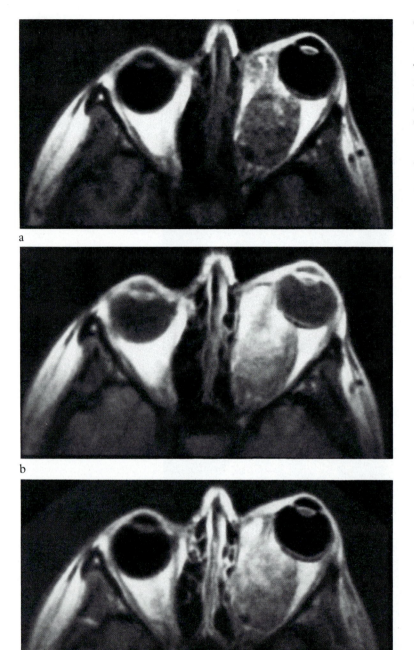

a

b

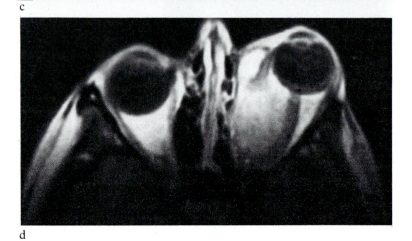

c

d

Figure 9.12

Tumor of left orbit. IR 1500/44/500 (**a**) and SE 544/44 (**b**) images before Gd-DTPA, compared with IR 1000/44/500 (**c**) and SE 544/44 (**d**) images after Gd-DTPA. Enhancement of the lesion, including the extra-conal component, is seen in (**c**) and the optic nerve is better defined in (**d**).

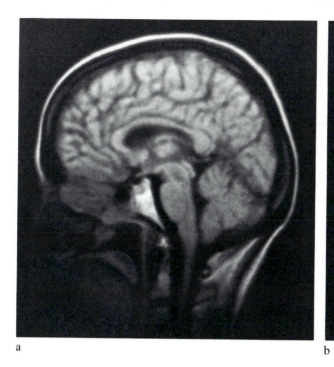

a

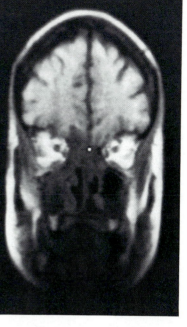

b

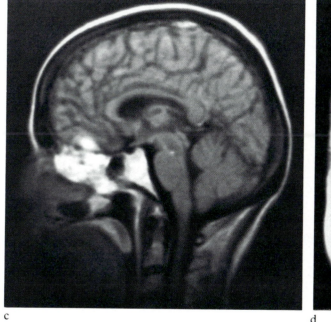

c

d

Figure 9.13

Carcinoma of the nasopharynx. SE 544/44 images before (**a–b**) and after (**c–d**) intravenous Gd-DTPA. The extension in the anterior fossa is best seen in (**c**) and (**d**).

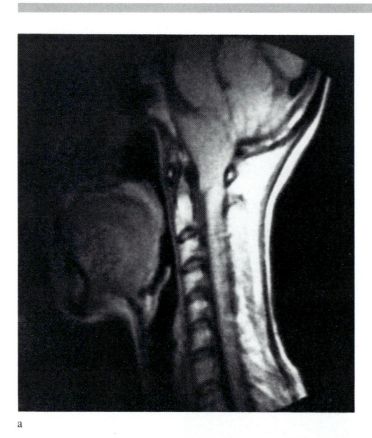

a

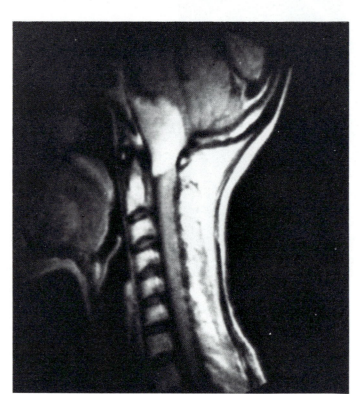

b

Figure 9.14

Meningioma. SE 544/44 images before (**a**) and after (**b**) Gd-DTPA. The tumor displays enhancement and is better defined in (**b**).

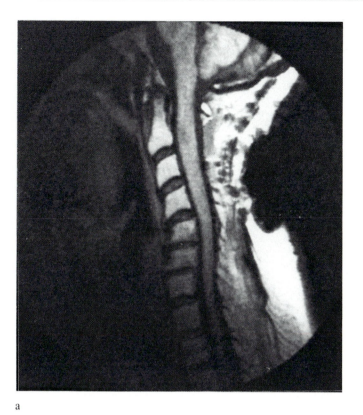

a

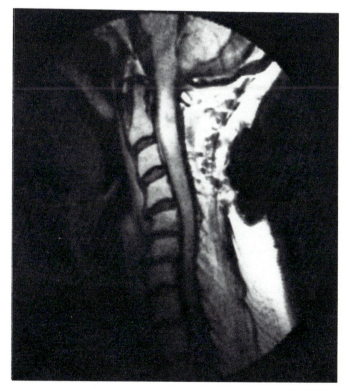

b

Figure 9.15

Metastasis from carcinoma of the nasopharynx. SE 544/44 images before (**a**) and after (**b**) Gd-DTPA. The tumor is seen within the expanded cord in (**b**).

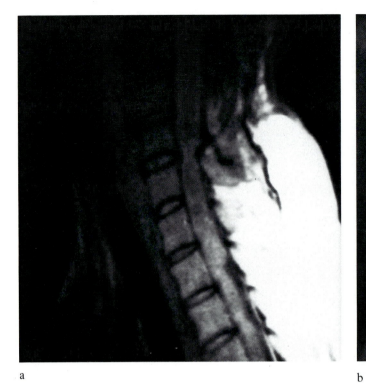
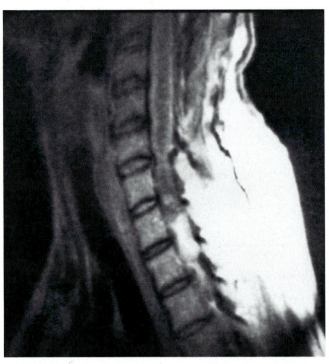

a

b

Figure 9.16

Neurofibroma. SE 544/44
images before (**a**) and after (**b**)
iv Gd-DTPA. The tumor is
best seen in (**b**).

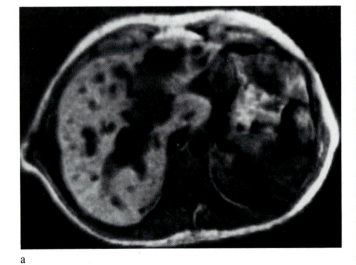
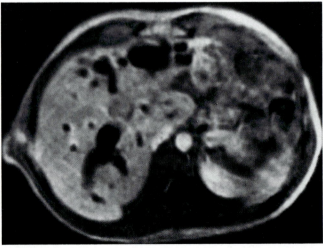

a

b

Figure 9.17

Adenocarcinoma at the hilum
of the liver. IR 1400/13/400
images before (**a**) and after (**b**)
Gd-DTPA. The tumor displays
enhancement with much of it
becoming isointense.

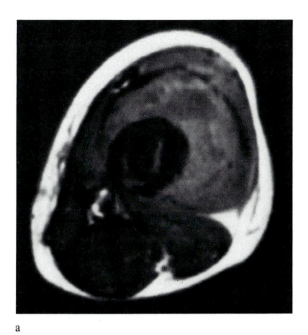

a

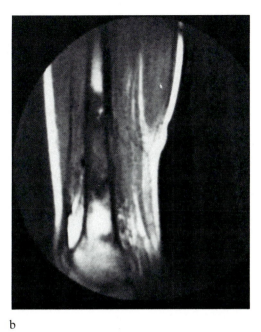

b

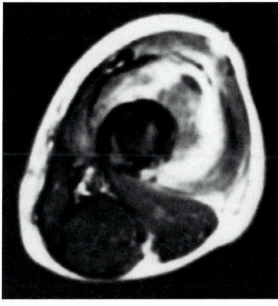

c

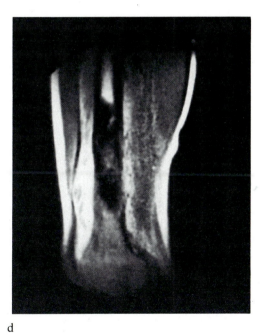

d

Figure 9.18

Osteosarcoma. SE 544/44
images before (**a–b**) and after
(**c–d**) Gd-DTPA. Enhancement
is seen within and around the
tumor (**c–d**).

10

Pediatric brain

Graeme Bydder

Introduction

The success of magnetic resonance imaging (MRI) of the brain in adults has provided a strong stimulus for use of the technique in children. Avoidance of ionizing radiation has also been important and with more experience it has become clear that it is possible to sustain adult-level image quality even in the smallest premature infant by use of appropriately sized receiver coils.

Other techniques including ultrasound and X-ray computed tomography (CT) are much better developed in terms of ease of operation, simplicity, and speed, but the image quality available with MRI is now fully competitive and the range of image parameters available provides a wide variety of options for different clinical problems, the potential of which is yet to be explored in depth. Several general reviews of MRI of the brain in children are now available and they provide a guide to what has been achieved so far, although the overall numbers are still relatively small.[1-6]

There are several important differences of technique in MRI of children and these are discussed first, followed by a brief description of normal appearances, then a review of MRI appearances in a variety of clinical conditions.

Technical aspects

For major illness such as cerebral tumor, general anesthesia is acceptable for immobilization of infants and children, but for less severe illness and repeated examinations it is necessary to use other methods. In neonates (who may also be brain-damaged) sedation can be avoided by beginning the examination during natural sleep after a feed. Neonates usually sleep better on their sides and this position is also more satisfactory in terms of the risk from inhalation of regurgitated milk or vomit. From about 3 months to 4 years of age oral chloral hydrate is reasonably successful, and from about 4 years upwards it is often possible to secure the child's cooperation. A respiratory monitor can be used throughout the procedure.

Significant improvement in image quality has been obtained by use of spherical receiver coils made in different sizes to fit the range of head sizes from small neonates to large children.[7] The coils are fitted like space helmets, shown in Figure 10.1 and are well accepted by children.

The neonatal brain contains a higher proportion of water (92 to 95 per cent) compared with the adult brain (82 to 85 per cent) and this is associated with a marked increase in T_1 and T_2.[2] T_1 may be increased by up to 300 to 400 per cent, and this requires a modification in the basic pulse sequences in order to obtain comparable appearances during the first two years of life. In fact all of the parameters TR, TI, and TE need to be increased, as shown for inversion recovery (IR) sequences in Table 10.1. With increasing age the brain water content drops to adult levels.

With satisfactory sedation to keep the child still, improved signal-to-noise ratio with better coil design, and age-matched sequences it has proved possible to increase the spatial resolution from 128×128 to 256×256 and decrease the slice thickness from 10 mm to 5 or 7 mm, whilst maintaining satisfactory control of

326

noise and soft tissue contrast. There has consequently been a considerable improvement in image quality since the first low-resolution (128 × 128) pediatric images were published in 1982.[8–10]

This machine development sometimes creates problems, both in the appearance of normal controls (used for reference) and in follow-up examinations on patients where early images become technically obsolete and are no longer comparable with current images.

Each of the major pulse sequences used in practice has undergone significant development. The options available with the partial saturation (PS) sequence have been extended by variation in the flip angle (θ), as well as extension of the echo time (TE) to increase the T_2 dependence of this sequence.[11] In doing so the sensitivity of the sequence to susceptibility change is increased, making it of considerable value in the detection of hemorrhage.[12] In addition to this effect, two PS sequences of different TE values can be used to construct a phase map which produces changes that can be directly related to susceptibility.[13]

Table 10.1 Age-related inversion recovery sequences.

	TR (msec)	*TI* (msec)	*TE* (msec)
0–3 months	3000	1000	44
3–6 months	2400	800	44
6–24 months	1800	600	44
24–	1500	500	44

The scope of the IR sequence has been increased by use of the short inversion recovery (TI) variant of this sequence. This sequence has many features in common with the spin-echo (SE) sequence, except it produces greater gray/white matter contrast.[14] It is of value in the demonstration of myelination and periventricular changes where the CSF signal can be kept less than that of brain.

Variants of the SE sequence have been used with TE values up to 200 msec and TR values up to 2400 sec (at 0.15 Tesla). These images display increased contrast, but there is considerable difficulty in keeping the signal intensity of CSF less than that of brain. In addition, by using bipolar gradients it is also possible to obtain flow-dependent sequences.[15] Phase maps produced in this way can be modified to detect flow rates of the order of 1 mm/sec, reflecting tissue perfusion.

Normal appearances

There are several particular features which differ from those of adults. During the first two years of life the pediatric brain changes rapidly and this change continues at a slower rate into the second decade.

As mentioned previously, the neonatal brain is notable for its very long T_1 and T_2. If adult-type sequences are used, the brain may appear noisy (IR) or featureless (SE). In addition, the periventricular regions containing unmyelinated white matter initially have an increased T_1 and T_2 beyond that of gray matter. The unmyelinated subcortical white matter also has a T_1 longer than gray matter, so that on medium TI IR scans the cortical mantle is highlighted between the long T_1 of CSF outside the brain and the unmyelinated white matter inside the brain.

The T_1 of unmyelinated white matter decreases and by about 3 to 6 months is equal to that of gray matter, so that the 'edge-enhancement' appearance of the cortex is lost and both tissues appear isointense with the IR scans.

The process of normal myelination, illustrated in Figure 10.2, also begins in the neonatal period, proceeding in a stereotyped manner with sensory tracts myelinating before motor tracks, and the internal capsule preceding the great commissures and the lateral hemispheres.[16] These features are all well demonstrated by MRI;[17,18] they are not seen so well with other techniques.

Establishing a range of normal appearances has its difficulties. The question of consent for normals is more difficult in children than in adults, and even when scans are performed they need to be obtained with the same technique as for the patient. When the technique evolves these controls may become obsolete so that an active programme of recruitment is necessary. Twins of the patient are a useful source of age-matched controls since they often have a documented medical history (including physical examinations), even when they are completely normal (apart from being twins). We still have insufficient information to assemble an atlas (comparable to that for bone age) for normal development of the human brain, but the correspondence with pathological descriptions of myelination has been very good so far.

Intracranial hemorrhage

In general terms, the appearance of hemorrhage parallels that seen in adults, however there are several important differences. The pattern of hemorrhage is different, being associated with anoxic damage and occurring frequently in the subependymal region on the germinal matrix. Also, hemorrhage in neonates occurs against a background of long normal values of brain T_1 and T_2 so that the T_2 of hematoma may appear distinctly shorter than that of the surrounding brain. Subdural and extradural hematomas have much in common with their adult counterparts. Intracranial hemorrhage may have important late consequences, including hydrocephalus and delays or deficits in myelination; these are considered later.

With T_2-weighted PS sequences, hemorrhage produces a loss of signal intensity as a result of a decrease in T_2 and susceptibility effects, as illustrated in Figures 10.3–10.6. This technique provides a high degree of sensitivity in subarachnoid, parenchymal, and intraventricular changes and may function as a marker of previous hemorrhage years after the event.

Infarction

In the neonatal period, infarction is usually manifest as an increased T_1 and T_2 region and there may be difficulty in distinguishing these areas from unmyelinated white matter areas normally present in the brain, although cystic areas are well shown. These appearances are also seen at later stages, but other more subtle features are also seen. There may be a loss of gray/white matter contrast in a focal area, with or without a slight increase in T_1. Border-zone areas of infarction may also be seen symmetrically within the parietal occipital lobes with essentially the same features. With increasing age, some porencephalic cysts decrease in size while others remain the same size, but the increasing size of the brain makes them appear smaller. Associated hydrocephalus with porencephalic cysts communicating with the ventricles may produce an apparent increase in the size of cysts, shown in Figures 10.7 and 10.8.

Ischemic anoxic encephalopathy is often associated with hemorrhage in the basal ganglia (Figure 10.9) and may lead to cerebral palsy (Figure 10.10). Precise correlation with the clinical syndrome of ischemic anoxic encephalopathy (IAE) in the neonatal period is difficult. This syndrome produces an exaggeration of the normal appearances of increased T_1 and T_2 in the periventricular regions, and the differentiation between normal appearances and minor degrees of IAE is very difficult.

Cysts and periventricular leukomalacia

Periventricular cysts are well displayed at the periventricular margins in patients with a history of anoxic damage, illustrated in Figures 10.11–10.13. The changes can be quite extreme. Sometimes these cysts appear to coalesce and become continuous with the adjacent ventricles, producing hydrocephalus. The appearance of severe or moderately severe cysts in infancy is frequently associated with a delay or deficit in myelination and four cases of this type have been documented in detail.[19]

Hydrocephalus

Hydrocephalus can arise in a number of circumstances in children.[20] It is possible to recognize periventricular edema with both SE and IR sequences, shown in Figures 10.14 and 10.15, and this may regress following satisfactory ventricular shunting. Likewise, it has been present in cases of shunt malfunction.

The ventricular size can be readily assessed and MRI has obvious advantages in the establishment of a baseline and in the long-term follow-up of children with shunts.

The short TI IR sequence displays periventricular changes in some cases of hydrocephalus, probably indicating transependymal spread of fluid. However, similar changes may be seen in other diseases such as periventricular leukomalacia and the changes are probably not specific.

Cases of hydrocephalus such as aqueduct stenosis and obstruction at the foramen of Monro are generally well displayed with MRI.

Congenital malformations

Brain development follows a well-defined sequence and disturbance at any particular time may affect one or more stages and result in a development anomaly.[21–23]

Dorsal induction occurs during the third to fourth week of gestation when the nasal plate folds to form the nasal tube. Failure to close caudally results in myelomeningocele and failure to close at the cephalad end may result in anencephaly, encephalocele, etc. In the next stage the mesencephalon divides to face the telecephalon. Failure at this stage produces prosencephaly.

Normal proliferation then follows, in which the germinal matrix forms the neurons that form the cortex. Neurons may fail to form the normal cortical layers or stop along their path, resulting in heterotopia.

Agenesis of the corpus callosum is thought to be a disorder of migration, illustrated in Figure 10.16.

Neurofibromatosis, tuberous sclerosis and Sturge-Weber disease are the common neurocutaneous diseases occurring in children. Magnetic resonance imaging is of considerable value in tumor demonstrations, but it may also show hematomas or gliotic regions in these disorders, as in Figure 10.17. Calcification in tuberous sclerosis is poorly shown but may be seen, as demonstrated in Figure 10.18.[24]

Obvious anatomical deformations are readily shown, including anencephalopathy, holoprosencephaly, Dandy Walker syndrome, and other conditions. The sagittal plane lends itself to demonstration of many of these conditions including, for example, agenesis of the corpus callosum (Figures 10.19–10.21).

White matter disease

As Figure 10.22 shows, diffuse abnormalities are seen within white matter in leukodystrophy. The changes are usually extensive and not confined to the periventricular region. In other forms of white matter disease, such as Alexander's disease, changes may be confined to the frontal lobes. A variety of other abnormalities have been described in different forms of leukodystrophy, some of which are illustrated in Figures 10.22–10.24.[25] We have also seen periventricular abnormalities associated with intrathecal methotrexate therapy in leukemia.

Infection

Cerebral abscess displays an increase in T_1 and T_2. Edema is well displayed, but the exact margins of the abscess may be difficult to define.[26]

Calcification associated with abscess is poorly demonstrated in comparison with CT, but soft-tissue changes are well seen, as in Figures 10.25 and 10.26.

In two cases of brainstem encephalitis, changes have been seen with very little associated mass effect. This has been the main distinction between tumors on the initial examination, and regression on follow-up examination provides strong support for the diagnosis, although a certain amount of caution is necessary as the patients are frequently treated with steroids, which may result in some regression of edema associated with a tumor.

Delays or deficits in myelination

Reference to normal controls provides a means of assessment of the degree of myelination in children.

The most rapid phase of myelination occurs in the first two years of life. Delays are difficult to recognize before about 6 months, since relatively little myelin is present. Conversely, after two years of age there is time for cases of delayed myelination to 'catch up'. Delays or deficits are most obvious from 6 to 24 months of age (Figure 10.8). With only limited information about the normal range, we have preferred to use age-matched controls (twins if possible) and diagnose delays only in the absence of myelination of named tracts or commissures where these are present in the control and both examinations have been performed with the same technique.

Delays or deficits in myelination have been recognized following probable intra-uterine rubella infection, in posthemorrhagic hydrocephalus, after ischemia anoxic encephalopathy, and in cystic leukomalacia. Figure 10.27 illustrates such delay or deficit in myelination.

Tumors

In general, the features of tumors in children parallel those in adults. However, there is a higher incidence of tumors in the posterior fossa and embryogenic tumors are more common.[27] The high incidence of midline tumors lends itself to sagittal imaging and the clarity with which the posterior fossa is seen is also an advantage.

Most tumors display an increased T_1 and T_2, providing high contrast with long TE long TR SE sequences, although distinction between tumor and edema may be difficult (Figures 10.28–10.30). Differentiation between brainstem and cerebellar site is reasonably easy. Craniopharyngiomas and various other lipid-containing tumors may show characteristic features.

Hamartomas may not display a significant change in T_1 and T_2 and may then need to be recognized by their indirect signs.

In two cases, hypothalamic tumors have been recognized when poorly seen by CT.

Other disease

Certain other conditions are worth reviewing, although they are quite rare.

Delays or deficits in myelination have been recognized in Hurler's disease and these may be reversed following successful bone marrow transplantation.[28]

Hallervorden-Spatz disease is of particular theoretical interest as a condition in which there is abnormal iron deposition in the brain, and in one case abnormalities have been seen in the basal ganglia.[2]

In Wilson's disease, abnormalities are seen in the lentiform nucleus and within the thalamus.[29]

In a case of juvenile Huntington's disease the head of the caudate nucleus was atrophic.

Follow-up examinations

This is an important aspect of pediatric practice. The normal appearances, including the values of T_1 and T_2, the presence of periventricular long T_1 areas, the degree of myelination, as well as the size and shape of the brain, all change with time. Pathological changes must be assessed against this changing background.

The lack of known hazard is a strong incentive for pediatric MRI. Follow-up examinations in conditions in which long-term survival is expected, without accumulation of significant X-ray dosage, are important.

Nevertheless, there are problems in achieving MRI scans at the same level and angulation as in the initial studies. There is also a theoretical problem in using age-adjusted sequences since the machine parameters are different. Genuine advances in technique can also make comparison difficult.

Conclusion

Developments in pediatric MRI lag behind those of adults, but it is possible to extrapolate findings in adults to children to a fair degree.

There are some problems, however. A population of normal controls is necessary and with rapid improvements in image quality these are likely to become obsolete quite quickly. Establishing the range of normal is even more difficult.

Clinical correlation has been progressing but the correlation is not precise and some children may have very large lesions with relatively small clinical deficits. Large unsuspected lesions have been found where the clinical signs are quite subtle.

The capacity for repeated examination without cumulative radiation dosage problems has been of value in the study of the natural history of a variety of neonatal insults.

Several new developments now used in adults have yet to be applied to children. One of these is the intravenous contrast agent gadolinium-DTPA,[21] which has been of value in defining benign tumors as well as separating edema from tumor in malignant cases.

The versatility of MRI with its basic image parameters ρ (proton density), T_1, T_2, chemical shift, flow, susceptibility, and diffusion effects provides a wide variety of options for the various clinical problems encountered in clinical practice and only a small number of these options have yet to be employed.

References

1 SMITH FW, The value of NMR imaging in pediatric practice: a preliminary report. *Pediatr Radiol* (1983) **13**:141–7.

2 JOHNSON MA, PENNOCK JM, BYDDER GM et al, Clinical NMR imaging of the brain in children: normal and neurological disease, *AJR* (1983) **141**:1005–18 and *AJNR* (1983) **4**:1013–26.

3 HAN JS, BENSON JE, KAUFMAN B et al, MR imaging of pediatric cerebral abnormalities, *J Comput Assist Tomogr* (1985) **9**:103–14.

4 DIETRICH RB, LUFKIN RB, KANGARLOO H et al, Head and neck MR imaging in the pediatric patient, *Radiology* (1986) **159**:769–76.

5 COHEN MD, *Pediatric magnetic resonance imaging*, (Saunders: Philadelphia 1986).

6 ZIMMERMAN RA, BILANIUK LT, Applications of magnetic resonance imaging in disease of the pediatric central nervous system, *Magn Reson Imaging* (1986) **4**:11–24.

7 BYDDER GM, BUTSON PR, HARMAN RR et al, Use of spherical receiver coils in magnetic resonance imaging of the brain, *J Comput Assist Tomogr* (1985) **9**:413–14.

8 LEVENE MI, WHITELAW A, DUBOWITZ V et al, Nuclear magnetic resonance imaging of the brain in children, *Br Med J* (1982) **285**:774–6.

9 BYDDER GM, STEINER RE, YOUNG IR, Clinical NMR imaging of the brain: 140 cases, *AJR* (1982) **139**:215–39.

10 BARKOVICH AJ, Techniques and methods in pediatric magnetic resonance imaging, *Seminars in US, CT and MR* (1988) **9**:186–91.

11 BYDDER GM, PAYNE JA, COLLINS AG et al, Clinical use of rapid T_2-weighted partial saturation sequences, *J Comput Assist Tomogr* (1987) **11**(1):17–23.

12 EDELMAN RR, JOHNSON K, BUXTON R et al, MR of hemorrhage: a new approach, *AJNR* (1986) **7**:751–6.

13 YOUNG IR, KHENIA S, THOMAS DGT et al, Clinical magnetic susceptibility mapping of the brain, *J Comput Assist Tomogr* (1987) **11**(1):2–6.

14 BYDDER GM, YOUNG IR, MRI: clinical use of the inversion recovery sequence, *J Comput Assist Tomogr* (1985) **9**(4):659–75.

15 BRYANT DJ, PAYNE JA, FIRMIN D et al, Measurement of flow with NMR imaging using a gradient pulse and phase difference technique, *J Comput Assist Tomogr* (1984) **8**(4):588–93.

16 YAKOVLEV PI, LECOURS AR, The myelogenetic cycles of regional maturation in the brain. In: Minkowski A, ed. *Regional development of the brain in early life.* (Blackwell Scientific: Oxford 1967) 3–69.

17 DIETRICH RB, BRADLEY WG, Normal and abnormal white matter maturation, *Seminars in US, CT and MR* (1988) **9**:192–200.

18 MCARDLE CB, RICHARDSON CJ, NICHOLAS DA et al, Developmental features of the neonatal brain: MR imaging part 1 gray white matter differentiation and myelination, *Radiology* (1987) **162**:223.

19 DUBOWITZ LMS, BYDDER GM, MUSHIN J, Developmental sequence of periventricular leukomalacia, *Arch Dis Child* (1985) **60**:349–55.

20 KITZ CR, Disorders of ventricles and CSF spaces, *Seminars in US, CT and MR* (1988) **9**:216–30.

21 BYRD SE, OSBORN RE, RADKORVOSKI MA et al, Disorders of midline structures: holoprosencephaly, absence of corpus callosum and chiari malformations, *Seminars in US, CT and MR* (1988) **9**:201–15.

22 POLLEI SR, BOYER RS, CRAWFORD S et al, Disorders of migration and fulcation, *Seminars in US, CT and MR* (1988) **9**:231–46.

23 CRAWFORD SC, BOYER RS, HARNSBERGER HR et al, Disorders of histogenesis: the neurocutaneous syndromes, *Seminars in US, CT and MR* (1988) **9**:247–67.

24 BRAFFMAN BH, BILANIUK LT, ZIMMERMAN RA, The central nervous system manifestations of the phakomatoses on MR, *Radiol Clin North Am* (1988) **26**:773–800.

25 NOVELL MA, GROSSMAN RI, HACKNEY DB et al, MR imaging of white matter disease in children, *AJR* (1988) **151**:359–65.

26 DAVIDSON HD, STEINER RE, Magnetic resonance imaging of infections of the central nervous system, *AJNR* (1985) **6**:499–504.

27 PETERMAN SB, BYDDER GM, STEINER RE, NMR imaging of brain tumors in children and adolescents, *AJNR* (1984) **5**(6):703–9.

28 JOHNSON MA, DESAI S, HUGH-JONES K et al, Magnetic resonance imaging of the brain in Hurler syndrome, *AJNR* (1984) **5**:816–19.

29 LAWLER GA, PENNOCK JM, STEINER RE et al, NMR imaging in Wilson disease, *J Comput Assist Tomogr* (1983) **7**(1):1–8.

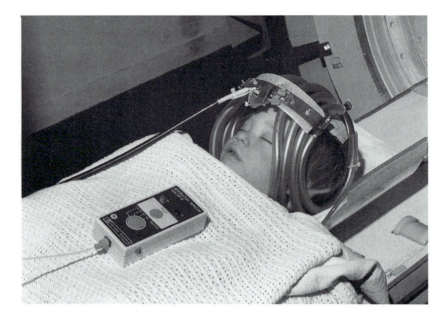

Figure 10.1

Sedated infant with head in a quasi-spherical receiver coil. The respiratory monitor is also shown.

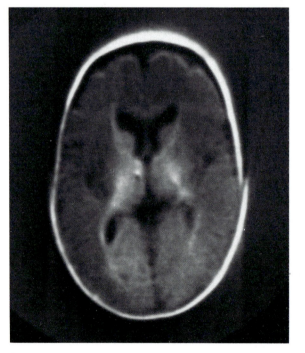

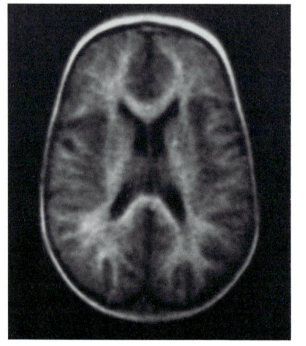

a   b

Figure 10.2

Normal myelination. IR 1800/13/600 (**a**) image at 6 weeks and IR 1400/13/400 (**b**) image at 20 months. There has been a marked progression in the level of myelination.

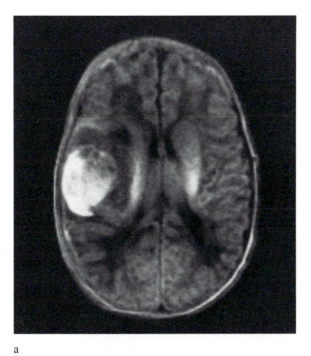

a

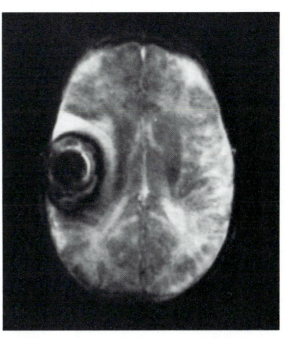

b

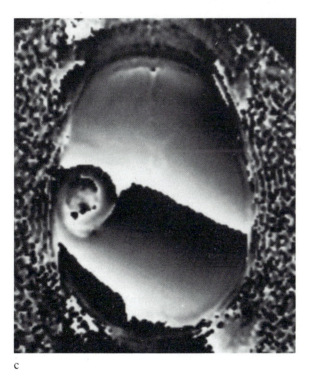

c

Figure 10.3

Subacute parenchymal
hemorrhage. IR 1800/44/600
(**a**), PS 500/193 (**b**), and phase
maps (**c**). The central
hemorrhage has a high signal in
(**a**) and a low signal in (**b**).
Marked susceptibility changes
are seen in (**c**).

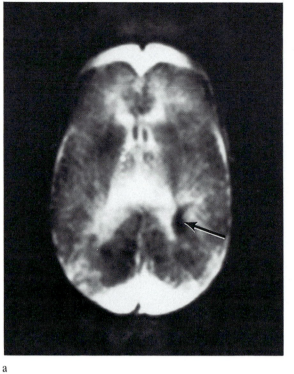

a

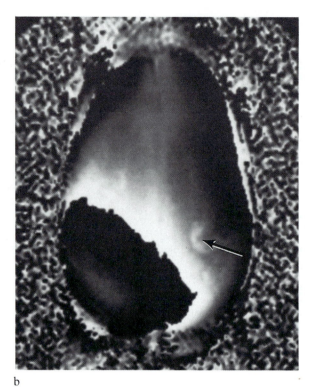

b

Figure 10.4

Subacute hemorrhage. PS 500/
193 (**a**) and phase map (**b**). A
parenchymal hemorrhage is
seen in the left hemisphere
(arrows).

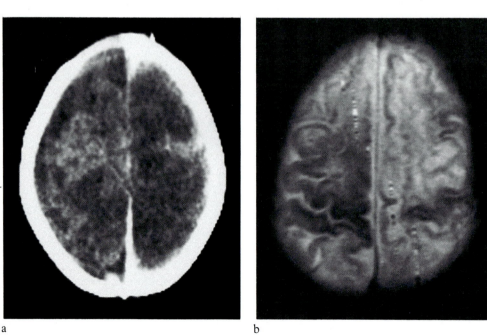

a   b

Figure 10.5

Chronic hemorrhage: CT (**a**)
and PS 500/193 image (**b**)
Decreased signal intensity is
seen in the parenchyma and
over the surface of the brain
in (**b**).

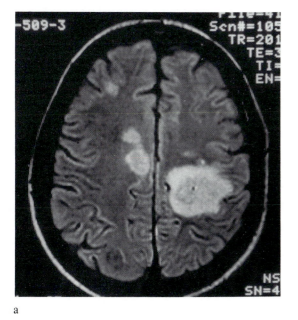

a

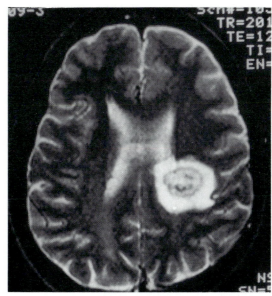

b

Figure 10.6

Subacute hemorrhage. SE
2010/120 (**a**) and SE 2010/32 (**b**)
images are seen. The central
hematoma has a high-signal
intensity on the T_2-weighted
spin echo sequence (**b**).
*(Courtesy of Meredith A
Weinstein MD, Cleveland, Ohio)*

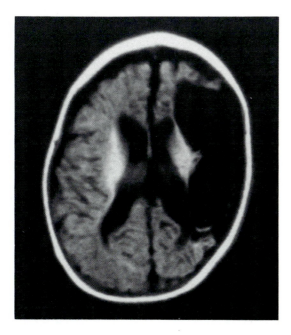

Figure 10.7

Porencephalic cyst (IR 1800/44/
600). The cyst appears similar
to CSF.

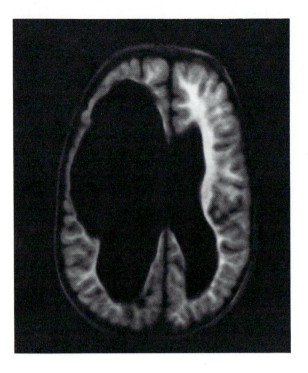

Figure 10.8

Infarction (IR 1800/44/600).
More myelin is evident on the
left (more normal) hemisphere.

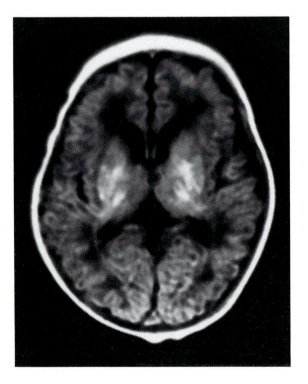

Figure 10.9

Ischemic-anoxic
encephalopathy in full-term
neonate (IR 2400/44/800).
Some exaggeration of the
decreased signal in the frontal
and occipital regions is seen, as
well as increased signal
intensity in the basal ganglia.

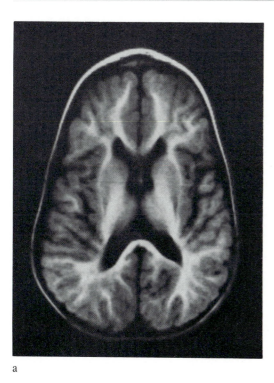

a

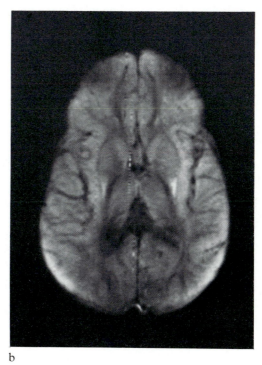

b

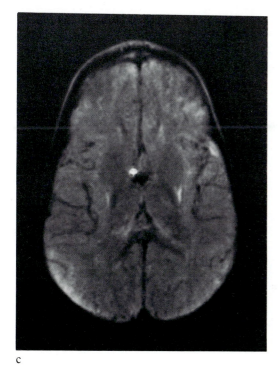

c

Figure 10.10

Cerebral palsy. IR 1800/44/600
(**a**), IR 1500/44/100 (**b**), and SE
1500/120 (**c**) sequences.
Decreased signal intensity areas
are seen in the posterior
lentiform nuclei in (**a**). These
areas have increased signal in
(**b**) and (**c**).

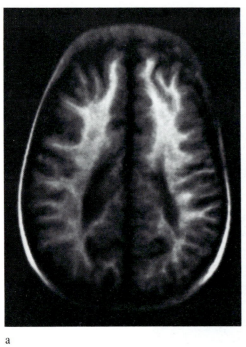

a

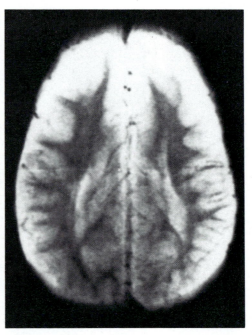

b

Figure 10.11

Periventricular leukomalacia. IR 1800/44/600 (**a**) and IR 1500/44/100 (**b**) sequences. Less myelin is seen posteriorly in both hemispheres.

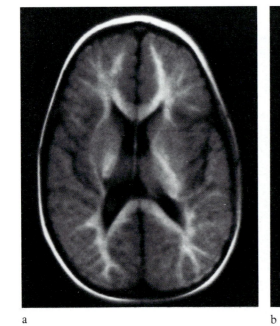

a

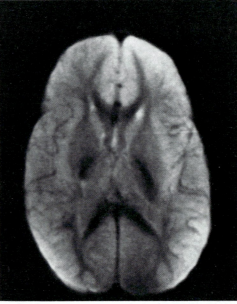

b

Figure 10.12

Periventricular leukomalacia. IR 1800/44/600 (**a**) and IR 1500/44/100 (**b**) sequences. Increased signal intensity is seen in (**b**).

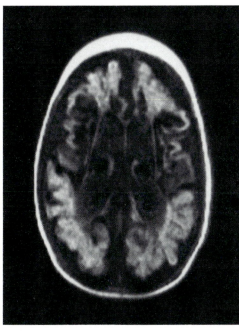

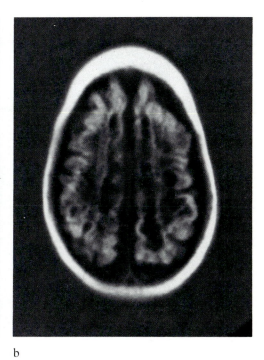

a

b

Figure 10.13

Periventricular leukomalacia. (**a–b**) IR 1800/44/600 images. Extensive cysts are seen with little evidence of myelination.

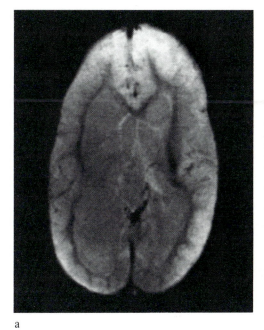

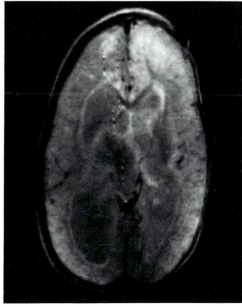

a

b

Figure 10.14

Hydrocephalus. IR 1500/44/ 100 (**a**) and SE 1500/200 (**b**) images. Periventricular changes are better seen in (**b**).

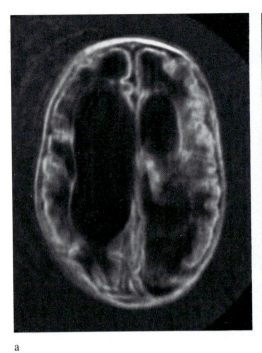

a

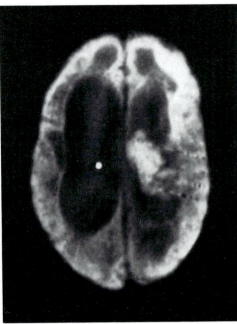

b

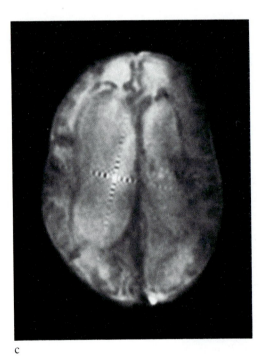

c

Figure 10.15

Hydrocephalus with intraventricular clot. IR 2400/44/800 (**a**), IR 1500/44/100 (**b**), and PS 500/193 (**c**) images. Evidence of hemorrhage is seen in the ventricles and at the ventricular margin.

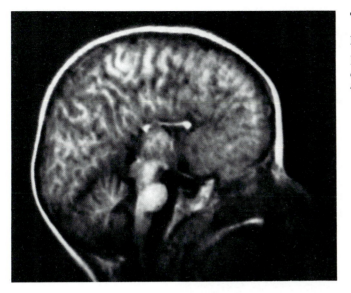

Figure 10.16

Partial agenesis of the corpus callosum sagittal scan (IR 1500/44/500).

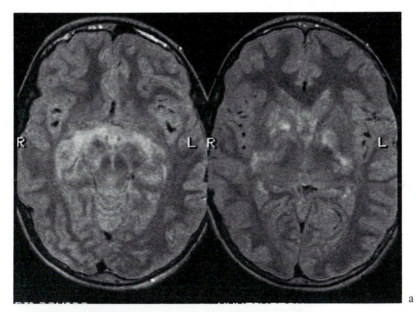

a

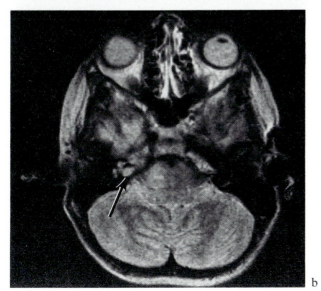

b

Figure 10.17

Neurofibromatosis. (**a–b**) SE 2000/80 images. Gliotic changes are seen in (**a**) and an acoustic neuroma in (**b**) (arrow).

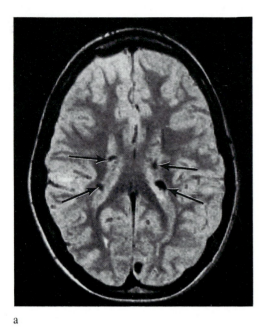

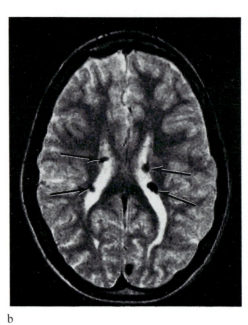

a

b

Figure 10.18

Tuberous sclerosis. (**a–b**) SE 3000/40 images. Low-signal areas are seen at the ventricular margins (arrows).

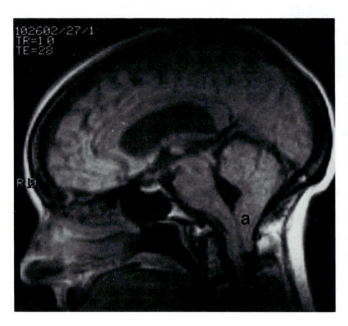

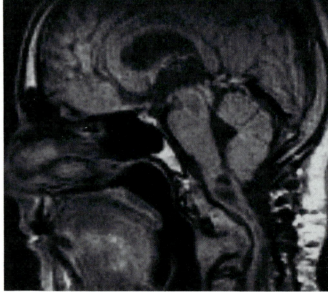

Figure 10.19

Arnold Chiari malformation (SE 1000/28). The cerebellum extends below the foramen magnum (**a**). The IV ventricle is seen (**b**).

Figure 10.20

Syringiobulba (SE 1000/28). Cysts are seen in the lower medulla and cord.

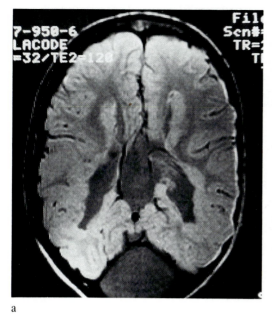

a

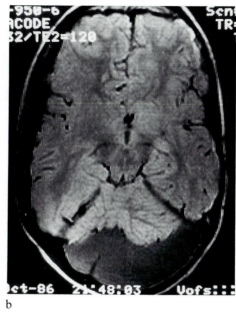

b

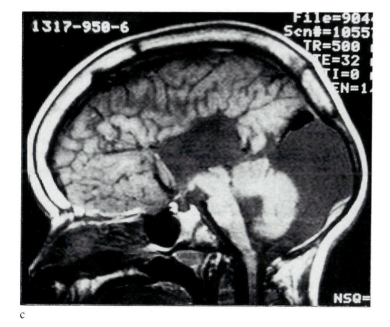

c

Figure 10.21

Dandy Walker syndrome with agenesis of the corpus callosum. SE 2000/32 (**a–b**) and SE 500/32 sagittal (**c**) images. *(Courtesy of Meredith A Weinstein MD, Clevland, Ohio)*

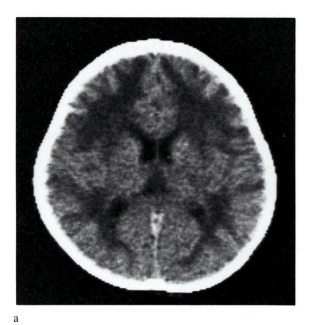

a

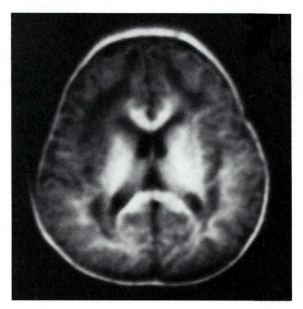

b

c

Figure 10.22

Leucodystrophy. CT (**a**), IR
1800/13/600 (**b**), and SE 1160/
120 (**c**) images. Extensive
abnormalities are seen in white
matter.

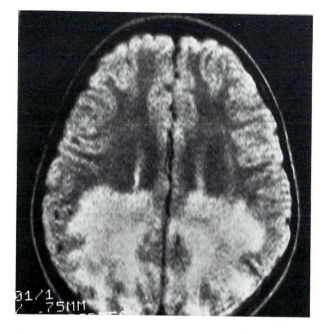

Figure 10.23

Adrenoleukodystrophy (SE 1984/84) (courtesy Dr RB Dietrich). Areas of increased signal intensity are seen posteriorly in both hemispheres.

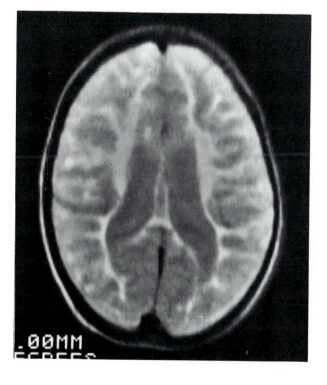

Figure 10.24

Pellazeaus Merzbachers (SE 1984/84) (courtesy Dr RB Dietrich). Extensive changes are seen in the white matter.

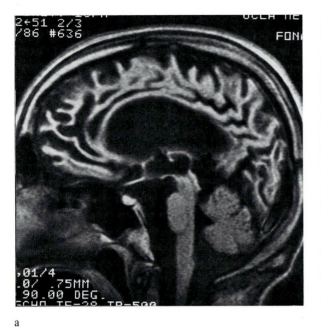

a

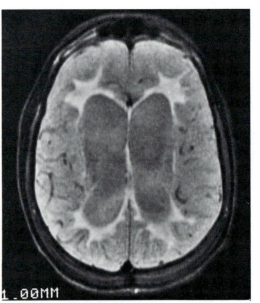

b

Figure 10.25

Subacute sclerosing porencephalitis. Sagittal SE 500/28 (**a**) and transverse SE 2000/84 (**b**) images (courtesy Dr RB Dietrich). Extensive atrophic and white matter changes are seen.

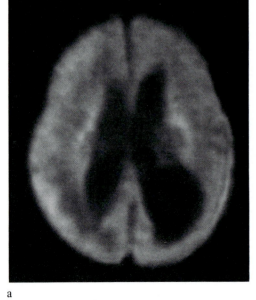

a

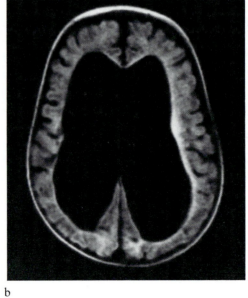

b

Figure 10.26

Toxoplasmosis. SE 1160/120 (**a**) and IR 1800/44/600 (**b**). Periventricular areas of increased signal intensity in (**a**) have been followed by hydrocephalus in (**b**).

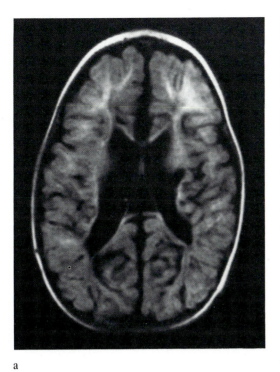

a

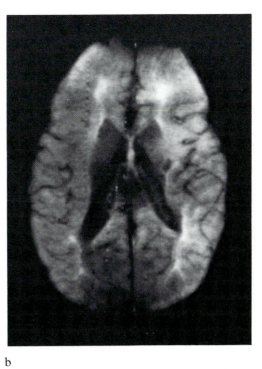

b

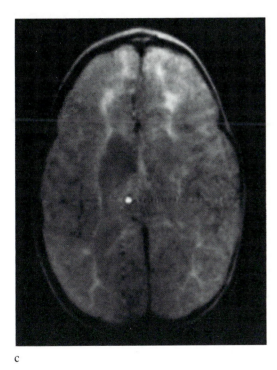

c

Figure 10.27

Delay or deficit in myelination.
IR 1800/44/600 (**a**), IR 1500/44/
100 (**b**), and SE 1500/200 (**c**)
images. Less myelin is seen
posteriorly.

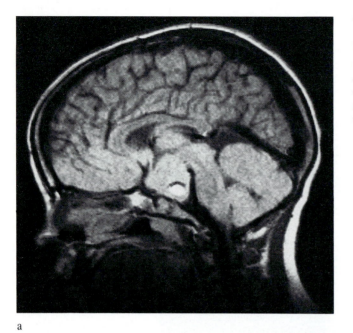

a

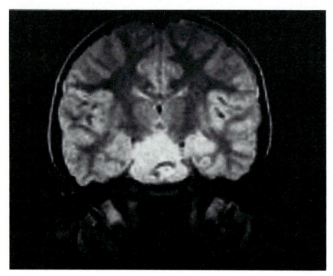

b

Figure 10.28

Hamartoma of the tubar cinereum. Sagittal SE 2000/56 (**a**) and coronal SE 1000/40 (**b**) images. The tumor contains a subacute hemorrhage.

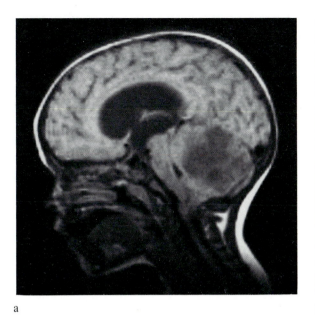

a

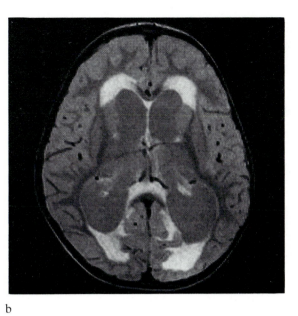

b

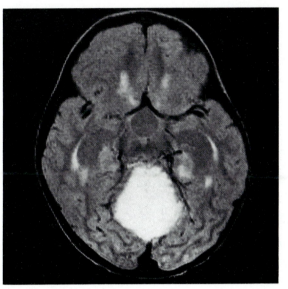

c

d

Figure 10.29

Astrocytoma I. Sagittal SE 500/
40 (**a**) SE 3000/40 (**b**) and SE
3000/80 (**c–d**) images. The
tumor is seen in the cerebellum
and is associated with
periventricular edema.

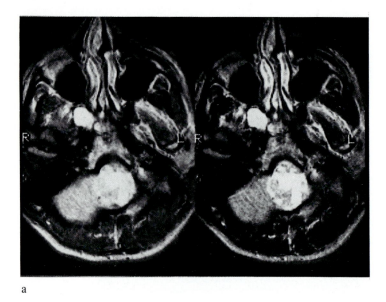

a

b

Figure 10.30

Hemangioblastoma. SE 3000/
40 (**a**) and sagittal SE 500/40 (**b**)
images. The tumor is seen in
the region of the medulla and is
expanding posteriorly.

Index

abscesses, 186, *198–9*
  in children, 329
  Gd-DTPA enhancement, 307
acoustic neuromas, *129-30*
  Gd-DTPA enhancement, 306, *315*
  IR sequence for, 66
  and obstructive hydrocephalus, 268, *287*
acquired immunodeficiency syndrome (AIDS), 186, *197*
adenocarcinoma, Gd-DTPA enhancement, 308, *324*
adenomas, pituitary, 119–20, *140–1*
adrenoleucodystrophy in children, *345*
agenesis, corpus callosum, 328, *341*
Alexander's disease, *192–3*, 329
aliasing, 8, *34*
aneurysms, 209, *246–8, 249–53*
  basilar artery, misdiagnosis, 75, *108*
  giant: Gd-DTPA enhancement, 307, *318*
    simulating hemorrhagic neoplasms, 210, *259*
  intracranial, even-echo rephasing, 72, *93*
  left middle cerebral artery, 77
angiography, for aneurysms, *252*
angiomas, 210, *260–3*
  cavernous, 117
  venous, even-echo rephasing in, *95*
anoxic disease, multiple sclerosis differentiation, 185
aqueductal obstruction, and obstructive hydrocephalus, 267, *284*
arachnoid cysts, *27, 142*
Arnold Chiari malformation, *342*
arteriovenous malformation (AVM), 209–10, *248, 254–9*
  and encephalomalacia, *258*
  phase mapping, *57*
  PS sequence for, *43, 54*
  signal loss from, *79*

artifacts
  chemical-shift, 9–10
    and echo delay time, 40–1
  motion, 8
    suppression, 41
  wraparound, 8, *34*
aspect ratio and image generation, 8
astrocytomas, 113–4; *see also* glioblastoma multiforme
  cystic: and obstructive hydrocephalus, 268, *286*
    and ventricular obstruction, 267, *279*
  Gd-DTPA enhancement, 30
  grade I: in children, *349*
    IR sequence for, *48, 63*
  grade II, *123*
    edema/tumor differentiation, *64*
  grade III, phase mapping, 44–5, *58*
  grade IV, Gd-DTPA enhancement, 307, *316*
  hemorrhagic, 210, *259*
  imaging, 5, *22*
  PS sequence for, *54*
atrophy, 269–70, *294–6*
  hydrocephalus differentiation, 265–6, *281*

bandwidth and spatial resolution, *34*
basilar artery: aneurysm, misdiagnosis, 75, *108*
  thrombosis, *160, 162*
bladder: carcinoma, 77
  Gd-DTPA enhancement, 308–9
blood, appearance, 3 *see also* phase mapping;
hemangioblastomas; hematomas; hemoglobin oxidation; hemorrhage
brainstem: encephalitis in children, 329
  hemorrhage, *225*
  infarcts, 145, *164–5*
butterfly glioma, *124*

calcification, 6, *33*
  in astrocytomas, CT versus MRI detection, 114
carcinomas: bladder, 77
  choriocarcinomas, 118
  of choroid plexus, 117
  embryonal, 118
  Gd-DTPA enhancement:
    adenocarcinoma, 308, *324*
    metastatic, *122*
    nasopharynx, 307–8, *321, 323*
carotid disease; and cerebral infarction, 145, *156–9*
  stenoses and global ischemia, 146
Carr Purcell Meiboom Gill (CPMG) spin-echo sequence, 71, *89*
caudate body simulating interstitial edema, 266, *276*
cavernous angiomas, 117
central nervous system: infections, Gd-DTPA enhancement, 307
  tumors, 112–42
    of blood vessel origin, 116–17, *136*
    of choroid plexus, 117, *137*
    classification, 112, 113
    of cranial nerves, 115
    intracranial, MRI features, 112–13
    local, 119–20, *140–1*
    maldevelopmental origin, 118–19, *139–40*
    mesodermal, 115–16, *132–4*
    metastatic, 120–1, *141*
    of neuroglial cells, 113–14, *123–8*; *see also* astrocytomas
    of neuronal cells, 114–15
    non-neoplastic mass lesions, 121, *142*
    pineal region, 117–18
    reticuloendothelial, 116, *135*
central pontine myelinolysis, 145, *166, 185, 192*
cerebral palsy, 328, *337*
cerebrospinal fluid; *see also* hydrocephalus

cerebospinal fluid (*cont*)
  flow, 74–5, *101–11*
    in hydrocephalus, 270–1, *298–300*
    modelled, 271, *301*
    normal, 270, *297*
  imaging, *32*
    versus brain, 5, *23, 24*
    and water hydration, *17*
    and water relaxation time, 4
cerebrovascular disease, lacunar infarction, 146, *174, 185, 191*
Charcot–Bouchard aneurysm rupture, 147, *175*
chemical shift artifact, 9–10
  and echo delay time, 40–1
children, 326–31, *332–50*; *see also* hydrocephalus;
pediatrics, IR sequence in
  astrocytoma, *349*
  congenital malformations, 328–9, *341–3*
  cysts and periventricular leukomalacia, 328, *338–9*
  follow-up examinations, 330
  hamartomas, 329, *348*
  hemangioblastomas, *350*
  hemorrhage, intracranial, 327–8, *333–5*
  infarction, 328, *336*
  infection, 329, *346*
  ischemia, global, 146, *168*
  myelination delays/deficits, 329, *347*
  normal appearances, 327, *332*
  rare conditions, 329–30
  sclerosis, tuberous, 329, *342*
  technical aspects, 326–7, *332*
  thalamic iron deposition, 210–11, *264*
  tumors, 329
  white matter disease, 329, *344–5*
cholesterol imaging, 4, *15–16*
chondromas/chondrosarcomas, 120
chordomas, 120
choriocarcinomas, 118
choroid plexus papillomas/carcinomas, 117, *137*

colloid cysts, 117, *138*
compensated hydrocephalus, 266, *277–8*
computed tomography/MRI compared, 1, 3
  contrast agents, 303
  image interpretation, 39, *51*
contrast agents, 302–3; *see also* gadolinium-DTPA
  for multiple sclerosis, 184
  paramagnetic, 4, *19*, 302
  susceptibility, 303
contrast enhancement, IR sequence in, 49
corpus callosum, 6, *25*
craniopharyngiomas, 119, *140*
cysts; *see also* syringiobulba
  arachnoid, *27, 142*
  in children: and periventricular leukomalacia, 328, *338–9*
    porencephalic, 328, *335*
  colloid, 117, *138*
  dermoid, 118
  epidermoid, 118, *139*
  mucus retention, 6, *31*
  and obstructive hydrocephalus, 266, *282–3*

Dandy Walker syndrome, 268, *343*
demyelinating disease/infection, 182–7, *188–200*; *see also* multiple sclerosis; white matter
  abscesses, 186, *198–9*
  acquired immunodeficiency syndrome, 186, *197*
  central pontine myelinolysis, 145, *166*, 185, *192*
  ear/nose/throat, 186, *200*
  encephalitis, 186, *196*, 329
  enhancement with Gd-DTPA, 307, *319*
  gray/white matter contrast, 182, *188*
  leucodystrophy, 185, *192–3, 324–5*, 329
  meningitis, 186, *200*
    and communicating hydrocephalus, 268, *288–9*
    and infarction, 146
  and methotrexate treatment, 185
  periventricular changes, age-related, 185
  post-infectious, 185–6, *193–5*
  radiation damage, 185, *193*
dermoid cysts, 118
diastolic pseugogating, 73–4, *100*
  and CSF flow, 75, *111*

echo delay time (TE), and image contrast, 40–1
edema: cytotoxic/vasogenic differentiation, 144, *149–50*
  interstitial, 266–7, *274–81*
    image, and water hydration, *17*
  tumor differentiation, IR sequence for, 48, *64*
embryonal carcinomas, 118
encephalitis, 186, *196*
  brainstem, in children, 329
encephalomalacia; and arteriovenous malformation, *258*
  in ischemia, 145, *155, 159*

encephalomyelitis, acute disseminated, 186
encephalopathy: arteriosclerotic, and multiple sclerosis, 185, *192*
  ischemic anoxic, in children, 328, *336*
  subcortical arteriosclerotic, 145, *165*
ependymitis granularis, 266, 276
ependymomas, 114, *128*
epidermoid cysts, 118, *139*
epidural hematomas, 208, *233–5*
epilepsia partialis continua, phase mapping, *56*
état criblé, 147, *177*

fat: and chemical-shift artifact, 9–10
  lipoma, *28*
ferritin deposition, 210
FLASH fast scanning, 305
  and flow related enhancement, 71
flip angle, and image contrast, 41, *51*
flow phenomena, 32, 68–76, *77–111*
  combined phenomena, 74
  cerebrospinal fluid, 74–5, *101–11*
    in hydrocephalus, 270–1, *298–300*
    modelled, 271, *301*
    normal, 270, *297*
  irreversible phase effects, 73, *97–8*
    Reynolds relationship, 97
  reversible phase effects, 71–3
    even-echo rephasing, 72–3, *91–6*
    odd-echo dephasing, 71–2, *89–91*
  stagnation, 73–4, *98–100*
    diastolic pseugogating, 73–4, *100*
    very slow flow, 73, *99*
  time-of-flight effects, 68–71, *80–8*
    flow-related enhancement, 69–71, *81–8*
    high-velocity signal loss, 69, *80*
fluorinated contrast agents, 303
free induction delay (FID), 2, 3, *14*

gadolinium-DTPA enhancement, 6, *30*, 302–10, *311–25*
  in the body, 308–9
  cerebrovascular disease, 307, *317–18*
  CNS infections, 307
  demyelinating disease, 307, *319*
  distribution/excretion, 303–4
  effects: general, 303
    net, 304–5
  nasopharynx/neck tissue, 307–8, *321*
  orbit, 307, *320*
  and signal intensity, 304, *311*
  spinal cord, 308, *322–4*
  and tissue relaxation rate, 304, *311*
  toxicity, 309
  tumors: benign, 305–6, *313–15*
    malignant, 306–7, *317*

ganglioneuromas/gangliogliomas, 115
gargoylism, 329
germinomas, 117–18
glioblastoma multiforme, 114, *124–7*; *see also* astrocytomas
glioma, *see also* neuroglial cell tumors
  butterfly, *124*
  hemorrhagic, *244–5*
  gangliogliomas, 115
glomus tumors, 120, *130*
GRASS fast scanning, 305
  and flow related enhancement, 71, *88*
gray/white matter contrast, 182, *188*

Hallervorden–Spatz disease, 329–30
  ferritin deposition, 210
hamartomas, 119
  in children, 329, *348*
hemangioblastomas, 116, *136*
  in children, *350*
hematomas: epidural, 208, *233–5*
  intraparenchymal, 205–7, *213–29*
  subdural, 207–8, *230–3*
    Gd-DTPA enhancement, 307, *317*
    imaging, signal loss, 4, *21, 22*
    and obstructive hydrocephalus, 266, *284*
hemoglobin oxidation, hemorrhage appearance and, 204–5, *213*
hemorrhage
  appearance, 201–12, *213–64*
    CT versus MRI, 201–2
    epidural hematomas, 208, *233–5*
    and hemoglobin oxidation, 204–5, *213*
    hemorrhagic neoplasms, 209, *243–5*
    intraparenchymal hematoma, 205–7, *213–29*
    subarachnoid hemorrhage, 208–9, *238–42*
    subdural hematomas, 207–8, *230–3*
    vascular abnormalities, 209–10, *246–63*
  in infarction, 144, 146, *151–4*
  intracranial, in children, 327–8, *333–5*
  PS sequence for, 42–3, *52, 53*
  subacute, imaging, 4, *29, 32*
    versus brain, *19*
  subarachnoid: and communicating hydrocephalus, 268, *289*
    and infarction, 146
hemosiderin, 2, 206, 207, *216, 229*
  siderosis, superficial, 207, *227–8*
  staining, 210
herniation, and infarction, 146
Hounsfield number, 39
Huntington disease: in children, 330
  ferritin deposition, 210
Hurler's disease, 329
hydrocephalus, 265–73, *274–301*, 328, *339–40*; *see also*

atrophy
  atrophy differentiation, 265–6, *281*
  communicating, 268, *288–9*
    and CSF flow, *105*
  CSF flow in, 270–1, *298–300*
  intersitial edema, *17*, 266–7, *274–81*
  nomenclature, 265
  normal pressure, 268, *290–3*
    and CSF flow, 75, *106–7*
  obstructive, 267–8, 274, *281–7*
hydrogen nucleus spin, 1, *12*; *see also* proton relaxation enhancement

image generation, 6–8
  reconstruction algorithms, 7
  spatial resolution determination, 7–8
image interpretation, CT/MRI compared, 39, *51*
infarction, *see also* ischemia/infarction
  cerebral, phase mapping, 44, *55*
    in children, 328, *336*
  white matter, 147, *165, 176*
    and atrophy, 270, *296*
    in children, 146, *168*
    and normal pressure hydrocephalus, 269, *291–3*
    and radiation therapy, 147, *178*
intraparenchymal hematomas, maturation, 208, *236–8*
iron deposition, 210–11, *263–4*
  thalamic, 210–11, *264*
    and ischemia in children, 146, *168*
ischemia/infarction, 143–8, *149–81*
  large vessel disease, 145–6, *156–73*
  pathophysiology, 143–5, *149–55*
    edema, cytotoxic/vasogenic differentiation, 144, *149–50*
    encephalomalacia, 145, *155*
    hemorrhage, 144, *151–4*
  small vessel disease, 146–7, *174–80*
  statistics, 143
  venous disease, 147–8, *181*, 206, *218*
ischemic anoxic encephalopathy in children, 328, *336*
isomorphic glioses and infarction in elderly brains, 147

jugular vein, positional slow drainage, 99

kidney, Gd-DTPA enhancement, 308

lacuna infarcts, 146–7, *174*
  multiple sclerosis differentiation, 185, *191*
Larmor frequency, 2
  and relaxation time, 4
leucodystrophy, 185, *192–3*
  in children, 329, *344–5*
leucoencephalopathy, progressive multifocal, 185, *193–4*

leukomalacia, periventricular
  in children, 328, *338–9*
  and ischemia, 146, *168*
  phase mapping, SE sequences
    for, 45, *59*
lipoma, *28*
liver, Gd-DTPA enhancement,
  308
  adenocarcinoma, *324*
lupus cerebritis, 147, *179*
lupus sclerosis, 147, *180*
lymphomas, 116, *135*

magnetite susceptibility agent, 303
magnetization, 2–3
  transverse, 2, *13*, *14*
mastoid infection, *200*
mediastinal masses, Gd-DTPA
  enhancement, 308
medulloblastomas, 114–15
melanoma, metastatic, 209, *243*
  malignant, *141*
meningiomas, 115–16, *132–4*
  and CSF flow, *103*
    transtentorial, *104*
  Gd-DTPA enhancement, 305–6,
    313–14
  spinal cord, 308, *322*
  intraventricular, 117
  IR sequence for, 49, *67*
meniingitis, 186, *200*
  and communicating
    hydrocephalus, 268, *288–9*
  and infarction, 146
metastases, 120–1, *141*
  IR sequence for, *65*
  melanoma, 209, *243*
    malignant, *141*
migraine, and white matter
  abnormalities, 147, *180*
motion artifacts, 8
  suppression, 41
mucus retention cyst, 6, *31*
multiple sclerosis, 183–5
  differential diagnosis, 184–5
    lupus sclerosis similarity, 147,
      180
  enhancement with Gd-DTPA,
    307, *319*
  features of, 182, 183–4, *188–90*
  imaging: partial volume effects,
    38
    and spatial resolution, 35–7
  and iron deposition, 210
  pulse sequences for, 184
  spinal cord lesions, 184, *191*
myelinolysis, central pontine, 145,
  166, 185, *192*

nasopharynx carcinoma, Gd-DTPA
  enhancement, 307–8, *321*
  metastasis, *323*
neck soft tissue, Gd-DTPA
  enhancement, 307–8
neoplasms, hemorrhagic, 209, *243–
  5*
neurinomas, 115
neuroblastomas, 115
neurofibroma, thoracic cord, Gd-
  DTPA enhancement, 324
neurofibromatosis, 119
  in children, 329, *341*

neuroglial cell tumors, 113–14; *see
  also* astrocytomas
  ependymomas, 114, *128*
  glioblastoma multiforme, 114
  oligodendrogliomas, 114
  neuromas, 115; *see also* neuronal
    cell tumors
    acoustic, *129–30*
      Gd-DTPA enhancement, 306,
        315
      IR sequence for, *66*
      and obstructive
        hydrocephalus, 268, *287*
    trigeminal, *131*
neuronal cell tumors, 114–15
nuclear magnetic resonance, 1
  spectrometer, *12*

oligodendrogliomas, 114
optic nerve glioma, *127*
orbit, Gd-DTPA enhancement,
  307, *320*
osteomas, 6, *33*
osteosarcomas, Gd-DTPA
  enhancement, 309, *325*
otic hydrocephalus, 268
otitis, malignant external, 72, *95*

panencephalitis, subacute
  sclerosing, 186
papillomas of choroid plexus,
  117, *137*
paramagnetic substances:
  contrast agents, 4, *19*, 302
  and proton relaxation
    enhancement, 203
paramagnetism, 2
  of deoxyhemoglobin, 204–5
parenchymal hematoma, 205–7,
  213–29
Parkinson's disease, iron
  deposition, 210
partial volume effects, 9, *38*
pediatrics, IR sequence in, 49; *see
  also* children
Pellazeus Merzbachers, *345*
periventricular changes, age-
  related, 185
perventricular lesions
  differentiation, 183, 184
phase mapping
  of arteriovenous malformation,
    57
  SE sequences for, 44–5, *55*
  leukomalacia, 45, *59*
pineal tumors, 117–18, *138*
  germ cell tumors, 117–18
  and obstructive hydrocephalus,
    267, *285*
  pineal cell, 118
pituitary tumors, 119–20, *140–1*
porencephalitis, subacute
  sclerosing, *346*
porencephaly and cerebral
  infarction, 146, *156*
posterior inferior cerebellar artery
  (PICA) infarction, *161*
progressive multifocal
  leucoencephalopathy (PMLE),
    185, *193–4*
protein in fluid, imaging and water
  hydration, *18*

proton relaxation enhancement,
  202–4; *see also* hydrogen
  nucleus
spin and paramagnetic substances,
  203–4
pulse sequences, 39–40, *51*
  IR, 45–9, *60–2*
  for multiple sclerosis, 184
  PS: clinical applications, 42–4,
    52–4
  and image contrast, 40–2
  SE, for phase mapping, 44–5

radiation: damage, 185, *193*
  therapy, and white matter
    infarction, 147, *178*
relaxation times: longitudinal, 3–4,
  13
  and signal intensity, 5–6
  transverse, 4–5, *20*
repetition time, 5
  and image intensities, 5–6
Reynolds: number, 73
  relationship, 97

saturation recovery, 41
schwannomas, 115
sclerosis, tuberous, in children,
  329, *342*
siderosis, *see* hemosiderin
signal-to-noise ratio, 8–9
  and averaging, 41
  and perceived image quality, 9
  and spatial resolution, 8–9
slice thickness and lesion
  detectability, 9
spatial resolution, 3
  and bandwidth, *34*
  determination, 7–8
  and image quality, *35–7*
  and signal-to-noise ratio, 8–9
spin-echo, 5–6, *14*
  initiation, 2–3
  intensity, 6
  sampling, 7
spina bifida, *see* Arnold Chiari
  malformation
spinal cord: Gd-DTPA
  enhancement, 308, *322–4*
  lesions, in multiple sclerosis,
    184, *191*
stenoses
  aqueductal, *102*
    and obstructive
      hydrocephalus, 267, *284*
  carotid, and global ischemia, 146
  even-echo rephasing, *93*
stroke, *see* ischemia/infarction
Sturge–Weber disease, 329
subarachnoid hemorrhage, 208–9,
  238–42
  and communicating hydrocephalus,
    268, *289*
  and infarction, 146
subdural hematomas, 207–8, *230–
  3*
  Gd-DTPA enhancement, 307,
    317
  imaging, signal loss, 4, *21*, *22*
  and obstructive hydrocephalus,
    266, *284*
syryngiobulba, *342*

tectal tumor, and aqueductal
  stenosis, *102*
teratomas, 118
thalami: of children, iron
  deposition in, 210–11, *264*
  infarct imaging, 26
  and ischemia, 146, *168*
thrombi, mural, 209, *246*, *249–50*
thrombosis: and communicating
  hydrocephalus, 268
  superior sagittal sinus, 218
toxoplasmosis in children, *346*
trauma: contusions, acute
  hemorrhagic, 206, *219–22*
  edema, *280*
  hematomas: epidural, 208, *233–
    5*
    subdural, subacute, 208, *231–
      2*
  and infarction, 146, *169–74*
  subarachnoid hemorrhage, and
    hydrocephalus, 268, *289*
trigeminal neuroma, *131*
tuberculosis, 186, *199*
tumors, *see also by specific tumor and
  site*
  imaging, 5, *22*
  in children, 329, *348–50*
  edema differentiation, IR
    sequence for, 48, *64*
  PS sequence for, 43, *54*
turbulence, 73

vascular disease: IR sequence for,
  additional lesions, *65*
  PS sequence for, 43, *54*
vasculitis, autoimmune/infectious,
  and infarction, 147
venous angiomas, *95*
venous infarction, 147–8, *181*, 206,
  218
von Recklinghausen's disease, *see*
  neurofibromatosis

water relaxation time and
  hydration, 4, *15*
  cholesterol imaging, *15–16*
  CSF imaging, *17*
  proteinaceous fluid imaging, *18*
watershed infarcts, 146, *164–5*, *167*
white matter: abnormalities, and
  migraine, 147, *180*
  disease
    in children, 329, *344–5*
    classification, 183
  gray matter contrast, 182, *188*
  infarction, 147, *165*, *176*
    and atrophy, 270, *296*
    in children, 146, *168*
    and normal pressure
      hydrocephalus, 269, *291–
      3*
    and radiation therapy, 147,
      178
Wilson's disease in children, 330
wraparound artifact, 8, *34*

X-ray computed tomography, *see*
  computed tomography/MRI
  compared